COMMUNITY HEALTH NURSING

HARPER & ROW, PUBLISHERS

PHILADELPHIA

Cambridge
Hagerstown
New York
San Francisco
London
Mexico City
São Paulo
Sydney

1817

CARL O. HELVIE, R.N., Dr. P.H.

Professor of Nursing
Old Dominion University
Norfolk, Virginia

with 2 contributors

COMMUNITY HEALTH NURSING

Theory and Process

East Washington Square, Philadelphia, Pennsylvania 19105
Printed in the United States of America
1 3 5 6 4 2

Library of Congress Cataloging in Publication Data

Helvie, Carl O
Community health nursing, theory and process.

Includes index.
1. Community health nursing. I. Title.
RT98.H44 610.73′43 80-22659
ISBN 0-397-54297-6

To two former teachers and friends who made learning exciting.

Ann Hill, R.N., M.P.H.

Formerly, Associate Professor of Nursing
University of California
San Francisco, California

and

Paul V. Lemkau, M.D.

Formerly, Professor and Chairman
Department of Mental Hygiene
Johns Hopkins University
School of Public Health
Baltimore, Maryland

Contents

Contributors

BRIAN ROBINSON, R.N., B.S.

U.S. Army Nurse Corps
Letterman Hospital
San Francisco, California

SHEILA SPELMAN, R.N., M.S.N.

Associate Director, Community Health Nursing
Virginia State Health Department
Richmond, Virginia

Preface

During the last 25 years there has been a knowledge explosion in the natural, behavioral, and nursing sciences. Often, this new knowledge has been added to nursing and prenursing courses as isolated concepts and facts that have left students frustrated with the amount of fragmented content to learn. The synthesis of these fragmented concepts and facts has often been left to students, and as a result, there has not always been a transfer of knowledge from one course to another. For example, students have not always transferred the principles and concepts of the small group from sociology to community health nursing, nor the concepts of interpersonal relationships from psychiatric nursing to community health nursing. This compartmentalization of knowledge has placed additional stresses on students and faculty and has affected the quality of nursing care to clients.

Many nursing curriculums have moved to an integrated approach where concepts, facts, and principles are synthesized and organized into a unified whole. This approach has facilitated student learning and improved the quality of nursing care. However, these programs are usually at the upper divisions level and are built upon foundations of the natural and the behavioral sciences. Because there is limited control by nursing faculty over the content and teaching methods in these science courses, the prenursing content has at times continued to be presented as isolated facts, concepts, and principles, which must be synthesized by students and incorporated into the nursing curriculum.

An important part of any nursing program is the nursing textbooks available for students that are appropriate for the particular curriculum design of the school. A limited number of nursing textbooks have been written that synthesize concepts, models, and theories of nursing. These books have been used in introductory courses in many nursing schools that have integrated curriculums to provide the foundation for subsequent nursing courses. However, these books have lacked the depth in content needed for most major nursing courses. Consequently, nursing faculty have often selected textbooks from each of the nursing specialty areas such as adult nursing, pediatric nursing, and community health nursing for use in major nursing courses in integrated curriculums. Students often retain these books throughout the nursing program and read specified content as it relates to the segment of the curriculum being learned. Other nursing programs that are organized in blocks around the medical-model approach may also use these same textbooks.

In my own specialty area of community health nursing, there have been no textbooks available to date that are organized around a theoretical framework. Some books have presented concepts and models useful in community health nursing but have not organized these into a theoretical framework. Others have presented concepts and processes used in community health nursing and some have presented selected aspects of theory, but none have presented in-depth concepts and models organized into a theoretical framework.

This textbook was written to fill this void and to facilitate student learning by presenting a theoretical framework onto which students can attach current and future concepts that relate to community health nursing. This should facilitate learning by providing the framework for organizing concepts, facts, and principles used in nursing care in community health nursing. The book also presents processes needed by students to approach and provide care for individuals and groups in a systematic, meaningful way, using theory and concepts. The application chapter demonstrates the use of theory, concepts, and processes with clients.

Initially, the book develops a theoretical base for community health nursing and the processes used in applying this theory with individuals, families, and communities. Later, selected concepts and models related to the theoretical framework are presented. Then, the theoretical concepts, models, and processes are applied to high-risk segments of the community population. The final section of the book looks at changes in society affecting health and includes the implications for community health nursing. Since many of these changes influence the quality and quantity of community-health nursing services, this section looks at ways to improve the quality and quantity of these services, which extends and strengthens community-health nursing services.

This book is intended for undergraduate nursing students in community health nursing in block or integrated design curriculums. In block design curriculums, students may read the text in-depth over one semester, whereas, in an integrated curriculum they may use the book over several semesters and read only content that relates to the particular segment of the curriculum. In the integrated curriculum design, students should initially read the overview of the theoretical framework in Chapter 1. Thereafter, they may use the chapters as needed, such as, theory related to individuals in one course, theory related to families in another, and theory related to communities in another, if the curriculum design progresses from an individual to a community focus. Processes and selected concepts related to theory in other chapters should be read whenever appropriate to the specific nursing course. Although the book is intended for nursing students in undergraduate curriculums it may be useful for practicing nurses who lack a theoretical framework for practice or graduate students who wish to review community health nursing for advanced preparation.

Carl O. Helvie, R.N., Dr. P.H.

Acknowledgments

Many individuals have contributed to the ideas expressed in this book. Community-health nursing families for whom I have cared, current and former professional colleagues in nursing, medicine, and the social sciences, and current and former students who have interacted with and challenged me have all contributed to the ideas presented in this book and continue to contribute to my development as a nursing educator.

Special recognition is given to the following individuals who made significant contributions to this book. Mrs. Johnnie Bunch, Assistant Professor of Nursing at Hampton Institute who reviewed the manuscript and made important suggestions for changes. Dr. John Phillips, Associate Professor of Nursing, New York University, who also read portions of the manuscript and offered many valuable ideas for revision. Special thanks is given to Mr. Brian Robinson, who, while a senior nursing student at Old Dominion University, read the manuscript from a student's point of view, gave valuable suggestions and provided a lot of support and encouragement throughout the writing process.

I am also indebted to the administrators at Old Dominion University who approved my research and development leave during the spring semester, 1979, which allowed me a block of time for writing. Recognition is also given to Mrs. Ellen LaBonte, Associate Professor of Nursing at Old Dominion University, for her continued support and encouragement; to Mrs. Colleen Wright, secretary, who typed the manuscript; and to Mr. William Burgower, former nursing editor of Harper & Row and Mr. David Miller of J.B. Lippincott Company for their assistance and encouragement. Special recognition is also given to Ms. Darlene D. Pedersen, manuscript editor at Harper & Row, for the excellent editing of the manuscript.

COMMUNITY HEALTH NURSING

PART I

THEORETICAL BASIS OF COMMUNITY HEALTH NURSING

1 Community Health Nursing and the Systems Approach

COMMUNITY HEALTH NURSING

Community health nursing is the synthesis of public health science and nursing science. It promotes the preservation of health and motivates populations to seek and maintain a high level of wellness. It focuses upon the total population and nursing activities directed toward individuals, and groups are valid only as they contribute to the health of the total community.[1]

This definition not only places the responsibility upon community health nurses for promoting and preserving the health of the community, but also recognizes the interrelatedness of individuals, groups, and community health. Thus, there is justification for working with individuals and groups if the outcome will benefit the community, and systems theory provides a framework for viewing these interrelationships.

The Western Interstate Commission on Higher Education in Nursing (WICHEN) adds additional components to a definition of community health nursing. This group says that community health nursing is the "engagement of a community health nurse with other people in a means–end action toward high level wellness in individuals, families and communities."[2]

This definition recognizes the involvement of the nurse with others to meet the goal of high level wellness. This may involve working with other health team members to provide care, either directly to families and groups who need health care, or by means of consultation and referral. It also involves working with and including families and groups in the planning and implementing of the change process. This concept is enlarged upon in Chapter 6 from the point of view of systems.

Both definitions go beyond prevention and health promotion to incorporate high level wellness of populations. Dunn defines high level wellness as "an integrated method of functioning which is oriented toward maximizing the potential of which the individual is capable. It requires that 'man' maintain a continuum of balance and purposeful direction within the environment where he is functioning."[3] Although Dunn defines high level wellness from an individual point of view, the concept is equally appropriate when viewing a family or community as a system. To help the system (individual, family, or community) maximize its potential and maintain a continuum of balance, community health nurses must assess the system's location on the health continuum and the factors influencing its location as a basis for interventions.

If the system is temporarily in balance, primary-prevention interventions may assist the system to maintain its health and balance or to attain a higher level of health. If the system is temporarily out of balance, secondary- or tertiary-prevention interventions may assist the system to regain its balance and health. Concepts of health and the levels of prevention are discussed in Chapter 9.

High level wellness may result from a wide spectrum of nursing activities such as teaching, counseling, or motivating people; manipulating the environment; giving physical care and emotional support; resocializing convalescing clients; or organizing community groups. The process of assessing the system's health or balance and planning, intervening, and evaluating the outcome of interventions are discussed in Chapter 6. Nursing activities helpful in assisting systems are discussed throughout the book.

Basic to any health-care plan is an assessment of the health conditions, environment, health-behavior patterns, resources, and location and factors responsible for placement at some point on the health continuum of a particular system (*e.g.*, individual, family, group, or community). The means of the "means–end action" portion of the WICHEN definition refers to this assessment by community health nurses and their plans to assist systems. It also refers to the relationship and communications between community health nurses and the particular system with which they are working. These processes are discussed in Chapters 6 and 7.

The community focus and efforts in community health nursing with individuals, families, and groups as a method of improving community health are based upon the recognition of the interrelationships among individuals, families, groups, and the community, and are an important aspect of systems theory. These relationships are conceptualized in Chapters 2, 3, and 4. Everyone in a community is a potential candidate for nursing services, but limitations of time and resources require that priorities of high-risk families and groups be established at a particular time and place (*i.e.*, those most likely to influence total community health). This process of identifying high-risk families and groups is discussed in Chapter 6, and some of the commonly accepted categories of high-risk systems (individual, family, communities) presently in American society, are discussed in Chapter 11.

The WICHEN definition specifies the engagement of a community health nurse. This implies that the community health nurse is a unique person on the health team. Some of the unique activities of the community health nurse within nursing, based upon a synthesis of concepts and philosophies from nursing and public health, have previously been identified by me.[4] Community health nurses are also unique members of the community health team because of their nursing background. For example, community health nurses are the only professionals on the community health team who provide continuous health care (*i.e.*, preventive, curative, rehabilitative) to all family members in the home or to groups in various settings over an extended period of time. Consequently, they are the only professionals who evaluate changing health conditions and patterns within families and groups as a basis for ongoing interventions. Nurses evaluate the changing biologic, social, psychological, and cultural conditions in families and groups, the changing resources (family or community) to meet the resulting health needs created, and the health patterns emerging from the total interaction. Other professionals may see the client periodically for medical care, social or nutritional counseling, but this kind of care does not allow for assessment of the changing forces affecting families nor assessment of family resources for meeting any health needs. Consequently, nursing is the one discipline on the health team that is in a position to make a dynamic assessment of health needs, to evaluate a family's or any other system's resources (*e.g.*, financial, intellectual, psychological, physical) to meet these needs, and to develop and implement health-care plans for supplementing a family's resources. Some health needs may require skill and knowledge beyond the nurse's area of competence, and the family or group may need to be referred to another resource within the areas of medicine, nutrition, or social work for periodic, intensive care. However, because nurses follow clients over a period of time and can reevaluate health needs and resources, they are in the best position on the health team to coordinate services to clients. The process for viewing forces impinging upon a specific family's or group's system, the reaction to these forces, and the nurse's role as coordinator, where indicated, are discussed in Chapters 6 and 7.

USES OF SYSTEMS THEORY

Systems theory provides a useful framework for viewing individuals, families, and communities and for viewing the interrelationships among these systems as they influence health. It is also useful for looking at nursing as it interacts with and influences the health of these systems. When used in conjunction with nursing processes, systems theory provides the framework for assisting systems (*e.g.*, individual, family, community) to attain, maintain, or regain an optimal level of health.

Chin discusses systems theory and says that the same model can be applied to different human interactional units such as the individual, the group, the organization, and the community.[5] He relates concepts of systems theory to these various units.

Using one theory such as systems theory that is pertinent to the various levels of clients seen in community health nursing facilitates learning for the practitioner and allows comprehensive care. Until recently, a theoretical base for community health nursing practice has not been available, and we have worked with a variety of concepts, facts, and principles. Thus, this theory provides a framework onto which these concepts and future concepts can be attached so that the practitioner can relate facts and principles to each other rather than view them as isolated or fragmentary pieces of knowledge.

Further justification for theory in general is offered by Auger who says, "one of the greatest practical values of theories is their use in the process of decision making. A valid theory . . . will provide a framework for predicting the potential effects of changing one or more dimensions upon the other dimensions of the phenomena."[6] Thus, theory will allow community health nurses to see the possible outcomes of interventions and will facilitate decision making about the best course of action, prior to the initiation of change with clients.

An overview of systems theory follows. Chapters 2, 3, and 4, relate this theory to individuals, families, and communities as systems.

SYSTEMS THEORY

DEFINITIONS OF SYSTEMS

Various authors have defined systems. Von Bertalanffy defined a system as "a complex of elements in interaction."[7] Buckley in two separate publications defined a system as "a whole which functions as a whole by virtue of the interdependence and its parts" and "a complex of elements or components directly or indirectly related in a causal network, such that each component is related to at least some others in a more or less stable way within a particular time period."[8,9] Rappaport defines a system as "a whole which functions as a whole by virtue of the organized interdependent interaction of its parts."[10] Hall and Fagan define a system as "a set of parts or components which have relationships between the parts and between the properties of the parts."[11]

Community health nursing texts have also begun using a systems approach. Archer and Fleshman use Banathy's definition of a system as "an entity comprised of parts which is designed and built by man into an organized whole for the attainment of a specific purpose."[12,13] Hall and Weaver define a system as "a set of components or units interacting with each other within a boundary which filters both the rate of the flow of input and output to and from the system."[14] Braden and Hebran use Buckley's definition, cited earlier.[15]

Although there seems to be agreement in definitions of systems in the general literature as just cited, there is less agreement in the community health nursing literature. Banathy's definition used by Archer and Fleshman is narrowed to man-made systems and fits such systems as automobiles or other machines and relates more to closed systems than it does to systems in general. Systems theory as used in community health nursing should go beyond this definition to include other than man-made systems (*i.e.*, individuals, families, and communities which are the focus for nursing care). Hall and Weaver's definition of systems presents another point of view. As compared to Byrne and

Thompson, Hall and Weaver's definition relates only to open systems rather than to systems in general. Byrne and Thompson say, "a closed system is one that is self contained, totally isolated, and therefore not affected by any changes outside its boundaries . . . an open system is one that is directly affected by happenings or changes in other systems."[16] On the other hand, Auger says, "it is possible to characterize various systems on the basis of their degree of interaction with the surrounding environment. Systems may be classified as open or closed, depending upon the degree of porosity of the boundary-maintaining mechanism, with the more open systems resulting in greater contact with the surrounding environment . . . the term closed system is used in a relative sense since the demonstration of a totally closed system is unknown at this time."[17] Braden's definition, which is taken from the general literature, reflects an adequate definition of a system that is either open or closed.

Because of the confusion in the nursing literature in defining systems and the lack of distinction between open and closed systems, it is important then to define systems as it is used throughout this book. We use the Buckley definition of "a whole which functions as a whole by virtue of the interdependence of its parts."[18] This definition seems to include the other definitions and is not limited to either system (open or closed). This definition implies that the whole of the system is distinguishable from its environment or other systems and that it has parts which have interdependent functions. It also states that the functioning of the interdependent parts is responsible for the functioning of the whole. Since the system acts as a whole, malfunctioning of a part causes a disturbance of the system rather than the loss of a single function.

OPEN VERSUS CLOSED SYSTEMS

Although the nurse deals strictly with open systems (individual, family, group, community) in community health nursing, we differentiate between open and closed systems at this point to facilitate an understanding of open systems. Following this chapter, the book focuses exclusively on open systems.

The essential difference between an open and closed system is whether or not the system exchanges matter, energy, and information with the environment. For this book we accept the concept that closed systems do not exchange information or energy with the environment. Examples of closed systems include rocks, pictures, clocks, statues, atoms, or molecules. An object that is a closed system is "self-contained, totally isolated, and therefore not affected by any changes outside its boundaries."[19] An open system, on the other hand, is a system that exchanges matter or energy with the environment. Examples of open systems are humans, families, groups, communities, and societies, which are all living systems and belong to the realm of community health nursing. All are "directly affected by happenings or changes in other systems."[20]

HIERARCHY OF SYSTEMS

Boulding proposes a hierarchy of systems that begins with the most fundamental closed system and progresses to the most complex open system.[21] At level I, a closed system, he proposes that the world of things includes pictures, statues, atoms, and molecules. Levels II and III are also closed systems of a more complex nature. Level IV introduces open systems, such as the cell; further levels progress through plants, animals, humans, social organizations, and transcendental systems. Although his view is basically the same, Miller looks at only open systems and uses a slightly different hierarchy.[22] He begins with cells and progresses through organs, organisms, groups, organizations, societies, and supernational systems. Both models present a hierarchy that moves from the most simple to the most complex of systems, in which each system exhibits similar characteristics and behavior.

BOUNDARY OF A SYSTEM

The boundary of a system can be conceived as that part of the whole system that stands between the system and its environment. This boundary can be identified because of the greater concentration of energy within the system or mass than is immediately around it, or is between the system and its environment. In other words, there is a greater interchange among the parts of the system (subsystems) than between the system and the outside. The boundary of a system may refer to that aspect of a system that is observable such as the outline of a rock, or a clock, or an individual. Or it may be conceptualized such as that of a family or as an energy field around a system through which exchanges take place. Auger says it is "helpful to visualize a boundary as a filter which permits the constant exchange of elements, information or energy, between the system and its environment."[23] As systems are defined in this book, a filter for screening exchanges with the environment would pertain only to living systems because closed systems do not exchange energy with the environment, nor are they affected by the environment. However, the concept of the boundary as a filter is useful for viewing living systems. The boundary in an open living system is dynamic, and the density of the filter will vary over time depending upon the status of the system. At times the filter will expand allowing for increased exchange, and at other times it will contract reducing the exchange. For example, during the grieving process the human system may contract to shut out external stimuli as it focuses exclusively upon the lost object, or the premature child may expand its boundary and eat more food than a normal-birth-weight child to arrive at the same weight at a later period in life as the normal weight child. Likewise, a family or community may expand its boundaries at one time to increase membership within the system and contract them at other times. These maneuvers are efforts to reduce a particular stress and strain felt by the system and is closely related to the concept of equifinality discussed later in this chapter. Stated another way, these maneuvers prevent overload or underload of the system's dynamic balance and provide purposeful direction within the environment. See the High Level Wellness concept in Chapter 9.

Boundary-maintenance functions (contracting and expanding) vary over time because of the varying goals and needs of the system as it develops. For example, individuals at different stages of their life have differing needs for food intake, sound in the form of information, social interaction, and so forth. In addition, their situational context may influence a need to contract or expand their boundaries. Loss of a loved object, as mentioned earlier, may require contraction of a human system boundary in order to facilitate the grief process. Various boundary function changes (contracting and expanding) can be predicted based upon the established norms of growth and development (see Negentropy, this chapter), and concepts such as grief and crisis, which are discussed in Chapter 10.

STRUCTURE OF A SYSTEM

Because the system has a boundary that distinguishes it from other systems or the environment, it must therefore be a discrete phenomenon, with structure. Hall and Weaver define structure as the "static arrangement of a system's parts at any moment in three-dimensional space."[24] Auger says structure is the "arrangement and nature of organization among the parts of the system."[25] Both definitions are in agreement and will be accepted for this book; they say that there are interrelated parts that function together to maintain the whole system. Thus, the structure of a clock (a closed system) would comprise the frame, the face, the hands, and the moving parts. The structure of the human open system would include the boundary, or body (mass), which can be observed, or the energy field around the body, and internal parts such as organ subsystems (circulatory, digestive, respiratory). These interrelated parts make up the whole of the system. As we move up the hierarchy of systems, interlocking roles and relationships may also be added to the structure. For example, the structure of the family consists of not only its individual members, but also of their interlocking roles and relationships, which maintain the family and assist in meeting its goals. One member may provide income, another may cook and clean, and so forth to provide for the family's needs.

In open systems we usually refer to these interrelated parts as subsystems, and consequently it is important to identify the specific system being used. Any one of the open systems identified in the hierarchy could be viewed as a system, from cells to supranational systems. Lower-order systems are always subsystems or subordinate systems of the next higher-order system. For example, the cell is a subsystem of its particular organ system; an organ is a subsystem of the entire organ system; the organ system is a subsystem of the individual as a system; and the individual is a subsystem of the family as a system. Likewise, each higher order system is a superordinate system of the system below it. Thus the community is a superordinate system of the family, the family a superordinate system of man, and so forth. To understand a system adequately, it is important to see the system in relation to its subsystems and its superordinate system. Thus if we are studying an individual as our system, we should also know about the individual's subsystems (organ subsystems, such as circulatory, urinary, respiratory) and his superordinate system—the family. (See the section titled A Focal Point on Systems later on in this chapter.)

If we look at the system as made up of mass, energy, and information we can identify three kinds of energy within the system. They are as follows: (1) organized energy; (2) kinetic energy, or energy in motion; and (3) potential, or stored energy.

Organized energy includes all matter in space, such as the material substances that make up the cellular structure of humans, animals, plants, microorganisms, and other living matter. In the higher forms of life this energy is not only organized but also specialized in that certain cells form the liver, some form the heart, and so on for the various other parts of the mass. Through the process of anabolism and catabolism this organized energy renews itself and grows more organized (negentropy). At some points in the life span, the breakdown process may exceed the buildup process and entropy occurs (see Entropy, this chapter).

Kinetic energy encompasses communication and the expendable energy of the system and is identified as energy in motion which maintains the homeodynamic energy needs of the system (organized energy) and allows movement of the total energy field. For example, in the individual, this energy facilitates all internal processes such as the conversion of glycogen to glucose needed to maintain a constant blood sugar level, and it facilitates the transmission of messages up and down the spinal cord. In addition, it allows for movement of the individual through space by working through the musculoskeletal and nervous systems. Kinetic energy in a family would relate to the functions performed by members and the system of checks and balances in the family. For example, kinetic energy would relate to who does what, who is accountable to whom, and to other role behaviors as well as to the overt and covert rules about behavior and the homeodynamic range of acceptable behaviors. These behaviors *in toto* facilitate the movement of the family as a group toward realizing family goals and help them evolve through the stages of family development.

Kinetic energy may come from within the system, that is, through conversion of potential energy (such as fat deposits or glycogen in the liver in the individual) to kinetic energy, or it may be drawn from outside sources. For example, in the process of digestion, humans convert the organized energy of plants and animals to kinetic energy, or they may use external kinetic energy such as heat, light, and sound directly. Likewise, a family may be able to meet the needs of a sick member or a newborn, or they may rely upon outside assistance.

The third type of energy is **potential energy** or stored energy. Within the individual this includes storehouses such as fat deposits, and also glycogen in the liver. In the individual's environment there are many sources of potential energy. A building has the potential for falling and creating sound (kinetic energy). It also has the potential to keep out heat and to block out light and sound. Work was done before this potential was realized; that is, energy was used to erect the building. In a similar vein, an electrical outlet has the potential for light, an automobile has the potential for motion, and a stove with fuel has the potential for giving off heat. Many of these are man-made conversions of energy for later use by individuals.

Potential energy in a family refers to the knowledge, attitudes, and skills that are available to the family for meeting its needs as a unit. Although some of these energies in the system relate to process rather than to structure, they have been presented here to identify energies within a system.

PROCESSES IN A SYSTEM

Dorland's Illustrated Medical Dictionary defines process as "a series of operations, events, or steps leading to the achievement of a specific result."[26] This section looks at the systematic actions of a system and the end result of these actions. Although both open and closed systems have processes, these processes and the end result of the processes vary because closed systems do not exchange with the environment. A contrast of these processes and the end results are presented to facilitate a better understanding of open systems. Auger refers to process as function, and Hall refers to process as dynamics.[27,28]

Exchange with the Environment. To present a somewhat systematic sequence of the processes in a system, we begin with the exchange between the system and the environment although this exchange takes place only with open systems.

Open systems exchange energy, matter, and information with the environment (see also Homeodynamics or Steady State later in this chapter). From conception until death the open system (individuals, family, community) continually take in energy, matter, and information from the environment and release energy, matter, or information back into the environment. These exchanges could be categorized in various ways depending upon the point of view. One category could include chemical, physical, biologic, and psychosocial energy as well as mass and include information under the psychosocial or sound category. Another might utilize autonomy, health, and resources where each of these is used in the broadest sense. For example, resources would include the previous category as well as financial, intellectual, and manpower resources, and so forth. Braden categorizes exchanges in another way and includes "spatial, sociologic, cultural, physiologic, psychologic, economic and political factors."[29]

These exchanges are elaborated upon in Chapters 2, 3, and 4, but an example here may help to clarify the concept of exchange in an open system. Probably the easiest exchange to grasp is the food cycle, which is a chemical exchange between individuals and their environment. Humans require an adequate quantity and quality of food from plant and animal sources. During the process of digestion, food undergoes physical and chemical changes and is made ready for absorption. Following transportation to the cells, food is utilized for energy, for building or repairing cell structure, and for the regulation of cellular processes. Excesses of food may be stored for future use as potential energy, or it may be excreted. The residue excreted by humans becomes energy for other living systems (organisms, plants).

What comes out of a system is different from what goes into it. In addition to the transformation of energy, information, and matter which is taken into the system (food broken down into energy), there is a decoding process that is consistent with the goals and purposeful direction of the system. Thus, energy from the ingested food is retained by the system to meet its goal of maintenance and growth (negentropy). In addition, waste products (output) are different from the food originally taken in. This also meets the system's goal of maintenance and growth by removing products that could be toxic to the system.

At another level, information taken into the system of a nursing student will come out differently in the form of work output in the clinical setting and may also come out differently on a pencil-and-paper examination, depending upon the meaning of the information input for that particular student (system). Thus in a group of students there is usually a range of grades for both theory and clinical performance depending upon the meaning of the information input, the amount of retained information, and the goals of the individual students.

Information as one kind of input into the system has been defined by Hazzard as "the degree of freedom that exists in a given situation to choose among symbols, messages or patterns that have been transferred."[30] She also says, "information processing or communication is the change of information from one state to another or its movement from one point to another over space." Because systems have a choice regarding the reception of messages transferred over space, the meaning of the information to the system as it is related to its goals is important if information is to be allowed into the system (input). This information may be decoded and responded to immediately (output), or it may be retained in the system as potential energy for future use.

In addition, the information that enters the system (input) will vary from that which comes out (output) because of transformation, decoding, and combining with already stored information (potential energy). For example, the written material in this book (input) may vary from your interpretation of it (output). You will perceive and interpret it based upon your goals, past experience (stored information), and current condition. If you need the information for practice, are rested while reading, and have a background in systems theory, your interpretation or learned behavior (output) will be closer to what I am writing (input) than if you lack one or another of these variables. Also, if we could discuss the material, toss ideas back and forth, and relate it to something that is meaningful to you, the output would become closer to the input because of the feedback process.

System Control of Multiple Exchanges. In reality there are many exchanges taking place concurrently between an open system and its environment, which can be controlled to some extent by the system. Earlier, we discussed the boundary that filters the rate and flow of energy, matter, and information to and from the system, causing the flow to vary from time to time. In addition, the feedback from this exchange process will monitor the input and output of the system to prevent system overload or underload. (See Feedback Process, this chapter).

Some of the overload is prevented from entering the system by containing certain energy, information, and matter within the environment. Containment is the holding, within fixed limits, of energy, information, and matter within the environment. Thus, the system (individual, family, or community) may contain or exchange with the environment depending upon the meaning of the energy, information, and matter in relation to the purposes of the system at that particular time. For example, if you talk with me about engineering and I have no need for this information or background in this area, I may block out the information by thinking of something else or I may listen to you but not retain the information. However, if my goal or need is to develop a closer relationship with you by sharing something that is important to you, I may receive this information but need a lot of interaction (feedback) in order to understand and exchange with you in the future to meet my goal (relationship).

Containment is also necessary to prevent disorganization (entropy) of the system because it focuses on behavior that will meet its goal. For example, in the area of sound I must block out the ticking of the clock, the noise of radiators, street traffic, and so forth to focus on writing this book (goal).

What is contained by the system will vary over time depending upon the goals of the system, the learned behaviors in meeting these goals, and the particular needs at the time. Goals, behaviors, and needs change over time as the system becomes more organized (negentropy). (See Boundary Maintenance, this chapter, for further discussion of this idea.)

Containment is a process similar to boundary contraction and is introduced here because it is part of a model of exchange presented by Bredemeier, who says that the process of adaptation consists of obtaining energy, information, and matter from the environment, disposing of energy, information, and matter to the environment, containing energy, information, and matter within the environment and retaining energy, information, and matter within the system.[31] These four aspects of adaptation are discussed in Chapter 2 and are useful in comparing the system's exchanges with established norms based upon age, stage of development, goals, needs, and conditions.

Internal Processes—Subsystem Change. In any system (open or closed) the interrelated parts function together to maintain the whole system and because the parts are interrelated, a change in one part (subsystem) will affect the other parts and therefore the whole system.

The process is complex in an open system because there is the continual exchange with the environment with increased order and organization of the system (negentropy). However, as the open system is acted upon by its internal or external environment, a change in a part of the system will also affect other parts and the system as a whole. For example, fluid intake (external exchange) would affect the subsystems and the whole system of an individual. To explain further, fluid intake (digestive subsystem) leads to an increased circulatory blood volume (cardiovascular subsystem) followed by a corresponding increase in urinary output (urological subsystem) and other changes needed to maintain the fluid balance of the system.

In the family system the parts (individual members) are joined together into the whole (family) by means of their interdependence and interaction. Behaviors such as cooking, cleaning, and providing income are patterned into roles for members to provide for the needs and goals of the family. These may be relatively fixed at times (steady state) because of overt and covert rules about roles and counteracting attempts by family members to maintain roles by reward and punishment when an individual member tries to change a role behavior. However, when change is introduced by either an external exchange (loss of job or illness of a family member) or internal changes (growth of individual with movement to a new stage of development) the family as a whole must change, or the individual may have to leave the family unit (*e.g.*, divorce). An example of an external change is the father as breadwinner becoming ill. The other family members must now take over the father's economic function as well as the function of caring for him during his illness. If the mother takes over this role, she will have less time to devote to the needs of the other members, and in addition, they may need to take over some of her role functions. If there is a decreased income as a result of the mother taking over the family's economics, other members may also need to forgo some of the previously attainable luxury items.

It should also be remembered that the family is an open system and exchanges energy and information with the outside community. Thus, if they are unable to provide for their financial and health care needs, they may turn to the community for assistance. However, even with this input into the system, the illness of the father will necessitate role changes. For example, the mother and children will need to use time previously used for other activities to visit him in the hospital. Likewise, if the family uses the community's welfare program during this period there will be less income (input) and a greater need to spend time budgeting, developing a plan for priority items, and so forth. Other role behaviors of the father, which may have been cutting the grass, driving the automobile, and paying bills, may also need to be taken over by other members. In addition, family members may well be emotionally upset and worried about finances as well as the father's condition, so there may also be a need for increased support of one another which increases the role behaviors of each of the members. This list of changes in family roles could be unending depending upon the particular family and circumstances.

In terms of internal changes affecting the family as a whole, it is useful to think of the developmental stages. While a child or adult is in a particular stage, the role behaviors are temporarily steady and fixed. However, as a member moves to another stage of development, all role behaviors must change to accommodate to the new needs of the individual members (see Chaps. 2 and 3).

The system, whether individual, family, or community, must be able to maintain a temporary steady state but also change its behavior at other times as it moves toward higher levels of order and organization (negentropy) as a result of internal (subordinate or subsystems) or external (superordinate) pressures. This process of maintaining a temporary steady state and moving toward a new steady state is accomplished by the process of feedback, which assists self-regulatory system processes. Feedback is discussed later in this chapter.

Internal Processes—Adaptive Processes of a System. The adaptive processes or temporary end result of the internal processes just conceptualized will differ for open and closed systems.

CLOSED SYSTEM ADAPTATION. In a closed system work must be done on the system before internal processes occur. Following this work, the interdependent parts work together until the process stops and there is no further tension on the system. Thus, the closed system moves toward homeostasis, which is defined as "the tendency of a system to seek equilibrium."[32]

This movement toward homeostasis is a characteristic of closed systems known as **entropy,** which is defined as the quantity of energy within a system that is not capable of conversion into work. We know from physics that whenever energy is transferred from one form to another, only a fraction of the internal energy change is available for doing useful work and the rest remains as heat energy of the molecule left at the completion of the reaction, or entropy. Because a great deal of energy is lost in transfer (entropy) and there is no further input into the process (mixing of sodium and chlorine), the processes are irreversible. This behavior is consistent with the second principle of thermodynamics, which states that in a closed system the process will proceed in one direction (irreversible) and the entropy must increase to a maximum and eventually the process comes to a halt, or state of homeostasis. Maximum entropy is the tendency toward maximum disorder within the system.

For example, heat will move in a definite direction from hotter to colder areas, and chemical reactions, likewise, follow this principle; thus, heat dissipates and chemical reactions become less and less effective and finally stop. The general trend of events is toward states of maximum disorder and the leveling of differences. The unwinding of the clock follows a similar pattern. It can go only in the direction of unwinding—doing less and less work—until it reaches a state of homeostasis when it stops. This second principle of thermodynamics is useful then to predict behavior in closed systems. However, this principle is invalid in predicting behavior in open systems, as we see now.

OPEN SYSTEM ADAPTATION. In an open system where ongoing exchange (input–output) of energy, information, and matter with the environment leads to increased order and organization of the system (negentropy), there can be no homeostasis and no freedom from tension because the system is continually adjusting to ongoing exchange. Thus, there is a homeodynamic adjustment of the system as the parts work together to keep the parts and the whole system within the normal range, such as a temperature around 98.6°F, a blood sugar within the range of 80 to 120 mg per 100 ml, and so forth. This process is known as the **self-regulatory mechanism,** adaptation of the system, or steady state. Sutterly, who calls this process a steady state, defines it as "the tendency of an open system to remain constant but maintain a continuous exchange and flow of components."[33] The process of maintaining this homeodynamic balance involves feedback, which is discussed later.

Auger defines equilibrium or steady state as a "hypothetical fixed point where opposing forces are cancelled out by one another" and says an example would be body temperature.[34] Equilibrium is reached when factors that result in the production of heat are precisely balanced by factors that result in the loss of heat; this point is somewhere between 97.6° and 100.6°F.

Entropy. In open systems there are both decreases and increases in entropy (disorganization) because open systems have both reversible and irreversible processes related to the ongoing exchange with the environment. Disorganization, or entropy, is always present because the parts of the system must continually adjust to the input and some energy is lost in the process of transformation and subsequent feedback. However, there is usually enough energy to go beyond entropy to do the system's work. For example, in the process of human digestion energy is lost and unavailable for work (entropy) in the energy transformation of food, but the body continually receives additional energy through inputs from the environment which are available for work. Braden says, "without the energy inputs . . . the existing energy level needed to run the system would be depleted quickly. Increased entropy leads to death of the system."[35]

As the system moves toward disorganization (entropy), it is less able to fulfill its goals because the parts are not functioning efficiently as a whole. This may relate to individuals, families, or communities as systems. Disease processes seen in individuals are examples of entropic processes. For example, in emphysema the individual has a disturbance in the oxygen–carbon dioxide exchange because of the decreased lung capacity. This change in the part of the system affects other subsystems such as the circulatory and nervous systems, which will accommodate but at a less efficient level. Because the whole system (individual) will be affected by these changes, the system is less able to meet its goal of maintaining itself and growing. Many nursing functions at the secondary and tertiary levels of prevention are aimed at counteracting these entropic processes.

As the system becomes less efficient, the parts work together less well to meet the goals of the whole system, and it theoretically moves down the health continuum toward death. Once this process begins, there is usually a need for outside assistance from nursing and other health professions because the self-regulatory processes are beginning to fail. Depending upon the degree of entropy, the system will survive or die. For example, if there is excess energy in the system (negentropy), it will grow and survive. If the entropic and negentropic processes balance each other, there will be a steady state, and if the entropic processes surpass the negentropic processes, there will be a breakdown and possible death to the system. Nursing interventions (input into a system) are geared toward preventing or reversing entropic processes. For example, the nurse may teach the harmful effects of smoking to prevent emphysema and other lung diseases (entropy), or the nurse may teach an emphysema patient to deep breathe. This will increase the client's lung capacity; it will have an effect on other interrelated parts (subsystems) and the whole system, and counteract to a degree the entropic process with negentropic processes (see The Nursing Process in Chap. 6).

Negentropy. When the system receives a sufficient input of energy, information, and matter to go beyond transformation (entropy), there is a tendency toward increased order and organization of the system (negentropy). Thus, negentropy, or negative entropy, is a characteristic of an open system (but not a closed system) and invalidates the second principle of thermodynamics for open systems.

Negentropy is energy that can be utilized by the system for work and is characterized by order and organization. From conception to death, humans as open systems exchange with the environment and utilize the energy and information to maintain themselves while moving toward increasing organization and order from a physical, psychological, and social point of view. The system becomes more complex with increased structure and processes that alter its state. For example, through the process of anabolism and catabolism the physical system of humans grows from infancy to adulthood. Sutterley discusses many other processes that lead to increased order and organization in systems.[36] Thus, the second law of thermodynamics, which was useful in predicting closed systems, does not pertain to open systems.

Likewise, from a social point of view, an individual as a system learns from exchanges with the environment and takes on increasingly complex roles in society. Many other examples of negentropy of open systems (individuals, families, communities) are cited in the following three chapters.

Because the open system grows in complexity (negentropy) and must alter its state to accommodate to this growth, the concept of homeodynamic adjustment and steady state is only one part of the self-regulatory processes of the system. Not only must the system be capable of maintaining a steady state for temperature, blood sugar, and other bodily functions as discussed earlier, but it must also be capable of moving away from a steady state to adjust to growth and increased organization (negentropy). Thus, self-regulatory processes involve two important functions to maintain the system's goal of maintenance and growth and are accomplished through the process of feedback. Because the system (individual, family, community) demonstrates increased order and organization as a result of exchanges and must alter itself at times, it is best to think of temporary steady states with systems.

Feedback. In open living systems, feedback facilitates self-regulatory processes. Feedback is the process whereby some of the output from the system is fed back into the system as input.

There are two types of feedback into the system: they are negative feedback and positive feedback. **Negative feedback** minimizes change within the system by decreasing deviations from what the system considers normal. When there is a deviation from the normal from internal or external changes, there is a counterreaction by the system to bring it back to a steady state, as discussed earlier. Using this process the system receives mismatched information from within and without the system, indicating a discrepancy (or divergence) between the system's behavior and some desired goal. Counteracting operations are triggered to bring the system's behavior back into congruence with its internal standards or goals. Examples of negative-feedback control from a physiologic point of view include the control of the electrolyte and fluid balance, the maintenance of blood sugar levels, and the maintenance of temperature and blood pressure in the individual within a normal range. Thus, although these variables may change in one way or another, when the system encounters internal or external changes, they will be acted upon by countering forces within the system to bring them back to a steady state. For example, Miller says, "depletion of body water increases the electrolyte concentration in extracellular tissues . . . which signals the osmoreceptors in the hypothalamus to send signals to the posterior pituitary to secrete vasopression, an antidiuretic that acts directly upon the kidney." This "increases the resorption of water by the kidney tubules into the blood stream and thus decreases the volume of urine by retaining water in the body."[37] Thus, any deviation in water intake is corrected, and there is a restored steady state of the water content of the body through regulation of the intake and output of water. An example of negative feedback from a sociological point of view includes the reward and punishment by families (overt and covert) of individual members who are deviating from accepted values, norms, or family roles.

The other type of feedback is positive feedback, which amplifies deviations from the steady state and facilitates learning and growth by forcing the system to change its internal steady state. **Positive feedback** has the opposite effect of negative feedback in that it moves a system away from a steady state instead of toward it, and once this effect is started, it tends to accelerate. This process can be disastrous or pathologic if not kept under control (entropy), but on the other hand, it is necessary for system maintenance and growth (negentropy). Positive feedback always begins with mismatched information between the system's behaviors and its internal goals and standards of external criteria. Subsequent operations increase the divergence or split between the system's status and its original goal. During this process the system will experience tension and conflict until the individual arrives at the next patterened set of behaviors that are consistent with the new goal, or decides to give up the goal. Some examples of positive feedback follow.

I have set for myself as a goal the completion of this book within a specified period of time. I have also been awarded a leave from my teaching position to accomplish this goal. Thus, it has been necessary for me to move away from the steady state of much interaction with students, faculty, and social acquaintances to spend long hours alone to read and write. When I deviate too far from this behavior—that is, spend too much time socializing—this information is fed back into my system, and produces tension and conflict. This tension and conflict can be resolved only by returning to the new patterns of reading and writing to meet my goal, or else I must change the goal and forgo writing the book. Another example is children who mature and grow out of their complete dependency role (physically, mentally, and emotionally) with their parents. They will need to move to another steady state and assume some responsibility for themselves by taking on some independent or interdependent roles (negentropy). Obviously, this will also necessitate changes in the roles of other family members (steady state) to accommodate to this role change.

An example of a social situation where the system may experience positive feedback that is disastrous for the system is a teacher who stereotypes a lower-class child as a slow learner when in fact the child is bright. If the child accepts this positive feedback, he will deviate even more from the ability he has; that is, he will perform as if he were slow even though he is actually bright. Scapegoating in a family or group can also lead to a similar phenomenon.

Whether or not a child accepts this positive feedback will depend upon the goals and maintenance needs of the child as he sees them, based upon his learning experiences. If the child has a goal of doing well in school and succeeding, he may counteract the teacher's positive feedback and continue to work up to his capacity, or, if the positive feedback produces enough stress and strain in the child's system, and if the child's goal is important enough, he will function extra hard and go beyond class expectations. Thus, one child may accept this type of feedback from the teacher, or scapegoating from the family, whereas another child will reject it based upon his goals and learned mechanisms of coping and maintaining a steady state.

Goals and maintenance needs as identified by the system are important aspects of feedback. If the individual (system) wants to do well in college (goal) but is in the habit of oversocializing with little time for homework he will need to move away from this state to one of long hours of study (positive feedback). The perceived difference between the set (new) goal with its change in the steady state and the current steady state will lead to stress for the system. If the individual persists toward the new goal the stress will lead to a new steady state of more studying and less socializing, or he may decide against the goal, and change it.

Without positive feedback there would be no growth or creativity for we would remain at a constant steady state. As anabolism exceeds catabolism in the individual system, growth occurs, and with it comes new steady states. We grow from the dependent child who is unable to walk or talk to the interdependent adult. Concurrent with the physical growth process, are other growth processes such as learning, creativity, and communication, which *in toto* continually lead to new steady states. Sutterley has looked at all of these conditions and their effects on the steady states of individuals as systems.[38] Some of these conditions are discussed in Chapter 2.

Learning is an aspect of feedback that facilitates this progression toward a steady state and is an important concept for community health nursing. Humans as systems learn ways of dealing with environmental exchanges to maintain a steady state or to move toward new goals and steady states. For example, in cold weather we learn to dress warmly when outside, or to heat our homes, with the goal of maintaining our systems' temperatures within a range of adaptability. Likewise for other exchanges such as food, light, and social relationships, we learn ways of maintaining a steady state. We also learn ways to reduce stress and strain when our goals are inconsistent with reality, and thus may move further away from the steady state toward the new goal, or we may change the goal.

Because individual systems are born and grow in different social and cultural groups and have different genetic and experience backgrounds, individuals will learn different ways of maintaining their systems and have different goals. Some of these learned behaviors and goals may facilitate the system's adaptation, and others may take it outside its range of adaptability. For example, if the individual learns to eat junk foods, he will probably be lacking in protein, vitamins, and minerals and move outside the range of adaptability, that is, outside the range where the body parts (subsystems) can work together to maintain the system because the system's reserves become exhausted, and there are insufficient external exchanges resulting from inadequate learning about nutrition. Illness (entropy) may result from this learning.

MULTICAUSATION

Because each system has its own learned ways of dealing with environmental exchanges and its own goals, it is impractical to look for single factors or cause–effect relationships for the states of the system being considered. Rather we should look for the underlying factors of multicausation for the state or behavior observed. The concept of multicausation is well accepted in community health, and we know there are multiple factors in humans, the disease agent, and the environment that influence health and disease processes. Leavell and Clark have presented a framework for viewing these relationships and have applied their framework to various health and disease processes.[39] We look at some of these in Chapter 9. Multicausation can also be applied to observed behavior. In an earlier article, co-workers and I developed the concept of interrelatedness to account for the multiple factors leading to specific behavior.[40]

CONCEPT OF EQUIFINALITY VERSUS FINALITY

Equifinality is defined as "the same final state of a system [that] can be reached from different initial conditions and in different ways."[41] Because of the transfer of energy and matter between open systems and the environment and available energy to the system for work (negentropy), the system can evolve toward increased order and organization. This order and organization in combination with the feedback process allow the system to grow and evolve while maintaining a series of steady states.

These steady states for an individual open system will vary from system to system because of the differing goals of each system and the learned behaviors that maintain the steady state discussed earlier. Thus the same final state of a system (a temporary steady state) can be reached from different points (initial conditions) and in different ways. For example, growth is equifinal; the same species final state can be reached in different ways. A normal individual can result from a complete ovum or from each half of a divided ovum (identical twins). Thus, open systems are equifinal; that is, they can attain a steady state independent of initial conditions and are determined only by the system's parameters.

This is in contrast to closed systems whereby the "final state of the system is determined by the initial conditions."[42] Closed systems exhibit finality. For example, the final product of chemical reactants depends upon the initial products. If one sodium atom is combined with one chlorine atom there will be one molecule of sodium chloride when homeostasis is reached.

Each equifinal state in an open system is maintained for an interval of time until the system sets new goals and evolves to a higher order of development. Again there is a new equifinal phase that is relatively stable. The concept of equifinality again specifies the need for viewing multicausal factors in behavior rather than cause–effect relationships. Individuals (systems) can become effective contributing members of the community in a variety of ways depending upon their goals. They may become professionals or unskilled workers. Likewise they may be active members of political parties and they may be members of charitable organizations. An individual's understanding of available approaches (learned behaviors) to meet a goal will partially determine the best decisions for meeting temporary steady states.

A FOCAL POINT IN SYSTEMS

Systems can be arranged in a hierarchy beginning with the simplest closed system and ending with the most complex open system. As we move up this hierarchy, the higher order system always includes the lower order system, as discussed earlier.

Most disciplines study or use in practice the behavior of a specific system. Behavior is a "response to a stimulus."[43] Ordinarily when we think of behavior we tend to think of a human's fight or flight (response) to a threatening situation (stimulus) or of the Pavlovian dog who was conditioned to salivate (response) to the sound of a bell (stimulus), which we learned in psychology. Or we may think of the behavior of groups of people such as the family which we learned about in sociology. However, these examples focus on only two levels of behavior (the individual and family) and behavior can be exhibited at various levels of the hierarchy discussed earlier.

"Behavior is the action or reaction exhibited as a particular unit—be it a cell, a human, or a business corporation—how it copes with stimuli originating from either an internal or external source."[44] Using our hierarchy, cellular behavior is the least complex behavior of the open living system. Next in complexity would be organs that are built from cells. Organs constitute body systems (respiratory, cardiovascular) which make up the next level of behavior, and individuals as the next unit of behavior are comprised of organ systems. Next we have families comprised of individuals, followed by communities comprised of families, and societies comprised of communities. As behavior is studied by means of a hierarchy, it becomes more complex and variable, and thus it is necessary to speak of levels of behavioral organization.

These various levels of behavior provide the focus for different disciplines in our specialized society. Each discipline focuses on the interactions between a structural unit of a specific system (cell, organ, organism, family, community) and its particular environment, and develops a comprehensive understanding of behavior at that level. Each discipline knows the conditions that will produce behavioral changes and can predict behavioral responses; it knows the norms for behavior at that level and the actions needed to produce change. Although each discipline will usually have a general knowledge of all levels of behavior (such as cells, organs, organism) as a basis for understanding its own level, this knowledge is not of the magnitude of the discipline itself.

Cellular behavior is the focus of the microbiologist and genetic worker. Physiologists focus on organs and organ systems' behaviors. Likewise, physicians and some allied health workers may specialize in one or another of the organ systems. For example, we have physicians in cardiology, dermatology, neurology, urology, and obstetrics, and in addition we have respiratory therapists, physical therapists, dental hygienists, and so forth. Organismic behavior is the focus of the psychophysiologist and the ecologist, and small-group behavior such as the family is the focus of the sociologist.

Behavior patterns of communities is the focus of health educators, sanitarians, and community organizers, and behavior at the societal level is the focus of sociologists and anthropologists.

FOCUS OF COMMUNITY HEALTH NURSING

In our definition of community health nursing, we indicated that the nurse works to improve the health of community populations by focusing on individuals, families, and communities. Thus, the nurse must have a knowledge of the individual, family, and community systems as unified wholes, that is, knowledge of the behavior of each system as it interacts with and is influenced by subordinate and superordinate systems. For example, the nurse must view individuals as a totality (see Chap. 2) with subordinate and superordinate systems which interact and influence their behavior. Likewise, the nurse must view the family as a system whose behavior is influenced by interaction with subordinate (individual members) and superordinate (community) systems.

Initially, the nurse must obtain knowledge about all levels of behavior in order to understand the behavior of the individual, family, and community system. As a student the nurse studies cell behavior in microbiology, immunology, and genetics, organ and organ system behavior in biochemistry, anatomy and physiology, and higher levels of behavior in psychology, sociology, and anthropology. However, once the student begins an intensive study of community health nursing, the primary focus should be on individuals, families, and communities as unified wholes with behavior resulting from interaction with subordinate and superordinate systems. At that time isolated facts and concepts from other courses should be synthesized and organized into meaningful wholes comprised of these relationships. Thus, from this point the student should look at the interrelationship among the system, its subordinate system, and its superordinate system as a basis for applying the nursing process.

In addition, community health nurses focus on all levels of prevention with systems (individual, family, community) and should therefore be concerned with preventing disease (entropy) as well as case finding and treatment. The levels of prevention are explained in more detail in Chapter 9.

REFERENCES

1. Executive Committee and the Standards Committee of the Division on Community Health Practice. Community Health Nursing. Kansas City, ANA, 1973
2. WICHE. Defining Clinical Content: Graduate Nursing Programs; Community Health Nursing, p 7. Boulder, University East Campus, 1967
3. Dunn H L: High Level Wellness. Arlington, R W Beaty, 1961
4. Helvie C, et al: The setting and nursing practice, part I. Nurs Outlook 16, No. 8: 27–29, Aug 1968
5. Chin R: The utility of systems models and developmental models for practitioners. In Riehl J, Roy Sister Callista (eds): Conceptual Models for Nursing Practice, pp 47–48. New York Appleton-Century-Crofts, 1975
6. Auger J: Behavioral Systems and Nursing, p 19. Englewood Cliffs, Prentice-Hall, 1976
7. von Bertalanffy L: General Systems Theory. New York, Penguin Books, 1973
8. Buckley W: Modern Systems Research for the Behavioral Scientist, p XVII. Chicago, Aldine, 1968
9. Buckley W: Sociology and Modern Systems Theory. Englewood Cliffs, Prentice-Hall, 1967
10. Rappaport A: Foreword. In Buckley W (ed): Modern Systems Research for the Behavioral Scientist, Chicago, Aldine, 1968
11. Hall A D, Fagan R E: Definitions of systems. In Buckley W (ed): Modern Systems Research for the Behavioral Scientist, p 81. Chicago, Aldine, 1968
12. Archer S, Fleshman R: Community Health Nursing Patterns and Practice, p. 5. North Scituate, Duxbury, 1975
13. Banathy B H. Instructional Systems, p 90. Belmont, Fearon, 1968
14. Hall J, Weaver B: Distributive Nursing Practice: A Systems Approach to Community Health. Philadelphia, J B Lippincott, 1977
15. Braden C, Hebran N: Community Health. A Systems

Approach, p. 5. New York, Appleton-Century-Crofts, 1976
16. Byrne M, Thompson L: Key Concepts for the Study and Practice of Nursing, p 6. St Louis, C V Mosby, 1972
17. Auger op cit, p 21
18. Buckley W, op cit
19. Byrne M, Thompson L, op cit
20. Ibid
21. Boulder K: General systems theory—The skeleton of science. In Buckley W (ed): Modern Systems Research for the Behavioral Scientist, pp 3–10. Englewood Cliffs, Prentice-Hall, 1968
22. Miller J: Living Systems, p. 4. New York, McGraw-Hill, 1978
23. Auger J, op cit, p 24
24. Hall J, Weaver B, op cit, p 20
25. Auger, op cit, p 22
26. Friel J P: Dorland's Illustrated Medical Dictionary, p 1257. Philadelphia, W B Saunders, 1974
27. Auger op cit
28. Hall J, Weaver B, op cit
29. Braden C, Hebran N, op cit, p 17
30. Hazzard E: An overview of systems theory. Nurs Clin North Am 6, No. 3: 388, Sept 1971
31. Bredemeier H C: Social Systems: Integration and Adaptation, New Brunswick, Rutgers University, 1962 (Unpublished paper)
32. Sutterley D, Donnelly G: Perspectives in Human Development, p 17. Philadelphia, J B Lippincott, 1973
33. Ibid
34. Auger J, op cit, p 11
35. Braden C, Hebran N, op cit, p 13
36. Sutterley D, Donnelly G, op cit
37. Miller J, op cit, p 456
38. Sutterley D, Donnelly G, op cit
39. Leavell H, Clark G: Preventive Medicine for the Doctor in his Community. New York, McGraw-Hill, 1965
40. Helvie C, et al: The setting and nursing practice, part II. Nurs Outlook 16, No. 9: 34–37, Sept 1968
41. Sutterley D, Donnelly G, op cit
42. Ibid
43. Byrne M, Thompson L, op cit
44. Ibid

2
The Individual as a System

In Chapter 1 an overview of systems theory and its justification in community health nursing is presented. In this chapter systems theory is related to the individual.

CONCEPT OF THE INDIVIDUAL

Consistent with the definition of a system, the individual can be conceived as a whole with interrelated parts that function together to maintain the whole system's balance and purposeful direction in the environment. Thus, the individual as a system is made up of interrelated parts (subsystems) such as the circulatory, respiratory, and musculoskeletal subsystems, which function interdependently to maintain the individual's balance. In addition, the brain as part of the neurologic subsystem assists in maintaining balance by reasoning and utilizing learning to influence exchanges with the environment. The brain is also used by individuals to set goals that influence behavior, although not all learning is rational. The individual interacts in social settings throughout life and learns certain psychosocial mechanisms to reduce stress and meet basic needs for love, belonging, and self-actualization. These learned behaviors may assist or interfere with the system's balance and purposeful direction. For example, some consistent emotional patterns may lead to psychosomatic illnesses, interfere with learning, or hamper coping with stress. The individual must therefore be conceived as a biopsychosocial being who interacts with an environment that is biologic, physical, chemical, and psychosocial.

INDIVIDUAL'S PLACE IN THE HIERARCHY

In the hierarchy presented in Chapter 1, the individual falls between the organ system and the family. The subordinate system (subsystem) of the individual is the organ system, and the superordinate system is the family. Thus, an assessment of the individual must consider not only the location of the individual on the health continuum, but also the influence of the organ system and the family on the noted behavior as a basis for nursing interventions.

BOUNDARY OF THE INDIVIDUAL

The boundary of the individual can be identified by the greater concentration of energy within the system than is immediately around it; that is, there is a greater interchange of energy among the parts of the individual than there is between the individual and the environment. The **boundary** is external to the skin, which covers the mass of the system, and can be conceptualized as the energy field surrounding the body. Interchanges within the system, which is discussed under processes, involve the various transformations of energy, information, and mass, which enter the system and are retained or disposed of by the system.

FILTER OF THE BOUNDARY

The individual's boundary serves as a filter for screening the exchange of elements, energy, and information with the environment, and, as noted before, can expand or contract to increase or decrease these exchanges. This allows the system to maintain a degree of balance in relation to the changing internal and external demands upon the system, and prevents overload or underload. Examples of boundary expansion include overeating to compensate for loneliness or frustration, increased oxygen exchange during jogging, or increased doses of vitamin C when the individual has a cold. Examples of boundary contraction include shutting out external stimuli when grieving or suffering from an illness, or withdrawing when hurt by a loved one. Some of these maneuvers are automatic on the part of the individual's system (*e.g.*, increased oxygen exchange) and others are consciously learned responses to overload or underload (*e.g.*, overeating or withdrawing). All serve to help the system maintain balance temporarily, but in the long run may lead to further stress and strain upon the system. For example, overeating may help the system compensate for loneliness and help maintain its balance temporarily, but this learned behavior may eventually lead to obesity and concurrent health problems if practiced regularly.

Throughout life, the individual's boundary contracts or expands depending upon the stage of growth and development. As individuals grow they take in greater amounts of information, energy, and mass, to meet the needs of the increasingly complex system (see Negentropy, this chapter).

ENVIRONMENT BEYOND THE BOUNDARY

The boundary of a system indicates that there is something beyond the system, and all, except for the largest systems, have suprasystems consisting of the system and its environment. The environment of the individual system is everything that is external to its boundary and is comprised of energy, mass, and information, which the system exchanges with its environment. Mass, or forms of organized energy such as humans, animals, and plants, can be seen with the unaided eye, while other forms of organized energy, such as bacteria, are so minute that they can be seen only with the help of a microscope. Some forms of energy in the environment are perceived through other sense organs of the individual system. For example, there is energy that travels through space in the form of waves, such as sound, heat, and light, and is perceived by way of the individual's skin, auditory, or optic sense organs. Information in the form of sound or the written word will register through the individual's auditory or optic sense organs. Thus, the individual's environment is made up of masses, energy, and information.

STRUCTURE OF THE INDIVIDUAL

The **structure** of the human system can be observed and is composed of the skin and sense organs, or body mass and internal parts, such as the organs, cells, and organ subsystems (circulatory, digestive, respiratory). These interrelated parts make up the whole of the system.

The individual as an open system is composed of energy, information, and mass, or energy, and information. Einstein's theory of relativity states that matter, or mass, is only a particular state of energy condensed in space. His formula $e = mc^2$ (energy = mass times the square of the speed of light) shows that mass and energy are only different forms of the same phenomenon. Thus, we can think of structure as mass or energy.

PROCESSES IN THE INDIVIDUAL

EXCHANGE WITH THE ENVIRONMENT

Because individuals are open systems, they exchange energy, information, and mass with the environment from conception to death. During the prenatal period this exchange takes place through the placenta and the exchange is between the fetus and the mother's body (environment). Following birth, the exchange is between the individual and the environment external to its boundary, as discussed earlier. These exchanges are in the form of input into the system and output from the system. Because open systems retain some input and also have stored (potential) energy, the output is different from the input.

These exchanges between the individual and the environment can be categorized as chemical, physical, biologic, and psychosocial. These categories and examples of each are presented in Table 2–1.

Chemical Exchanges

FOOD. The chemical exchange of food is mentioned in Chapter 1 and is elaborated upon here. If we consider the food exchange from an elementary point of view, that is, if we consider the cycles of plants and animals, without the help of other organisms which break down chemicals, we find certain chemical elements undergoing successive energy transformations from simple elements to complex products and again back to simple elements. Plants synthesize two or more inorganic chemical elements and store energy (potential), whereas animals, including the human individual, break down the complex products, use the released energy and return waste to nature as simple products. The green plant transforms energy from the sun into potential energy and stores it as chemical energy in the complex materials it produces. During digestion, the animal transforms this chemical (potential) energy into actual energy in the form of heat, motion, electrical impulses, and waste products. For example, carbon is a natural element present in nature in both organic and inorganic forms. From water in the soil, plants absorb carbon and transform it from a simple element to a complex product, which is known as a carbohydrate (carbon and water). Animals, including the human individual, feed on plants, separate the carbohydrates, utilize the released energy, and return the carbon to nature in the form of carbon dioxide (carbon and oxygen). Other plants pick up the carbon in this new form, combine it with water to form carbohydrates, and return oxygen to the atmosphere for use by humans. Plants also provide energy sources for animals, which are used by humans as a source of protein and fat. Thus, there is an exchange between individuals and their environment across the body's boundary.

OXYGEN. A second chemical exchange between the individual and the environment takes place during the oxygen-carbon dioxide cycle. Plants join water (hydrogen and oxygen) from the ground, with carbon, to form carbohydrates. During the process of digestion, humans break down carbohydrates into hydrogen, oxygen, and carbon. The last two substances are excess energy for the individual, and are given off through respiration as carbon dioxide. Carbon dioxide is then picked up by plants, which separate the carbon from the oxygen, and return the oxygen to the atmosphere for human use. This oxygen given off by plants is transported to the cells by way of the respiratory tract, and it is necessary for converting food into kinetic energy, which is done by the oxidation-reduction reaction. Oxygen combines with hydrogen in the cell to form water, or it combines with carbon products to form carbon dioxide. Survival

Table 2–1. Exchange Between Individuals and Their Environment

CHEMICAL	PHYSICAL	BIOLOGICAL	PSYCHOSOCIAL
Food cycle	Heat	Humans	Humans
Oxygen cycle	Cosmic forces	Animals	Animals
Man-made	Sound	Bacteria	
	Light	Viruses	
		Plants	

is threatened by any condition interfering with the intake of oxygen or the output of carbon dioxide.

OTHER CHEMICAL EXCHANGES. Many of the other chemical exchanges between individuals and their environment are related to human activities. Humans have learned to transform energy and to store it as potential energy for their use, as needed. Man's manipulation of energy has been of benefit to humans, but has often created other hazards because of the inability of humans, or their inventions, to utilize energy completely. For example, the automobile has decreased the output of human energy in transporting individuals from place to place, and it has given humans greater mobility and has shown further adaptability. However, the inability of the combustion engine to utilize fuel (energy) completely has introduced chemicals into the air that we breathe, creating new health problems. Likewise, modern drugs (chemical energy), which may calm some individuals and allow them to regain their equilibrium, may create disequilibrium in others when used indiscriminately.

New chemicals in medicine, agriculture, food processing, vermin control, the cosmetic industry, and so forth have increased at a tremendous rate. In addition, such products as bleaches, cleaning fluids, and detergents, are a common part of an individual's chemical environment. According to Jones an estimated 400 to 500 new potentially toxic chemicals are added to the market each year.[1]

Many of these chemicals have had a beneficial effect on humans, by increasing the food supply, improving methods of preserving and transporting food, by providing life-saving drugs at a time of body disequilibrium, or by the destruction of disease-carrying insects, such as mosquitoes. On the other hand, new drugs, insecticides, food additives, and other chemicals in the home, work setting, or community have often posed a threat to the survival of humanity, and have changed the pattern of disease processes.

NURSING ASSESSMENT OF CHEMICAL EXCHANGES. Community health nurses should assess the quality and quantity of food taken in (input) by individuals and also the waste products (output). The quality and quantity of food will vary by age, activity level, genetic factors, and other factors in the individual. For example, the intake of food will be higher for an active teenager than for an aged sedate individual, and the protein intake of a normal child will vary from that of a child with phenylketonuria. Acute and chronic illnesses may also alter the nutritional needs (intake) of individuals. A variety of these factors should be considered when comparing the observed behavior of the individual with established standards of behavior. The waste products (output) from the individual may also be assessed for evidence of blood, mucus, fatty acids, worms, or other abnormalities that may indicate an imbalance in the system. These products can also be compared with normal values.

The oxygen-carbon dioxide exchange should also be assessed. Are there factors that may interfere with this exchange and create imbalance, such as, chain smoking, poor posture, or abdominal breathing? Is there cyanosis of the skin, clubbing of the nails, or other indications of an oxygen-carbon dioxide imbalance?

Nurses should also assess the actual or potential exchange with man-made chemicals. What medications are taken by the individual? Are these prescribed or over-the-counter medications? Do any of the medications cancel out another or interact in a way to produce harmful side effects? Are there side effects to the prescribed medications? Does the individual know the signs and symptoms of toxicity? Are drugs and cleaning supplies accessible to children as potential poisons? Does the individual eat an excessive amount of processed foods containing chemicals? Does the child eat paint chips and plaster? If so, does the paint contain lead? Does the individual work with chemicals where employed? Are there systemic symptoms or skin lesions resulting from this exposure? Does the individual know methods for reducing exposure to chemicals at work? These and other questions may be evaluated as a basis for nursing interventions.

Thus, community health nurses assess the chemical exchange (input and output) of individuals as a basis for nursing interventions. If these exchanges are beyond the range of adaptability, interventions may be required to help the individual's system maintain or regain balance. Many of these interventions involve teaching the components of an adequate diet, correct posture, ways to reduce chemical exposure at work, ways to keep drugs and chemicals unaccessible to children in the home, and so forth.

Physical Exchanges

HEAT. Another exchange between individuals and their environment is heat exchange. This takes place primarily through the skin, although small amounts may be lost through excreta and expired air. As a result of metabolic processes, humans continually produce heat (see Entropy, this chapter) and must lose heat to maintain heat balance, although the body adapts to fairly wide ranges of temperature, for limited periods of time. This need to lose heat combined with evolutionary adaptability has probably led to the concept of an ideal climate. For example, Dubos says, "In the absence of clothing, housing, and other means of protection, a temperature of 29.4°C (85°F), with moderate humidity and low air movement, seems most satisfactory for his comfort and least likely to cause physiological disturbances."[2] This environmental temperature is lower than the normal body temperature of humans because of the need of humans to lose heat from entropic processes, during energy transformations, and because heat moves from an area of higher concentration to an area of lower concentration. In addition to environmental conditions, humans can increase heat production by exercise, increased food intake, and anger, or other emotions, which increase the flow of adrenalin; conversely humans can reduce heat production, by rest, light diets, meditation, or other states of peacefulness.

The major factor governing the individual's heat exchange with the environment is the temperature of the environment. Individuals can either gain or lose heat, depending upon the temperature of the air, the temperature of the surrounding objects, the relative humidity, and the amount of air movement.

Heat may be lost from the surface of the skin by three methods: (1) conduction-convection, (2) radiation, and (3) evaporation. These methods and the process of heat loss and heat gain are discussed by Guyton.[3]

Human inventions and the conversion of energy into other forms have reduced some of the energy exchanges between humans and their environment. For example, heating and cooling systems in houses have allowed a more consistent and ideal climatic environment for individuals. It seems possible that such environmental changes have lead to the current interest in saunas, steam baths, and whirlpools, which seem to have a calming effect on individuals, and probably allow for a greater range of physiologic processes, which involve heat exchange. Dubos sees a possible connection between the consistent temperatures of human environments and disease processes. He says, "Modern man is living under conditions that differ more and more from those under which he evolved. He heats and cools his dwelling in an attempt to obliterate as completely as possible the environmental changes associated with the seasons . . . these technological innovations certainly have profound effects on human physiology, and it would not be surprising if some of their effects played a part in the diseases characteristic of modern life."[4] However, with the advent of the energy crisis, whereby we are forced economically to reduce heating in the winter and cooling in the summer, we may be moving back to a broader range of heat exchanges.

COSMIC FORCES. Another exchange between individuals and their environment, which is recorded in the scientific literature, is the exchange with the cosmos. Humans evolved under cosmic forces that have a rhythmic or uniform pattern, and as a result, it is believed that human physiologic and behavioral responses follow this pattern. Day becomes night and then day again establishing a daily cycle related to the earth's rotation on its axis in relation to the sun, every 24 hours. Monthly cycles result from the moon's return to its previous position in relation to the earth and sun every 29.5 days, and seasonal cycles result from the earths revolution around the sun every 365 days. Dubos says, ". . . all the functions of his body continue to fluctuate according to certain rhythms linked to the movement of the earth and of the moon with respect to each other and to the sun. His hormonal activities in particular exhibit marked diurnal and seasonal rhythms, and probably other rhythms also linked to those of the cosmos."[5]

Energy received from the cosmos has a marked influence on humans, and because of the rhythmic nature of their responses, the term **biologic rhythms** appears in the literature. Although the mechanism in humans accounting for this rhythmic response is unknown, it is assumed that each organism possesses a number of internal clocks that indicate when a given biologic activity should begin. These clocks constitute anatomic and physiologic mechanisms of evolutionary adaptation to the rhythms of the physical world.

The most extensively studied biologic rhythm is the daily cycle, which coincides with the earth's rotation on its axis. This cycle occurs over a 23.6 to a 23.8 hour period, rather than 24 hour period as we normally measure time. Because of this slight variation in time, Franz Halberg coined the term circadian from the Latin *circa,* and *dies,* meaning, "about a day."

Circadian rhythms identified in humans include many physiologic and biochemical processes. Peaks and low points are reached daily in a consistent pattern for different blood levels of hormones; total plasma protein, sugar, iron, and such constituents as red and white blood cells; also, the urinary excretion of chloride, urea, and potassium; adrenalin output; epidermal mitotic activity, fibrinolytic activity of plasma; intraocular activity; and deep body temperature. In addition, the functions of the liver, lungs, heart, and other organs follow a similar pattern. For example, vital capacity of the lungs is greatest in the afternoon and lowest about 2 AM; cardiac output is highest from 6 PM to midnight, and lowest from 4 AM to 6 AM. Many of these findings are discussed by Luce.[6]

Biologic rhythms are not immutably set, but can be influenced by manipulating environmental stimuli. However, these changes may lead to physiologic disturbances. For example, there are definite periods of light and darkness during the 24-hour cycle. In animal research, when these periods are reversed (*i.e.,* the research creates an artificial night during the day, and vice versa) the usual cycle of body temperature gradually changes, and is completely reversed within 12 days. The pattern, or cycle, remains but the period of high temperature becomes the low period, and vice versa. Other bodily functions show similar changes, and during this process stress is greater for humans or animals than it is at other times.

In summary, humans receive energy in a cyclic fashion from the cosmos (*e.g.,* solar and lunar energy, background radiation, electromagnetic energy), which influences physiologic processes, and behavior. Individuals respond in a cyclic fashion with heat production, blood chemistry, and urinary changes. At one point during the cycle individuals give off a higher amount of heat and chemical energy than at other points. These cycles can be influenced by environmental stimuli or behavioral changes, but these changes may lead to physiologic disequilibrium.

Sound. Another energy exchange between humans and their environment is sound. Some sounds are from the physical world, such as thunder; others are from the biologic world, such as the sound of insects, birds, and animals; but many sounds are from the human world in the form of words, or are a by-product of human inventions (transformation of energy), such as the automobile, the airplane, the air conditioner, or other machines. Therefore, although sounds are a subcategory of exchanges within the physical world, they actually cut across many of the categories.

At an early age, humans learn to use their vocal cords to make sound, and to communicate with others. Sound is caused by compression waves that usually travel through air, but occasionally travel through liquids and solids. The transmitter (larynx) creates sound by alternately compressing air and then relaxing the compression. Energy waves follow from the compression of the air adjacent to the transmitter, and cause a build-up of extra pressure, which in turn causes the air beyond it to become compressed. Then, the pressure in the next region compresses the air beyond it as was done before, and the process continues until the wave reaches an ear, and is heard as sound.

Through an elaborate process described by Guyton, the ear converts sound energy into nerve impulses.[7] Sound energy has an effect on the energy level of humans, and is dependent upon the characteristics of the sound (pitch, quality, and intensity) and the individual's biopsychosocial set at the time. Humans may be stimulated intellectually by a challenging conversation and respond with further sound in the form of words, or they may respond with anger (noises or words) to what they perceive as an annoying sound (noises or words). Likewise, humans may simply withdraw without making further sound, and as a consequence, will lose energy because of suppressed feelings and a subsequent increase in the secretion of hormones, which puts stress on the human system.

Humans may also respond to positive feelings, as well as the sound expressed, and, on the other hand, they may damage their hearing from any of the negative characteristics of sound.

There is more about the effects of thoughts, and feelings, on other living things in the section on psychosocial energies, but here it seems worthwhile to mention some research on the effects of sound on humans. According to a television report on CBS, music can have a stimulating or a retarding effect upon the growth of plants.[8] Results of these effects were demonstrated by the use of time-lapse photography, and it was shown that plant growth was dependent upon the kind of music, or the vibration, or the energy, set in motion. The pieces of Debussy and Bach were found to encourage lush growth and harmonious plant structure, whereas constant exposure to the discordant vibrations of rock music caused healthy plants to shrivel and die.

Although little research has been done in this area, research presented in the section on psychosocial energies suggests the possibility of the existence of a crude emotional system in plants, and may connect the effects of sound with development to the endocrine system, which responds when emotions are activated. That is, sound that is disturbing to us may engender negative feelings, thus activating the endocrine system and subsequent energy loss from the system. This process, if continued, may lead to structural changes related to continued imbalance in the endocrine system, in the same way that the worried, busy, executive tends to suffer frequently from ulcers, and other structural changes, from the stress placed upon the endocrine system.

In addition, sound is the basis for much of our learned behaviors; that is, from talking with others we learn how to cope with environmental energies, and thus have more tools at our disposal for adaptation. We discuss this concept at greater length in another section.

LIGHT. The major source of light is the sun, although humans have learned to transform other energy sources into light. The sun emits radiant energy continuously giving us, in addition to heat, which was discussed earlier, light and color. All objects above absolute zero (solids, liquids, and gases) give off radiant energy in the form of heat. Although heat is the same energy as light, it is of a longer wavelength (infrared) and, thus, not visible to the human eye in its usual form. Humans have learned to heat objects and thereby reduce the wavelengths, moving them into the visible spectrum. For example, as steel reaches a temperature of about 1700°F, it gives off radiation at the red end of the visible spectrum. If it is heated further to 2100°F, it appears white from the emission of wavelengths throughout the entire visible range. For the mere purpose of lighting a home, the tungsten filament is heated, or electrical energy is discharged through mercury or neon gas. In the ordinary light bulb, the tungsten filament is heated to a temperature at which visible light is emitted. In fluorescent bulbs, mercury vapor is heated and the bulbs, which are lined with phosphorus, absorb the shorter wavelengths (ultraviolet), and reemit them as visible light.

The wavelengths of radiant energy, which stimulate the retina and produce the sensation of light, range from about 4000 to 7000 Å (400–700 mμ). Wavelengths shorter than visible light include x-rays, ultraviolet rays, and gamma rays, and wavelengths longer than visible light include infrared rays (heat). Improper lighting can have detrimental effects on vision. For further discussion of these wavelengths and their effect on humans, see Baetzer.[9]

Without sunlight, all life on earth would cease. Sunlight is required by plants to carry out their processes for building up the food supply for human use, as mentioned earlier under chemical exchange. Without food, humans would soon die. In addition, many bodily processes, social customs, and behaviors are built around the recurring periods of sunlight. For example, most humans eat, work, and play during light hours, and rest and sleep at night to replenish their energy supply. During daylight hours, many energy transformations are carried out within and between humans and their environment; at night these exchanges are at a minimum. Dubos has found that even slight deprivation of sunlight affects the hormonal activity of Eskimo women. He says, "Eskimo women are said neither to menstruate nor to conceive during the long polar nights; and similar statements have been made concerning Patagonian women of the Antarctic."[10] In addition to our dependency on the sun for food, light, and bodily activities, we are also dependent on it for heat, which was mentioned earlier.

Since light is responsible for color, the effects of color on humans should be mentioned. Different colors and shades have been found to influence human concentration and emotions. Light pastel colors assist concentration and also reduce glare from artificial light. Thus, these have been found to be ideal in classrooms and other school settings. In general, pastel colors or white tends to give the feeling of coolness and increased space; such shades also have a calming effect. On the other hand, dark colors, such as red, may increase physical activity, give a feeling of warmth, and tend to make a room look smaller.

An individual's output is in the form of heat given off from bodily processes and actions or thoughts, in the form of writing, given off as a result of mental processes stimulated through vision. Thus, there is an exchange between the individual and the environment about light and color.

NURSING ASSESSMENT OF PHYSICAL EXCHANGES. Community health nurses should also assess the physical exchanges between individuals and the environment. Is there adequate heat in the home and school or work setting during the winter months? Is there excessive heat exchange at work, such as in an industry, where the individual works with high temperatures to melt metal? If so, does the individual know ways to remain within the range of adaptability? Does the individual alter clothing and diet for the various seasonal changes in temperature? Are fans or air conditioners used during the summer months? Is there proper ventilation?

Does the individual attempt to stay within the cyclic patterns of the cosmos? Is there frequent traveling across time zones, and if so, does the individual adapt to the new times by adjusting his or her clocks before the trip or by arriving at the destination early before being required to perform at an efficient level for a long period of time? Does the person work nights and thus have a reversed pattern of physiological patterns? If so, are there adequate rest periods during the daytime hours? Does the individual burn the candle at both ends by using daylight and artificial light to extend the working day? Are medications being taken by the individual? Are these time-released or taken to coincide with biorhythms for maximum benefits? These and other questions may be asked about individuals' biorhythms.

Sound that affects the individual should also be assessed. Does the person stay within the range of adaptability of sound in the home, in school and in work settings. If individuals must work around damaging sounds, do they know about and wear ear plugs? Do children hear sounds within the family that are appropriate in quality and quantity to stimulate their intellect? Do they produce sounds that are appropriate for their age and physical condition? What type of music does the individual consistently listen to? Are there outward signs of nervousness and anxiety, or signs of calmness? How do individuals respond to sounds from the community health nurse? Are they able to provide feedback that indicates they have heard and understood the nurse? Do their behaviors indicate a change, which ensures that learning took place?

Is the lighting adequate in the home, school, or place of employment? Does this vary depending upon the kind of activity carried out? Is this within the range of adaptability? Are stairways and halls adequately lighted to prevent falls and accidents? What is the visual acuity of the individual? Do they wear glasses? Are glasses prescribed but not worn? These and other questions should be assessed for individuals.

After community health nurses make an assessment of the exchanges between the individual and the physical environment and compare these with established norms, they again develop plans to work with the learned behaviors of individuals. They may teach or help the individual solve problems regarding ways to adequately heat the home, to alter clothing and diet during different seasons, to reduce work hours and increase rest periods when working around processes requiring high temperatures, to reduce sound by wearing ear plugs, to increase the interaction with a child to stimulate the intellect, or to obtain or wear prescribed glasses. At times, individuals may lack the financial resources to adequately heat a home, to buy eyeglasses, ear plugs or other supplies or services that will help them stay within the range of adaptability. Nurses may then help them identify community or other resources which may be available to them.

Biologic Exchanges. Humans live in a world of many forms of life (organized energy), and they continually exchange energy with those around them or with those with whom they have been in contact. Some of these interchanges increase our energy level, whereas others deplete it, although usually within a range to which we can adapt. There is a great deal of energy exchanged through thinking, feeling, and speaking, which is discussed under psychosocial energies.

We also have contact with the animal world. A rat may frighten us, causing an increased output of adrenalin in the body and a readjustment of our internal parts because of the increased body metabolism and energy loss from heat. Becoming angry at a barking dog, or other sound-energy, when we are concentrating or trying to sleep, will set the same processes in motion. On the other hand, we may relate to a dog as a companion, which generates positive feelings and an uplifting feeling, or increased energy.

Our attitudes and feelings about plants and trees also vary from person to person and time to time, and we can be aware of them, be annoyed by their presence, or be awed by their beauty. These various reactions, which are conditioned by psychosocial development, will affect our energy level. In addition, it seems that we not only affect our own health by negative thoughts, but also the health of other plant and animal life in our surroundings. Findings from studies (reported in the next section on psychosocial energies) seem to indicate that thoughts and feelings are energies that may be perceived and reacted to by other life in the environment.

It is felt that cooperative behavior takes place among living forms in nature because it benefits all of us. Under such an arrangement an ecologic equilibrium is established, which provides for the survival of the greatest number of all species. Those most adapted within a species survive, and a built-in check-and-balance system maintains equilibrium. For example, most animals live in a predator–prey relationship. If too many animals that are prey die for natural reasons (lack of energy), there is a corresponding decrease in the number of predators. This is exhibited in the fluctuation of fur animals from year to year, reflecting the availability of rodents on which they feed. The size of the rodent population, in turn, is dependent upon weather conditions, disease, and the abundance or absence of food. Thus, there is a built-in system of energy exchange among animals, which maintains an ecologic balance (equilibrium). Only humans can use their minds to go outside this energy–ecologic system to create imbalances (see Chap. 9).

Humans, also, exchange energy with microbes, either directly or indirectly. Indirectly, microbes affect our energy levels by interfering with our food supply. These indirect exchanges may be positive or negative. For example, microorganisms add to our food supply by converting debris into humus, which fertilizes the soil and enhances the growth of crops. On the other hand, they can destroy the crops that we use for food. In addition, microorganisms contribute to many essential steps in the processing of food, but also spoil or decompose food if it is not stored under conditions that are outside their range of growth and adaptability.

The fetus seems to be free of bacteria before birth and receives indigenous bacteria from the mother at birth, or immediately after birth, and then later from the external environment. These bacteria reside within the gastrointestinal tract of the infant and adult. Studies show that lactobacilli of several species constitute one of the dominant groups, sometimes as high as 10^9 or 10^{10} viable lactobacilli per gram of intestinal content. Another commonly found bacteria in the gastrointestinal tract is the gram-negative, nonsporulating, anaerobic bacilli. A detailed account of this bacteriologic knowledge is presented in Dubos.[11]

These organisms, which have established an ecologic equilibrium internally with humans, probably assist them by synthesizing certain vitamins and amino acids. On the other hand, other indigeneous organisms can aggravate nutritional deficiencies either by competing with their host for available nutrients or by increasing nutritional needs through the physiologic disturbances they cause. An obvious example of nutritional competition is provided by infestation with helminths, which do not establish an equilibrium with the individual and derive their nutrients from the intestinal tract (see Chap. 9).

Indigenous microorganisms also have a morphogenetic influence on humans, affecting their anatomic and physiologic development. When laboratory-raised germ-free animals are compared with those animals in nature, the laboratory animals are found to have abnormalities that would probably hamper their survival in the real world. The laboratory animals' lymphoid tissue, which provides protection against foreign matter; is poorly developed, and their gamma-globulin level is abnormally low. In addition, their cecal sacs are grossly enlarged. These animals are more susceptible to all forms of stress when deprived of food. Dubos considers many of these physiologic adaptations in humans who are exposed to microorganisms, and concludes, "[that] while the mechanisms through which the indigenous microbiota exerts its protective effects are ill understood, the effectiveness of the protection it elicits has been experimentally proved repeatedly . . . it seems likely that . . . the indigenous microbiota play a useful role by increaasing resistance not only against pathogens but also against dangerous microbial species which would otherwise multiply extensively in the intestinal tract."[12]

Although these microorganisms are beneficial to humans, they are also capable of causing a wide range of pathologic disturbances under special conditions. These disturbances become obvious when individuals are placed under different conditions from those conditions established between host and microbes through evolution. Nutritional deficiencies, toxic agents, and physiologic stresses are a few of the factors that may upset the equilibrium and allow the microbes to multiply to the point of depriving individuals of energy. Because of these relationships, science now accepts a multicausational theory for disease, rather than the germ theory, this concept is discussed in Chapter 9.

In addition to a variety of stresses that may upset our equilibrium along with internal microorganisms, modern medicine has also caused disequilibrium in some instances. Through animal research it has been found that small amounts of penicillin, or other antibiotics, changes the microflora of the intestinal tract. There is a sudden disappearance of lactobacilli and anaerobic streptococci accompanied by an explosive and lasting increase in enterococci and gram-negative enterobacilli. Following the discontinuance of drug therapy, lactobacilli, anaerobic streptococci, and bacteroids slowly reappear in the intestinal tract and return to their initial level.

Other drugs and surgical procedures have been found to have similar effects, and in some instances enteritis and other disease processes have resulted from the change in intestinal bacteria caused by these treatments. Although such treatments may arrest the actual disease process, it is rare for the causal organisms to be eradicated from the body. For example, even after successful treatment of gonorrhea with penicillin or tuberculosis with isoniazid and streptomycin, some of the gonococci or tubercle bacilli remain within the tissue. It is probably the same with other organisms.

Other organisms that are not indigenous to humans may also cause disequilibrium. In such instances, pathologic processes are usually the outcome of exposure to virulent pathogens at a time of suceptibility. Diseases such as smallpox, yellow fever, syphilis, diphtheria, tuberculosis, typhoid fever, and malaria are examples of illnesses caused by exogenous microbes. In these diseases, there is usually a history of exposure to the responsible organism, and the pathologic process develops within a fairly predictable period of time. However, exposure to such pathogens does not always create disequilibrium. Thus, the multicausational theory applies to exogenous, as well as endogenous, organisms.

NURSING ASSESSMENT OF BIOLOGIC EXCHANGES. Community health nurses should also look at the biologic exchanges between individuals and their environment. Do they have a safe water supply? Do they have cooling facilities for foods? Do they utilize these facilities? Do they have habits of personal hygiene such as washing hands and covering the mouth when coughing that will reduce the spread of disease when present? Do they have adequate living and sleeping facilities in the home for isolating individuals when communicable illnesses are present? Are rodents, cockroaches, or insects present that can spread disease? Do individuals have rashes or skin lesions, which may indicate diseases caused by an excess of biologic energy? Do they know signs and symptoms of illnesses, ways to prevent and treat illnesses, and community resources that can assist them?

These and other areas may be assessed by community health nurses.

Psychosocial Exchanges. So important are psychosocial energies in the life of humans that (as studies reveal) we suffer physical, mental, and social disturbances without them. As newborns, we are completely dependent upon others and slowly assume responsibility for ourselves as we develop. The psychosocial energies (verbal and nonverbal communication including feelings) we receive during this process will affect our development (negentropy). These exchanges are perceived through the senses, interpreted, and responded to through the mental–affective processes of childhood, and influence how we think, feel, and act. For example, it has been found that children who lack social stimulation (verbal and nonverbal) during early life do not respond as well in intellectual activities as those who received much stimulation. If this process is prevented at an early age through programs such as Head Start, the child may function intellectually at an equal level with children who were socially stimulated. Likewise, children who do not receive love are later unable to form close relationships, and if deprivation is too severe they may be retarded physically, mentally, and emotionally, or they may wither and die. Under special circumstances, this process is reversible.

Depending upon our genetic background and environment (all exchanges including psychosocial), we learn to perceive the environment and react to it. We pick up family biases and values, and, thus, differ in our perceptions of situations from others. These perceptions lead to reactions that may vary from others. For example, Koos found that middle class families recognized backache as a symptom of illness, and subsequently sought medical care; whereas, lower class women did not recognize it as symptomatic of illness, and thus avoided it.[13]

We also pick up attitudes and feelings (psychosocial energy) in our environment that will influence our perceptions and reactions. If we see authority persons as threatening, or ourselves as inadequate, we may react by fear when approached by a policeman or a teacher. On the other hand, if we have received love from parents and learned to love others in authority positions, as well as ourselves, we shall react differently. Crisis theory (see Chap. 9) focuses more on these relationships; also, see Feedback Process later in this chapter.

From experiences, then, we learn to react to situations and to relate to others. Our reactions can take on a positive or a negative character, and either facilitate or hamper the efficient functioning of our internal parts. For example, several studies show that continuous negative feelings decrease our energy level, and may lead to structural changes (organized energy), which may be instrumental in causing disease. New research in the area of psychosocial energy reinforces the concept that thoughts and feelings have an effect on plants, animals, and humans.

White reviews the work of Cleve Backster, where Backster says, based upon his research, that plants are sensitive to the thoughts and emotion of humans.[14] Using a polygraph normally used to register emotions in humans, Backster found that plants register emotions, such as apprehension, fear, pleasure, and relief.

Vogel also says that "plants are sensitive to the emotions and thoughts of people" and has published experiments that can be replicated to demonstrate the reaction of plants to humans.[15] These experiments are outlined in Vogel's chapter.

Research on animals also confirms the existence of psychosocial energies between living things, when strong feelings are expressed. Research carried out on rabbits by Naumov in Russia, and reported by Ostrander and Schroeder, showed that when baby rabbits were killed in a submerged submarine, there was a response in the mother's brain (on shore) at the exact moment of each baby's death.[16] Likewise, Backster found that when tiny shrimp were killed, there was a reaction in other living things, such as the plants, in the surrounding area.[17] He concluded: "Nothing seems to be able to stop communication, not even lead shields."

Research on the human transmission of feelings shows consistent findings. Ostrander and Schroeder reported that in clinics mothers were often separated from their babies and could not possibly hear them; yet when the baby cried, the mother exhibited nervousness.[18] And in the same situation, if the infant was in pain (*e.g.*, the doctor taking blood), the mother showed signs of anxiety, although she had no way of knowing the doctor was with her child at that moment.

In a paper presented at a conference, Naumov concluded that a two-way hookup existed between mother and child.[19] For instance, if the mother is in severe pain, the baby senses it and cries. This communication was found in 65% of the cases studied.

Other researchers have looked at the effect of thoughts and feelings (energies) on our physiology (kinetic energy). Ostrander and Schroeder reported on the Naumov–Sergeyev–Pavlova team, which found that EEG records changed drastically when telepathic impulses had an emotional element.[20] Pavlova reported: "transmission of several successive emotions of a negative character called up the appearance of cross-excitation of the brain. It changed the spontaneous EEG character to the tired state of the brain, dominated by slow, hypersynchronized waves of the delta and theta type."

Pavlova also found that the receivers themselves experienced "unpleasant bodily sensations and strong head pains." In response to positive emotions (calmness, cheerfulness), the EEG normalized again within 1 to 3 minutes, and the unpleasant bodily symptoms changed to a calmness.

Strong emotions may also affect the circulatory system of the receiver. In 1956, Serov and Troskin found that following positive emotions, the number of white blood cells in receivers increased by 1500, whereas, following negative emotions, they decreased by 1600.[21] These cells are instrumental in defending humans against disease processes, and this finding led to the hypothesis that positive emotions, both within humans and their environment, may be instrumental in preventing disease processes or in speeding up recovery from illnesses.

It seems likely, then, that energy used in the mental-affective processes (thinking, feeling) is transformed into thought waves and sent out to be picked up by others. These energies may have a helpful or a harmful effect upon the receiver, and perhaps we are beginning to obtain a scientific basis for prayer and healing meditations, which have long been a part of the major religions.

If thoughts and feelings can be communicated and do have a psychophysiologic effect on other living things (the receiver and the sender), then there is a tremendous need for the community health nurse, who works with individuals and groups, to improve the level of health of the community and to help replace negative feelings with positive feelings and emotions. Perhaps this is not a new concept, for it has been recognized for some time that mental illness is a family rather than an individual maladaptation, and treatment must be geared accordingly. But if these findings about the effects of emotions on others are correct, do we deal only with the family, or do we work with other key persons, in schools, in industry, in police departments, and in other settings, who have an influence on large numbers of people? This is an important mental health concept that should be incorporated into community health nursing.

Many psychosocial energy exchanges, including sound, take place within the family. At other times, these exchanges take place within the community (*i.e.*, the political, educational, recreational, and economic subsystems of the community). These are elaborated upon in Chapters 3 and 4.

NURSING ASSESSMENT OF PSYCHOSOCIAL EXCHANGES. Community health nurses should also assess the psychosocial exchanges between individuals and others in their environment. Are there good interpersonal relationships between members of the family? Are they supportive of one another? Do they openly demonstrate love and caring? Can they freely express feelings and emotions? Are children loved and protected? Are they given freedom to grow and explore? Is a separation necessary in the maternal-child relationship? What provisions have been made to make this easier for the child? If there is a newborn, is the child held and loved while feeding takes place? Are other siblings loved and cared for to reduce sibling rivalry? These and other appropriate areas of psychosocial exchanges should be assessed and compared with established norms. In some situations community health nurses may work directly with individuals to bring about change whereas in other situations they may refer the individual to other helping professions in the community.

OTHER EXCHANGES

There are additional exchanges between individuals and their environment that have not been elaborated upon previously. For example, individuals pay taxes or tuition, and, in return, receive their basic education from the community. Or, they pay a fee and participate in community recreation programs. Many of these additional exchanges are elaborated upon in Chapter 3. Although these exchanges take place between the family and community, they are equally appropriate for individuals. Their placement within the family chapter is merely a matter of convenience and a way of minimizing repetition. See Family–Community Exchanges in Chapter 3.

It is important for community health nurses to be aware of these additional exchanges between the individual and the family or the community in the area of health. If individuals are unable to meet their needs, they may turn to the family or community for assistance. Thus, health and health resources are an important aspect of a community health nursing assessment, and nurses must continually relate the individual's health and health resources to those of the family and community.

MULTIPLE EXCHANGES

Bredemeier's concept of boundary-maintenance functions of a social system relates to multiple exchanges.[22] He says that social systems must do four things to be more or less successful at adapting. They must "obtain matter, nonhuman energy, information and human energy (or services) from the environment; dispose of some of them to the environment, contain some of them in the environment (*i.e.,* prevent them from entering the system); and retain some of them in itself (*i.e.,* prevent their moving from the system to the environment)."

Obtaining information and matter refers to the systems input, and disposing of information and matter refers to the systems output, which was previously discussed. For example, the individual takes in food, oxygen, and other chemicals from the environment and disposes of waste products. In addition, the individual contains some information, matter, and energy in the environment. Some containment is a result of the body's mass and is thus automatic. For example, certain bacteria and pathogenic organisms will not enter intact skin, and dust particles over 10 μ will not enter the lungs. On the other hand, some containment within the environment is a result of learned behavior that has developed from experience, social-cultural variables, peer pressure, and so forth. For example, teenagers often dislike vegetables and fruits and will not take them into their systems. Certain foods, information, and so forth may be contained within the environment. This containment may assist the individual momentarily to maintain balance and purposeful direction, but over the long run containment can create stress. For example, the typical teenager's diet may meet certain needs initially, but can lead to vitamin, mineral, and protein deficiencies if continued over a long period of time. If the community health nurse educates teenagers about increasing the quality and quantity of their food intake, they may alter their diets, as a result, or they may choose to continue with their poor eating habits.

In addition, the system retains certain information, energy, and matter. For example, we retain energy from the breakdown of carbohydrates and dispose of the waste products. Likewise, we may retain information we receive, especially if it is presented in a manner acceptable to us and is useful in solving a problem. This fact has led to many efforts in education to identify principles of learning that involve the active participation and readiness of the learner, the climate of the setting, and so forth, which are discussed in Chapter 7.

NURSING ASSESSMENT AND MULTIPLE EXCHANGES. Although the exchanges between individuals and their environment have been separated into categories, these exchanges are not discrete. Thus, there are multiple exchanges influencing individuals continuously. Community health nurses must always be aware of these multiple exchanges between individuals and their environment and the effect of change over time. Thus, assessment is an ongoing process when visiting the individual, family, or other groups. One model for assessing these exchanges that is based upon the dynamic interaction between the individual, disease agent, and environmental factors is presented in Chapter 9.

Community health nurses should also be aware of both potential and actual imbalances of individual systems interacting or exchanging with the environment. For example, if an individual continues to consume an inadequate diet, is nervous and high strung, receives a limited amount of sleep and rest, and has poor personal hygiene habits, there is a strong potential for imbalance if these patterns are not changed. Intervention may be directed toward changing any one or more of these patterns before the individual and disease agent interact to produce illness and create an imbalance. The concept of multicausation of diseases, a theory for intervening at various levels in the health continum, and concepts of intervention at each level to prevent, detect, and treat diseases or imbalances in individuals is presented in Chapter 9.

INDIVIDUAL EXCHANGES AND NURSING INTERVENTIONS

Because some of the processes of obtaining, disposing, retaining, and containing involve learned behaviors based upon sociocultural and other factors, they will vary from individual to individual, and will vary over time with the same individual. These processes for a particular individual can be compared with established standards to determine if the observed behaviors will continue to maintain balance for the individual or if the balance established is temporary and precarious. Standards also will vary throughout the individual's life because of the increased order and organization (negentropy) of the individual as well as the physical condition, activity level, and other factors. The assessment of exchanges between the system and the environment allows community health nurses to intervene to prevent imbalance or to restore balance when an imbalance is assessed.

Community health nurses work with whole individuals and, thus, do not assess organ systems, organs, and cells as discrete units. Rather, they assess entire individuals for indications of potential, or actual, internal imbalances by observing input and output and comparing with acceptable standards for individuals of different ages at different activity levels. This assessment gives an indication of which exchanges are contained and which are retained. For example, a dietary history or an observation of eating habits may reveal a protein deficiency (contained), and a stool specimen may reveal abnormal mucus. (Abnormal mucus in the stool indicates an imbalance in the internal body parts [improper retainment]). If the protein reserves of the individual are being depleted because of the length of the containment, there will likely be an imbalance of internal parts, which can be further assessed by observing the body and the actions of the individual. However, if this is a recent dietary pattern and the body has a reserve supply of potential energy, there is a potential imbalance if the pattern is continued. Thus, nursing interventions may reverse the process.

Besides assessing the input and output from systems, community health nurses should assess the body and actions of the individual system for indications of imbalance. The eyes, ears, nose, skin, and other aspects of the structure should be assessed and compared with established norms. Likewise, the gait, posture, tone of voice, and so forth should be assessed. For example, if the individual gives a history of an inadequate quality and quantity of food for his age, sex, and activity level, and the nurse observes a lack of subcutaneous fat, poor skin turgor, poor muscle tone, pallor, rough skin, bad posture, a red tongue, corneal and conjunctival changes, and a rapid heartbeat malnutrition should be suspected. Thus, an assessment of the input and output as well as the body and actions of the individual is necessary to adequately identify imbalances.

Community health nurses' interventions are usually directed toward the learned behaviors of individuals (systems) in an effort to help them maintain or regain balance. Nurses may teach individuals about diet, growth, and development, signs and symptoms of health and disease, preventive and treatment aspects of disease, and community resources. If there is a severe imbalance within an individual's system, nurses may work with the learned behaviors of significant others in the environment as a way of reducing external stimulation and output, until the body heals itself. For example, individuals with hepatitis may require special diets, reduced activities, isolation precautions, and so forth. In order to meet the individual needs, family members or significant others may need to learn to care for the individual. Or, if this arrangement is not possible, community resources, such as a hospital or home health service, may be used to meet the individual's needs.

If nurses intervene before an imbalance has occurred in the individual system, they use primary-prevention interventions. If an imbalance has occurred in the individual system, they will use secondary- or tertiary-prevention interventions. These levels of preventive intervention are discussed in Chapter 9.

Factors identified in the exchanges between the system and environment are included in the assessment guides in Chapter 6. The process of adaptation to these exchanges is discussed later in this chapter, and the accepted standards for exchanges (input and output) are found in other nursing texts, such as Sutterley.[23]

INTERNAL PROCESSES

SUBSYSTEM CHANGES

In the individual, as in any system, the interrelated parts function together to maintain the whole system, and because these parts are interrelated, a change in one part will affect all other parts and, therefore, the whole. Any change that affects a part of the system may be the result of internal or external change. For example, there are interrelated processes that tend to keep the body's temperature at 98.6°F. When exposed to internal or external factors, which tend to change body temperature, the parts work together to maintain a constant temperature. When the external temperature of the individual increases, information is sent to the hypothalamus of the brain by way of circulating blood and sensory receptors. In the hypothalmus, the information is interpreted and converted into nerve impulses that initiate behavior at other levels, which increases or decreases the rate of body heat loss and production. For example, stimulation of the anterior hypothalmus initiates sweating and dilatation of the surface blood vessels to prevent overheating of the body. Dilatation increases circulation by bringing heat from the core of the body to the surface, and this causes heat loss from the skin, through conduction and radiation. If peripheral vasodilation leads to a fall in blood pressure, the body usually compensates by increasing the pulse rate and redistributing the blood. A dilution of the blood may result, leading to increased blood volume and blood pressure. If the external temperature continues to increase beyond this point (through conduction and radiation), then sweating comes into play. Thus, there are many interrelated parts within the individual system that work together to maintain a constant body temperature for the whole system.

We have said that a change in any one of the parts will affect the whole system. An injury to the hypothalamus will cause a failure of the temperature-regulation mechanism of the body, and the temperature will continue to rise until external assistance is given to the body. During this process the body is moving toward disorganization (entropy). In addition to these automatic changes within the body, humans learn ways to assist the normal adaptations and, thus, reduce the demands made upon the body.

Some of the body's adaptive processes (related to categories discussed earlier) follow. These processes focus primarily upon adaptation when the body is faced with excesses or deprivation. Other adaptive processes, when the body is not faced with such extremes, can be found in most basic medical-surgical nursing texts.

ADAPTIVE PROCESSES OF THE INDIVIDUAL

Individuals are continually bombarded by various energies, and through evolutionary processes and experience have developed a wide range of adaptability to them. Beyond this range, either through excesses or deprivation, humans may experience changes in the organized energy of the system or they may die.

Individuals adapt to energies as total beings, and although we may talk about physiologic processes as part of adaptation, mental and emotional processes also participate in this process. For example, when individuals are confronted with drastic changes in temperature, certain physiologic processes help them adjust to the change. In addition, the energy moves through the internal circuits and stimualtes the brain to assist. Based upon learned responses, individuals may remove clothing, take a cold shower, turn on the fan or air conditioner, go to the seashore, and so forth to assist in adaptation. Learned responses to energies (adaptations) are based upon the past and current experiences of individuals and, thus, may vary from person to person. Whether these responses are based upon scientific principles or not, they are attempts by individuals to maintain a degree of balance and to meet their goal of health maintenance.

Nurses play a major role in helping individuals stay within their range of adaptability, or to increase this range, by working with clients to assist them in increasing or decreasing their energy exchanges within a range consistent with their current status and past experiences.

Although, in reality, individuals are bombarded with multiple energies concurrently, for clarity, we shall look at these separately, and shall use the same categories discussed earlier in relation to exchanges.

CHEMICAL EXCHANGE ADAPTATION

Nutrition. As with all energies, there is a range within which humans can adapt. Too much food leads to changes in the structure of the individual's organized energy or to changes in internal energy transformations (functions), caused by obesity, poor body alignment, improper functioning of the glands and organs, and a variety of illnesses ranging from diabetes to heart disease. Too little food can cause similar internal changes leading to diseases, such as malnutrition, kwashiorkor, rickets, beriberi, pellagra, and a variety of other diseases. Malnutrition occurs in the United States frequently, and the other diseases are occasionally seen. According to Jones, a large group of Americans are malnourished because of inadequate incomes, inadequate knowledge of nutrition, and inadequate eating patterns.[25] Jones found that there was an inverse relationship between income and diet. Thirty-six percent of the population at the very lowest income level had poor diets, 27% had borderline diets, and 36% had good diets.

At the highest level of income, 9% had poor diets, and 28% had borderline diets. Thus, malnutrition is a fairly common problem in the United States.

Therefore, there is an ideal standard set for the quantity and quality of food for humans (at various ages and under various conditions), which are within the range of adaptability. Beyond this range, in either direction, humans are unable to adapt; although this does not mean that individuals cannot deviate from the standard for limited periods of time. The human need for food is less acute than the need for a continual oxygen supply; this is because of the ability (physiologic) to store and draw upon this potential energy (food). The physiologic process of converting potential energy to kinetic energy (to supplement external energy from food) keeps the internal environment in a balanced state. However, unless the overall pattern of food intake meets more than established minimum requirements, growth, health, and productivity are threatened.

Research, reported by Birch, indicates that in the early years, deprivation of food (quality and quantity) may prevent individuals from reaching their full potential of physical growth and mental abilities.[26] He says, "Inadequate nutrition results in stunting, reduced resistance to infectious diseases, apathy and general behavioral unresponsiveness. . . . The evidence we have surveyed indicates strongly that nutritional factors at a number of different levels contribute significantly to depressed intellectual level and learning failure."

Likewise, it has been well established that in the special case of phenylketonuria, an inadequate diet at an early age leads to mental retardation. It seems likely that there are critical periods in our development in which deficiencies in exchanges, whether in the form of food, sensory stimulation, love, and so forth, have a lasting effect on our ability to adapt. The effect of the environment on human genetics is discussed in Chapter 9.

When there is a long-range deficiency of food and the individual's potential energy stores are used up, the body continues to attempt to adapt by using substances in the tissues for energy. First, carbohydrates are depleted within a time period of 24 to 48 hours. Next, fat is used (*e.g.*, in an individual who is made up of 15% fat, this process is completed in 5 to 6 weeks). Finally, body protein is used for energy, but human life can be sustained at this level for only a short time. If individuals are in poor physical condition, these periods of time are reduced.

When humans exceed the period when external sources of energy (food) are needed but are not received by the body, certain biochemical and physiologic factors are initiated to help the body maintain its balance. Hunger is accompanied by unpleasant gastric contractions, feelings of weakness, emptiness,, and sometimes headache and nausea. Gastric contractions result from a low blood sugar. These responses are correlated with metabolic and neurologic factors in the brain.

Physiologic processes help individuals adapt to energy needs for food, but their mind and emotions participate in this process and may help or hinder adaptation. In the process of growing up, humans learn to like and value certain foods and develop feelings around food that direct their behavior. This behavior, which helps maintain equilibrium temporarily because of its basis in values, customs, and habits, may lead to eventual physiologic maladaptation if the food intake (quality and quantity) is inadequate.

Oxygen. It was mentioned earlier that cells require a continuous supply of oxygen, water, and nutrients for their survival and functioning, and without cellular activities life processes stop. Oxygen must be supplied continuously to the cells; whereas, the need for food is less acute. Some cells are more sensitive to oxygen deprivation than others are, as are some individuals. For example, the cerebral cortex, the myocardium, and the kidneys are most susceptible to oxygen deprivation, and irreversible damage to cerebral cortex cells can result from a 4- to 5-minute oxygen deficiency. Individual variability in oxygen needs is dependent upon age, sex, anatomic and physiologic status, and other factors. These other factors may relate to the adaptation of individuals to a particular area, through evolutionary or experiential processes. For example, by "survival of the fittest," as described by Darwin, humans adapt to the particular atmospheric conditions in which they live. On the other hand, humans (especially in these highly mobile times) move to different areas that have varying atmospheric concentrations of oxygen, and may adapt within limits by rapid physiologic adjustments or by acclimation through slower processes.

In addition, humans use their minds and knowledge to facilitate survival. For example, the unacclimated human can survive only a few minutes at 25,000 feet above sea level because of the pressure of the surrounding gases. However, modern aircraft have pressurized cabins, which allows humans to move to higher altitudes. In addition to movement from one place to another (with varying atmospheric pressures), our oxygen needs will vary with body activities, such as, temperature, exercise, and metabolic rate.

In general, we have adapted through evolutionary processes to an atmospheric pressure close to sea level; that is, we can adapt to minor variations, but we cannot survive with very high or very low (excesses or deprivations of oxygen) pressure changes. The highest altitude at which we can live and work is about 20,000 feet, and at low altitudes (300 feet below sea level), we can work for only brief periods.

Our adaptability to higher altitudes is dependent upon the altitude reached, the rate of ascent, the duration of exposure, the degree of acclimation, and the ability of each individual to adjust to changes. At 22,000 feet the partial pressure of oxygen in the alveoli is 30 mm Hg, which is equivalent to breathing air containing 7% or 8% oxygen at sea level. In this instance, the blood is only 55% saturated with oxygen, as opposed to the usual 97% to 98% saturation at sea level, and symptoms, ranging from headache and dizziness to paralysis, coma, and death, may result. Within human limits of adaptability, a move to a higher altitude is followed by physiologic changes, known as acclimation. Initially, there is an increase in the rate and depth of respiration and an increase in pulse rate and cardiac output. This leads to an increased removal of carbon dioxide from the blood because deep breathing enlarges the alveoli, increasing their volume, or capacity to hold air. Following this increase in volume, the partial pressure of carbon dioxide in the alveoli decreases in accord with Boyle's law of gases, which states that when the temperature of a gas remains constant, its pressure varies inversely with its volume. This decrease in the partial pressure of carbon dioxide in the alveoli increases the gradient between the alveoli and the blood, creating alkalosis.

Following this initial process of adaptation to higher altitudes, there is an increase in red blood cells, and hemoglobin, overcoming the initial respiratory alkalosis through renal mechanisms that reduce the buffer base. The increase in hemoglobin and red blood cells is probably caused by contraction of the spleen, which allows more oxygen to reach the cells. The time required for this complete process of adaptation at 20,000 feet may take up to 2 to 3 months.[27] This process again demonstrates the effect of external changes on human systems (a change in one part leading to a change in all the parts and the whole).

When we are below sea level, the atmospheric pressure and the partial pressures of all gases in the alveoli increase, and more oxygen and nitrogen are absorbed into the blood and into the body tissues. Nitrogen is physiologically inert at sea level, but can exert an analgesic effect at 100 feet below sea level. Returning to sea level too quickly from areas of higher atmospheric pressure can cause severe symptoms, and death, from the development of nitrogen bubbles within blood vessels. Under increased atmospheric pressures, the increased nitrogen is absorbed by the blood, but rapid decreases in atmospheric pressure produces the opposite effect, leading to decompression sickness (the bends).

Oxygen at a higher partial pressure may also produce harmful reactions depending upon the pressure and the duration of exposure. Edema and atelectasis may result from pulmonary irritation, and at extreme pressures (280 feet below sea level), convulsions may occur. The mechanism of oxygen poisoning is believed to be related, in part, to the accumulation of carbon dioxide in the tissues and blood, and a disruption of enzyme activity.[28]

In summary, there seems to be a certain range of atmospheric pressures to which man can adapt. Beyond this range, death results from an excess or a deprivation of oxygen.

Additional information on these processes may be found in Baetzer, Beland, and Levin.[29,30,31] Such information is especially useful to community health nurses who work in industries where humans are required to work at high or low altitudes, such as, mines, or places that use deep-sea divers.

Chemicals. Other chemicals in the human environment are mainly man-made, and excesses or deprivations of these chemicals at various times may affect us directly or indirectly. The chemicals used to protect crops during growth and to preserve them during distribution ensure us an adequate food supply wherever we live. On the other hand, residue from insecticides, herbicides, and fungicides as well as food additives, if beyond the range of our adaptive ability, may lead to disease or death. Likewise, modern medicines such as penicillin and tetracycline may alter physiologic processes in some individuals and allow their bodies and minds to regain balance; in other individuals, these drugs may prove useless, depending upon the bodily needs of those involved and the amount of the drug. Deprivation of certain drugs (*e.g.*, vitamin D) in a sick individual, is as harmful (because of the body's inability to alter physiologic processes and allow the body to heal) as an excess of the same drug, which may create a toxic imbalance.

As a result of modern technology, humans are also exposed to a wide range of chemicals in industrial plants, in the fish and animals we eat, in the water we drink, and in the air we breathe. We are able to adapt to these chemicals within a certain range, but beyond this point our adaptive mechanisms break down. From experience with chemicals threshold limits for many drugs have been established, and new ones are always being evaluated, and old ones revised.

In general, chemicals in our environment may affect our skin, mucous membranes, respiratory tract (inhaled), gastrointestinal tract (swallowed), or may enter the blood stream and affect a variety of organs. Our ability to adapt is dependent upon the specific chemical involved, its rate of absorption, the character of the tissue reaction, the location of the action, and so forth.

Within the range to which we can adapt, certain processes come into play. Adaptation to chemicals entering the respiratory tract by way of dust droplets and aerosols begins in the upper respiratory tract (nose, trachea) and the bronchi and bronchioles, where 100% of the particles 10 μ in diameter and 70% to 80% of those 5 μ in size are removed. Some particles in the 1 to 2 μ range that enter the lung are later swept toward the pharynx by the ciliated epithelium. Upon reaching the pharynx they are swallowed, and other particles may remain in the pulmonary lobules. Particles between one and two microns settle out in the alveoli by gravity and smaller particles up to 0.5 μ are deposited on the walls of the alveoli where they may be removed by phagocytosis and carried into the lymphatic system.

The solubility of gases in body fluids determines whether or not gases will penetrate the respiratory tract. Those that are highly soluble are absorbed in the upper respiratory tract, whereas, the less soluble gases penetrate the deeper lung tissue. These latter gases enter the systemic circulation and move throughout the body before reaching the liver for detoxification.

Chemicals absorbed through the digestive tract may be removed or altered by the liver before reaching the circulatory system. These chemicals reach the digestive tract either by swallowing material deposited on the upper respiratory tract or by contamination of the mouth by way of food, water, and hands. Most of this material is excreted directly in the feces without absorption taking place. Whatever is absorbed is dependent upon its reaction with digestive secretions, with the byproducts of digestion, and so forth.

Other chemicals are absorbed through the skin. Substances that are fat soluble may be aborbed through intact skin, and almost any substance may be absorbed through damaged skin.

When chemicals are absorbed in the blood, they are taken up by the tissues and cells, depending upon their water:fat solubility ratio and their chemical properties. Some are excreted unchanged in the urine, feces, or expired air, while others are metabolized, and the end product is excreted.

Humans adapt themselves and their environments to protect themselves from chemicals. Various protective devices are available in industrial plants, and numerous organizations have set standards, and enacted legislation, to protect workers. Most recent among these efforts are restrictions for dumping industrial wastes into streams, antismog devices on automobiles, and stricter governmental control of drugs. In addition, there is increased attention given to lead poisoning in children and child safety caps on medications. Nurses should be aware of the chemicals that are in individual homes, in schools, and in the work environment.

PHYSICAL EXCHANGE ADAPTATION

Heat. As with all energies in the environment humans can adapt to a certain range of temperatures, but life is threatened by any extreme. The temperature range to which we can adapt is probably determined by both genetic evolution (Darwin's "survival of the fittest") and our life experiences. For example, genetic evolution probably accounts for the differences in body size in various parts of the world. There seems to be a relationship between body shape and the temperature and humidity of the area we live in. This is probably related to the body surface, whereby the smaller the ratio of body surface to body volume, the smaller the heat loss per unit time. In Africa, which is hot and humid, a tall, lean body helps to dissipate body heat; whereas, in Alaska, a short, stocky body covered with fat helps to retain body heat. In relation to experiences and how they affect our adaptation to heat, it is known that southerners in the United States, where temperatures are consistently higher, show greater ability to work in heat than northerners; with less rise in metabolic rate; less profuse sweating; and less expenditure of energy. On the other hand, northerners are better able to tolerate cold temperatures than southerners because of their acclimation and development in a colder climate.

Various researchers have studied the range of body temperatures to which humans can adapt. Dubos says that such adaptations are efficient with a body temperature between 34°C (93°F) and 41°C (105.8°F); although, the body may survive beyond these limits.[32] He sets the wider range between 74°F and 114°F for short periods of time. Guyton uses similar limits of adaptability and says that different tolerance limits depend upon the amount of activity, wind, and altitude conditions; physical condition of the individual; the amount of adipose tissue; age; clothing worn, and length of exposure.[33] However, above 106°F or below 93°F the temperature regulation may be lost or seriously impaired.

In addition to the influence of external conditions on heat adaptation, humans also influence these adaptive mechanisms through physical activity and strong emotional reactions. These adaptive maneuvers, in turn, affect all internal processes, as discussed earlier. In general, within the range of adaptability to heat—biochemical reactions within the cells are accelerated by increasing body temperatures, and slowed by decreasing temperatures. These reactions are accelerated 7% for 1°F of temperature elevation, as measured by the metabolic rate.

Within our range of tolerance to heat, adaptive mechanisms tend to keep the body at a fairly consistent temperature. (This process was discussed earlier.) If the external temperature is further increased beyond the capacity of the mechanisms of conduction and radiation discussed earlier, the backup adaptive mechanism of sweating comes into play. This process usually begins when we are at rest in an environmental temperature between 81°F and 88°F, or lower, if at work. When the sweat glands become active, evaporation accounts for heat loss, and up to 2 or more liters of sweat may be produced each hour. In addition to water loss, sodium chloride is lost and if the water and salt are not replaced, tissue dehydration results.

For long periods of temperature change, such as with the seasons, it is believed that hormonal mechanisms are activated. There may be an increase in aldosterone secretion, which leads to salt conservation, and a small decrease in the metabolic rate. According to Dubos, . . . "the size of the thyroid and of the adrenals is usually greater in the winter than during the summer in laboratory animals, and also that it can be altered almost at will by changing the environmental temperature."[34]

In a similar way, humans adapt to a range of cold temperatures. Initially, a center in the posterior hypothalamus is stimulated and causes shivering, increased muscle tone, and constriction of blood vessels. Such activities may prevent heat loss from the body or may increase heat production. Messages from the hypothalamus are sent to the body's surface through the nervous system.

Heat production, the first physiologic mechanism of humans when faced with a cold climate, is augmented by voluntary exercise, unconscious tensing of the muscles, and shivering. Baetzer says, "It is possible to increase the metabolic rate five to seven times for short periods by shivering but this increased rate cannot be maintained indefinitely."[35] On the other hand, Dubos feels adaptation to cold is independent of shivering. He says,

> . . . animals and men experimentally adjusted to cold exhibit an increase in heat production in the muscles without any electromyographic evidence of shivering. . . . Furthermore, cooling of the hypothalamus in animals produced within a few seconds an increase of metabolism in the rest of the body. Finally, liver tissues from animals acclimatized to cold has an increased ability to oxidize fatty acids. Taken together, these facts suggest that there exists some form of adaptive response to cold which is not related to shivering and which is probably controlled by the temperature of the thalamus.[36]

The second mechanism of adaptation when confronted with cold climates is constriction of the blood vessels in the skin and reduction in plasma volume. These two processes reduce blood flow to the skin so that less heat is lost by conduction and radiation.

When we go beyond our adaptive ability we may experience heat exhaustion, heat cramps, and heat stroke. In **heat exhaustion** there is a failure of the cardiovascular system and the individual may have mild symptoms of dizziness, fatigue, and headache, which may lead to unconsciousness and collapse. Treatment includes the use of intravenous saline and glucose, and cardiac stimulants. **Heat cramps** may follow profuse sweating during physical activity in areas where there are high temperatures. There is painful spasmodic cramping of the muscles that were used during the physical activity. A saline solution should be given orally, or by the intravenous route. **Heat stroke** is the most serious condition of high temperatures. There is often collapse followed by coma, convulsions and delirium, and a marked rise in body temperature usually between 107°F and 110°F. The fatality rate for heat stroke varies from 40% to 80%, depending upon the body temperature. Treatment involves methods to reduce the body temperature.

At the other end of the heat continuum, our adaptive mechanisms may break down when we are exposed to a cold climate. If this exposure is prolonged, and we cannot adapt through the mechanisms discussed earlier, body temperature continues to fall; pulse rate, blood pressure, and respiration also fall after an initial rise; glomerular filtration rate, renal blood flow, and urine volume decrease; and there is a general reduction of body metabolism in all tissues. The feelings of coldness and pain are replaced by a loss of sensation, muscular weakness, and a desire to sleep. According to Baetzer, coma sets in when the body temperature reaches about 80°F, and death usually occurs when the temperature falls to between 70°F and 77°F.[37]

Cosmic Forces. Humans, through evolutionary processes have adapted to the rhythmic energy forces of the cosmos. If we pattern our lives around these rhythms we are able to adapt successfully to the peaks and low points in physiologic processes, such as heat production, blood circulation, and chemical and hormonal components. However, when we try to go against this natural rhythm, we experience excesses or deprivation of energy and may not adapt successfully.

Little is known about the adaptive mechanisms that come into play when we move outside an established rhythm, but some individuals adapt more rapidly than others and come into the new rhythm with less stress and strain. During these periods of being out of phase, we experience tiredness and irritability, and are probably more susceptible to a variety of physical and psychosocial stresses. It seems possible that even crisis situations may be precipitated during this state, which might not occur if we were rested and in balance. During stressful periods we are more prone to have accidents, bad reactions to drug therapy, and so forth.

Humans may also use their intelligence to adapt to biologic rhythms. If we have knowledge of the various rhythms to which our body responds, we can plan activities to stay within this pattern. If we must deviate from an established rhythm we can allow for this in our planning.

An interesting book that describes the various rhythms, other than the circadian rhythm, is entitled *Biorhythm: Is This Your Day*.[41] Thommen, the author, believes that we have rhythms that fluctuate during the month, which influence our physical, emotional, and intellectual well-being. The 23-day cycle involves the physical rhythm, the 28-day cycle involves the sensitive rhythm, and the 33-day cycle involves the intellectual rhythm. During these cycles we have high and low points physically, emotionally, and intellectually. During the high points, we are resistant to stresses and can accomplish things of a physical and intellectual nature, and are sensitive to others. During low periods, we are more susceptible to environmental exchanges. In addition, Thommen feels that everyone can calculate these periods for themselves and, thus, know when things will go well and when we need to move cautiously. Charts and tables for such calculations are included in his book.

In summary, we adapt to cosmic forces and usually remain within an established rhythm. This rhythm is influenced by environmental factors, for example, light change, and we adapt to a new rhythm. During the process of changing, we are out of phase and experience greater physical, psychosocial stress, and maladaptation.

Sound. There is a range of sound to which humans can successfully adapt. This range is dependent upon the pitch and the intensity of the sound reaching our auditory system. **Pitch,** or frequency, refers to the number of complete waves, double vibrations, or cycles produced each second that the sound is vibrating, because sound is essentially waves of positive and negative pressure caused by the forward (compression of air molecules) and backward (expansion of air molecules) movement of the vibrating object (violin, vocal cord, and so forth). This can be represented simply as in Figure 2–1. **Intensity** at each pitch depends upon the amplitude of pressure of the vibrating body, and

Figure 2–1
Sound wave pattern of pressure. (Unpublished information drawn from lecture in Environmental Medicine, Johns Hopkins University, School of Public Health, Fall, 1965)

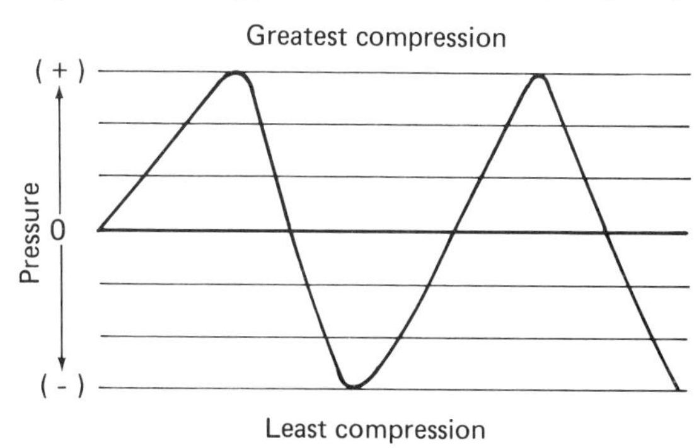

varies inversely with the distance from the source; that is, the greater the distance from the vibrating body, the lower the intensity, and vice versa. The differences in intensity of sound are shown graphically in Figure 2–2.

Frequency is usually expressed in cycles per second (cps) and intensity is expressed in decibels (db); a decibel is one-tenth of a bel, which is a unit named after Alexander Graham Bell. Baetzer says, "Most authorities agree that levels below 85 db in the frequency bands between 300 and 4,800 present little or no risk of damage to hearing, but more data on permanent hearing loss must be accumulated before higher levels can be fully evaluated."[42] As with other exchanges, the range of adaptability is dependent upon the duration of exposure, the pitch and intensity of the sound, the condition of the individual involved, and so forth.

Table 2–2 presents the intensity of common sounds in our environment. Within this range, the top three items can affect hearing depending upon the length of exposure to the sound, the distance from the source, and so forth; the next five items may also affect hearing depending on the pitch or frequency.

Figure 2–2

Sound waves differing in frequency and intensity. The sound waves in **A** and **B** are of the same intensity or pressure, while the sound waves in **C** are of greater intensity. In addition, **B** and **C** have the same frequency which is higher than in **A**. (Unpublished information drawn from lecture in Environmental Medicine, Johns Hopkins University, School of Public Health, Fall, 1965)

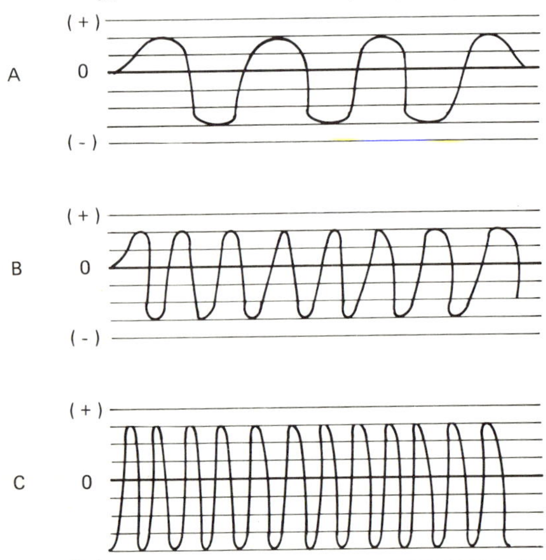

The human ear can perceive sounds within a pitch range between 15 cps and 15,000 cps, and some individuals can hear higher pitched sounds. The range of speech is usually between 500 cps and 5000 cps.

We adapt to the range within which we hear by a complicated process. Initially, sound energy passes through the outer ear into the auditory canal, which funnels the waves to the tympanic membrane. This membrane sends vibrations across the auditory ossicles (malleus, incus, and stapes) to a small membranous section of the cochlea. Vibrations travel from this membrane through the liquid-filled vestibular canal to the apex of the cochlea. Here, the vestibular canal joins the tympanic canal; at the roof of the tympanic canal is the basilar membrane, which separates the tympanic canal from the cochlear canal. Attached to the basilar membrane, but within the cochlear canal, is the organ of Corti. This organ consists of about 23,000 hair cells, which initiate neural impulses in the nerve fibers to which they are joined. These nerve fibers join together to form the auditory nerve that travels to the brain. This organ allows us to receive and to respond to sound.

Learned behaviors allow us to adapt to sound, which assists our physiologic processes. We may learn to cover our ears, with loud noises of short duration, or we may use earplugs, or earmuffs, if we work in a factory and are exposed to sounds for long periods of time. It is believed that earplugs reduce noise levels between 25 db and 35 db for high-pitched sounds. In addition, we are continually bombarded with sounds in our environment, and we learn to use our minds to focus on the tasks at hand, to block out any extraneous noises. Without this mechanism, we would be continually responding to noises without ability to organize our thoughts or performances. It is believed that hyperkinetic children may not have this adaptive mechanism and cannot screen out these incoming stimuli.

When sound is beyond our range of adaptability (excesses or deprivation), we suffer periods of disequilibrium, which may result in permanent damage to our system (organized [structure] or

Table 2–2. Noise Intensity of Common Environmental Sources Near Their Source

COMMON ENVIRONMENTAL SOUNDS	INTENSITY IN DECIBELS
Jet airplane	140*
Drop hammer	130*
Loud thunder	120*
Loud motorcycle	110
Boiler Shop	105
Subway train	105
Pneumatic drill, 10 ft away	90
Truck or bus	90
Heavy street traffic	80
Industrial noise	80
Average automobile	70
Ordinary conversation, 3 ft away	60
Vacuum cleaner	50
Quiet office	40
Average residence	35
Low whisper, 3 ft away	20

* May affect hearing, see text

kinetic [function]). The effects of sound-deprivation have been well-documented. Dubos concludes his discussion on sensory deprivation (sound, light, and so forth) by stating the following:

> . . . whatever the precise mechanism involved, sensory restriction can exert two deleterious effects. In young organisms, it prevents the orderly development of essential mechanisms and patterns of responses without which adaptability is severely handicapped throughout the rest of life. In adults, it can bring about a disintegration of the personality, and this disintegration can be permanent if the sensory deprivation is prolonged.[43]

The effects of excesses of sound-energy have also been documented. Exposure to high noises may cause either temporary or permanent hearing loss. When we are exposed to continuous steady noise, there is a temporary reduction in the ability to hear. The magnitude of this shift is related to the level, or intensity, the frequency, and the duration. Hearing loss increases progressively with noise frequencies up to about 4000 cps.

Intermittent exposure to noise is not as harmful as continuous exposure, but permanent hearing loss may result from continuous or intermittent noise over prolonged periods of time (*e.g.*, repeated impact noise from drop hammers, or from single short exposures, such as gunfire). Permanent hearing loss usually results after 5 to 10 years of exposure, and occurs about one-half octave above the predominant tone of the noise itself. Sounds above 120 db may be painful as well as heard.

In addition to physical changes resulting from noise outside of our range of adaptability, there may be immediate physical and psychological changes. When sound exceeds 135 db to 140 db, and the frequency is between 200 cps and 1500 cps, we may experience nausea, vomiting, nystagmus, dizziness, and an unsteady gait. If continued, fatigue, apprehension, and irritability appear, but these symptoms are reversible, with cessation of the noise. In addition, continued noises may create lower work efficiency and fatigue, and sudden noises may cause a rise in blood pressure and a reduction in salivary and gastric secretions and in stomach contractions. These last changes are probably related to fright and the fight or flight response.

Light. Humans are able to adapt to light within a range beyond which there is deprivation or excess of this energy. Wave lengths stimulate the retina and produce the sensation of light, which ranges from about 400 mμ to 700 mμ. When the duration or intensity of light is beyond our range of adaptability, we may experience periods of disequilibrium. Several studies have shown the effects of light deprivation, and Dubos reports on several of these studies.[44] He says, "Most forms of sensory deprivation, especially during the early phase of life, thus seems to prevent the organism from developing essential mechanisms and patterns of response without which adaptability is severely handicapped throughout the rest of life." Other authors frequently refer to critical periods of development in which a deprivation in the environment during a critical period leaves lasting defects.

A variety of studies have shown that deprivation of stimuli, including light, affects all age groups. Results from these studies show removal of sensory stimulation leads to disorganized thought and an inability to concentrate. Symptoms such as restlessness, irritability, disorientation, and anxiety, often reaching a panic state, are common.

Vivid imagery, illusions, and hallucinations are frequent and, in general, sensory deprivation leads to experiences similar to those following the taking of psychotropic drugs.

On the other hand, excesses of light increase sexual activity in all animals by affecting the anterior lobe of the pituitary. This phenomenon has been studied in chickens, which are often placed in nocturnally illuminated hen houses to increase egg production.

Dubos says,

> Until the last century, man lived in the dark for long hours during the winter months and this is still true in many primitive societies. Modern man, in contrast, is exposed to bright light for 16 hours a day throughout the year. In view of the fact that light rays can affect several hormonal activities, and that many, if not most, physiological functions are linked to circadian and seasonal cycles, it seems possible that this change in the way of life will have long-range consequences for the human species.[46]

Excesses in the form of light intensity create a variety of harmful conditions also. These are usually from ultraviolet radiation or infrared radiation, which are the part of the light rays beyond our visibility. Ultraviolet radiation is absorbed entirely by the surface of the body, and its effects, therefore, are on the superficial organs, such as, the skin and eyes. Any injury is caused by distruction of protein and nucleic acid. First, there may be injury to the skin from extensive exposure to ultraviolet rays. Baetzer has discussed this process.[47] The body may attempt to prevent this damage by the formation of melanin—the pigment responsible for suntans. Following exposure, melanin migrates from the malpighian layer to the corneum, and more melanin is formed. This darkening of the skin may provide protection from the damage of further ultraviolet rays, depending upon further duration and exposure. In addition, it seems likely that repeated exposure to ultraviolet radiation may cause skin cancer; several epidemiologic studies confirm this finding. Other effects of excess ultraviolet light energy may be experienced by the eyes. Conjunctivitis accompanied by photophobia and eclipse blindness have been reported. In the first condition, there may be pain and the feeling of a foreign body in the eye, followed by necrosis, edema, opacities, and ulcers of the cornea depending upon the duration and intensity (which is a result of the wave lengths absorbed by the conjunctiva and cornea). In the second condition, blindness probably results from heat coagulation of the protein by infrared radiation from the sun. Recovery is usual in both conditions.

Deprivation of light is the possible cause of rickets from a vitamin D deficiency. Vitamin D is formed by the interaction of ultraviolet radiation on 7-dehydrocholesterol, or some closely related compound.

Humans use their intelligence to remain within the range of light exposure to which they can adapt. For example, we use protective glasses and skin oils to screen out harmful wavelengths when exposed to ultraviolet or infrared rays, either at work or out of doors; we may select times for working in the garden, going to the beach, and so forth, when the sun's rays are less intense.

Within our range of adaptability to light rays, certain mechanisms of the eye assist in light adaptation. Light passes through the pupil to the retina; in dim light, the pupil enlarges and in bright light it becomes smaller to protect the retina. The retina contains receptors, known as rods and cones, which are sensitive to light. Rods are more sensitive to light than cones and are responsible for visual perceptions in dimly lit or dark places. When light is more intense the cones take over. Optic nerves run from each eye to the occipital lobe of the brain, crossing over at the optic chiasma and traveling to the side of the brain that is opposite from the eye from which it originated. From this center, perceived data is interpreted and causes a response.

BIOLOGIC EXCHANGE ADAPTATION

Humans also adapt to the energies of the biologic world within a certain range; such adaptations may be based upon genetic and experiential factors. For example, during a widespread epidemic, when a new potent organism is introduced into a population, the most susceptible die; whereas, those who survive are genetically endowed with a high level of natural resistance. This resistance is passed on to the offspring in what Darwin termed "the survival of the fittest." This type of adaptive mechanism is seen among Blacks living in Central Africa who exhibit the sickle-cell gene, which may be associated with a form of anemia. Because the incidence of sickle-cell anemia has not decreased in recent times, it is felt that there must be some survival advantage. Recently, it was found that children exhibiting this trait had a high degree of resistance to malaria, which was widespread in the area. After groups move from areas where this disease is prevalent, (*i.e.,* Africa, Southern Italy, Sicily, Greece, Turkey, and India) to areas where it is uncommon, the incidence of the sickle cell anemia decreases. Genetic changes are also taking place in the world of microbes to favor the survival of both man and microbes as they establish an ecologic equilibrium (see Chap. 9).

Excesses and deprivations of biologic energy beyond the human range of adaptability leads to disease and possible death. Several examples of deprivation of biologic energy were given in an earlier section where we discussed the fate of germ-free animals, the effects of drugs on the intestinal flora of humans, and the effects of bacteria on the food cycle. On the other hand, excesses may affect us directly or indirectly. Indirectly, biologic organisms may destroy our food supply and contaminate our water. Numerous examples from the literature document the direct effect of excess biologic exchanges with humans.

The severity of the threat to humans from these other forms of life is influenced by previous contact with these organisms. When a population is exposed to a pathogen, with which it has had no previous experience, exposure may bring about severe disease in many of its individuals. The generalized epidemic, over time, brings about adaptive changes in both the host population and the infective agent, which brings about an ecologic equilibrium between both organisms. The infective agent may remain widely distributed in the community, but its presence need not be associated with any injurious effects. Disease, when it occurs, is due to a change in the conditions under which the ecologic equilibrium evolved. These changes may be of a varied nature. In humans, the provocative cause of microbial disease may be a disturbance in any of the factors of internal, or external, environments, such as, weather conditions, available food supply, working habits, economic status, or emotional stress.

Humans may upset the balance of energies established with the biologic world and create imbalances that are not always in their favor. This is usually a result of a lack of understanding of the laws of energy, which we continually try to manipulate to improve our adaptability. For example, drugs produced by modern technology to control disease may actually change the internal environment of man and lead to other diseases. Or, when humans cut down trees and replace them with freeways and apartment complexes, this may lead to flooding or soil erosion following heavy rains, because of a lack of trees.

Humans have a variety of mechanisms that assist them in adapting to the biologic world. The organized energy of the body (*e.g.,* bones that protect vital organs; intact skin and mucous membranes) provides some protection against assaults and foreign matter. Other barriers include the sensory receptors, which are stimulated by conditions in the external environment; mechanisms for conditioning air and removing foreign particles from the alveoli, which were mentioned earlier; and mechanisms for rejecting irritating substances from the gastrointestinal tract. In addition, the stomach contains a highly acid fluid in which few organisms can survive, and movement of mucus out of body openings keeps the body relatively clean of foreign matter. These protective actions constitute the preliminary mechanisms of adaptation

The response of the body to insult or injury is a complex interaction of many physiologic functions; some are chemical functions and others are cellular. Each individual's body possesses its own unique proteins and the ability to distinguish its own from any others. This discrimination is coupled with a rejecting response, so that "foreign" proteins are met with efforts to exclude them. This ability to discriminate and reject foreign proteins is developed by exposure to the environment. Laboratory and germ-free animals do not have such adaptive abilities. The ability to reject foreign proteins that are not innate to the organisms is called **immunity** and continues throughout life, so that, within limits, new exposure to strange proteins is met by the development of an immunity response.

New organisms in the bloodstream stimulate

the formation of specific antibodies to eliminate them. The production of specific antibodies, once begun, may continue after the stimulus has been removed; and, as long as the specific antibody continues to circulate in the bloodstream, the individual is immune to the specific microorganism. This ability to develop a defense against new organisms provides the rationale for immunization. Deliberate exposure to a modified specific organism calls forth the antibody defense system and, thus, serves to protect the individual during any subsequent exposure to the organism, as long as the antibody remains in the bloodstream. Some antibodies are blood-borne and remain only as long as the blood continues to carry the antibodies; whereas, others are tissue-borne and may confer lasting immunity.

Since the effectiveness of antibody defense is dependent upon the presence of antibodies in the bloodstream or tissues, and requires time to develop when the microorganism has not previously been encountered, the leukocytes or white blood cells react instantaneously to help the body to adapt. These cells, which are formed in the hematopoietic tissues, are motile and therefore capable of moving to the invasion site. The supply of these cells is dependent upon the health of the tissue producing them.

In addition to physiologic adaptations to the biologic world, humans have learned behaviors that help protect them from harmful organisms. For example, it is known that proper diet, rest, relaxation, exercise, and a variety of other activities offer some protection from illnesses. Even simple handwashing and other hygienic patterns may offer protection. The problem is one of making this information available to the community in a way it can and will be utilized.

In addition, humans have learned to manipulate the environment so that they rarely come into contact with organisms with which they have not developed a biologic equilibrium. For example, malaria has been controlled in this country not by eradicating the malarial parasite, but by reducing the number of mosquitoes (the carrier), by draining, or disinfecting, stagnant ponds where they multiply. Many of the environmental sanitation activities to be considered in Chapter 9 have been geared toward breaking the weakest link in the cycles that cause disease.

PSYCHOSOCIAL EXCHANGE ADAPTATION

Human perception of and adaptation to psychosocial exchanges in the environment is probably strongly influenced by the genetic equipment as well as the various experiences of the individual. If we are born with limited mental faculties, we will be less able to interpret and respond to environmental challenges, than if we have average mental faculties. Likewises, since we are almost completely dependent upon others for our exchanges during early life, we learn to preceive and respond to future energies, based upon how these needs are met. For example, if the infant and preschooler are deprived of love, whether through lack of or separation from the source, they are unable to form close emotional relationships later in life; that is, they develop mechanisms of withdrawal, which serve as a psychological defense against being hurt. The process whereby this occurs has been observed and documented.

Likewise, our attitudes, feelings, and self-concept regarding new situations and people are influenced by how our early needs are met. If we are of average body and mind and are encouraged and supported emotionally as we face new experiences on our path to becoming independent, we will probably continue to face new situations well, and will develop more healthy adaptive mechanisms (defenses), with a higher threshold for stress, than if we are not supported. In the latter instance, a lack of psychosocial energies in the form of emotional support and encouragement may lead a person to perceive each new situation as a threat and cause a low threshold for stress, because of a defective perceptual apparatus and a poor defense mechanism.

Most humans have a comparable perceptual apparatus that includes taste, smell, touch, vision, and hearing. However, stimuli received through these receptors are sent to the brain for interpretation and response. Responses are influenced by the intellect and emotions, and these condition future perceptions and responses to similar situations. Thereafter, patterns of perception and response (internal and external) are established, which attempt to maintain balance for the individual. These patterns include our defense system, and, as mentioned before, are determined by how our early exchange needs are met by our parents or our caretakers (emotional level, knowledge, skills, intellectual level, and so forth). Parents or caretakers, in turn, are conditioned by their own genetic endowment and experiences.

At any point in time, all people could theoretically be placed on a perception adaptation continuum that would plot likely responses to environmental stimuli. Those with a low genetic endowment and nonsupportive experiences would fall at the low adaptation end; whereas, those with an average genetic endowment, supplemented by a supportive psychosocial environment, would fall at the other end of high adaptation. Various combinations would fall somewhere between these two extremes (*e.g.*, low genetic endowment and supportive experiences in a child with phenylketonuria who is treated with the proper diet in a supportive environment and suffers no mental retardation or inappropriate defenses). Depending upon a person's placement on the continuum, a person would theoretically tolerate more or less stress reactions when confronted with similar situations. Stress and crisis will be discussed in Chapter 10.

Human responses and adaptation levels are not as fixed as implied above. Humans are always encountering experiences, some of which are familiar, while others are new. Our reactions to these challenges will be based upon (in addition to patterns derived from the past) our present state of balance, our needs, and the support (psychosocial energies) in our environment. For example, adolescents who have always adapted well to environmental exchanges prior to adolescence may need additional support at times or else suffer maladaptive behavior because of physical and psychosocial changes in their life, which influence their internal balance and external relationships. In addition, situations, such as, pregnancy, or the death of a loved one, may require increased needs for psychosocial energy if a person is to remain adapted. A situation always looks bleak when we are tired (not quite in balance), whereas, it seems to improve when we are alert and rested. Thus, our state of balance (physical, mental, and emotional) and the support in our environment will determine how we perceive a situation. Therefore, the combination of genetic factors and our experiences influence how we adapt to psychosocial exchanges.

It is clear, then, that much of our adaptation to psychosocial energies is learned and relates to activities of the mind and emotions. We use our sense organs to perceive the external environment and the mind incorporates and integrates these experiences. Patterns that evolve serve to direct and regulate our reactions to the environment. However, in addition, we have a memory for past situations and previous responses, and will often react and adapt even when no actual stimulus is present. For example, we may relive an earlier experience that we perceive as threatening. We may then experience bodily discomfort from the increased adrenalin in our system brought on by the thoughts of the feared stimulus. We may also react psychologically by getting angry at the person or situation and bring into play mental processes of retaliation, retreat, and so forth. These may lead to other thoughts of ways to avoid the person, or to gain an upper hand in the next encounter. These, in turn, may affect our immediate environment for we may then project our anger onto our spouse rather than the threatening person, which in turn may have personal ramifications. All of these processes may be patterned ways of adapting to real or imagined threats, and are based upon past and current happenings. It is likely that such adaptations are a total response of the organism (physical, emotional, mental) and affect the total organism, in return. Likewise, remembering a positive experience may influence our behavior in a positive way.

Humans, then, adapt to a range of psychosocial energies in their environment and this range will vary greatly from person to person depending upon past and current factors. Within our range of adaptability we may use a variety of psychological defense mechanisms, such as, projection, reaction formation, repression, and denial, which are learned and help us to adapt. If we are placed within a situation that we preceive as too threatening for our psychological defense system, we may withdraw physically, psychologically, or both.

Society tends to vary its definition of what is adaptive and maladaptive behavior from time to time and place to place, but usually we are considered maladaptive if we withdraw totally from the environment or behave as a closed psychosocial system. Some withdrawals may be labeled normal. For instance, Anna Freud believes that adolescents use their defense system to withdraw from former love objects (the parents), when they begin to experience an increase in the intensity of their sex drive.[48] When there is this additional strain, their defense system may be inadequate to deal effectively with the sex drive so, instead, they deny their need for their parents and withdraw their attentions from them and direct them toward their peers. There is still physical and psychosocial contact with the parents, but the relationship changes and is of a different nature. This behavior is considered adaptive and sets the stage for humans to experience normal grieving in later life. A lack of this behavior results in symbiotic relationships and is considered abnormal adaptation. Such behavior may be encouraged by either the adolescent or the family (suprasystem), or both.

On the other hand, if humans encounter situations in which they are unable to cope, because of an inability to use defense mechanisms to maintain a balance, they may become confused intellectually, and exhibit a variety of behaviors and symptoms. These symptoms may include an inability to perceive and interpret accurately what is going on around them, irritation with others, depression or anxiety, and these symptoms may become so dominant that the person cannot carry on with normal activities. The degree to which these behaviors and symptoms are expressed and dominate other activities probably determines which behaviors society considers normal or abnormal, for adaptation. For example, confusion, anxiety, inability to carry on usual activities, and other symptoms often coincide with a crisis situation and, with the exception of grief following the loss of a loved one, usually disappear within a 6-week period, which is considered normal. (See Crises in Chap. 10.) On the other hand, long-term symptoms and behaviors, which interfere with what society considers normal functioning, usually are considered maladaptive behavior.

Definitions of maladaptive behavior will vary with groups at any point in time and within a group over time. In general, maladaptive behaviors are usually considered to be **psychoneurotic** if there is a disturbance of personality that causes intense anxiety, or behaviors are labeled **psychotic** if there is a gross derangement of mental processes and an inability to evaluate external reality correctly. Psychoneurosis is common and experienced by most people at one time or another, and is usually not considered abnormal enough to require treatment, unless it involves an acute disruption of life patterns. Symptoms during a difficult period depend on the way the person has learned to handle anxiety. The anxiety may be diffuse and uncontrolled, or it may be focused upon a specific fear (phobic reaction). It may also be expressed organically as a conversion reaction, such as, paralysis (*e.g.*, "glove" anesthesia, which does not follow the sensorimotor nerve distribution) or tics, as a depressive reaction, with feelings of guilt, or as an obsessive-compulsive reaction involving a persistence of unwanted ideas or repetitive impulses to perform nonrational acts.

Another area considered by society as maladaptive involves adaptations that lead to psychosomatic illnesses where there are obvious manifestations of physiologic malfunctioning, without apparent organic cause. A great deal of research has been carried out in this area. Although we may all react at times to stress with transitory physical discomfort, such as, a headache, an attack of diarrhea, skin rash, rapid heartbeat, dry mouth, wet palms, and other relatively mild symptoms, some people have symptoms so severe that there are marked structural alterations (in organized energy). As mentioned earlier, humans have a mind and can remember as well as anticipate. If we are fearful of speaking in public we may think about our fear prior to an appearance and vicariously experience the feelings, causing a physiologic reaction, without any actual stimuli, except for our anticipation of the event. The mechanism for dealing with fearful situations in past generations probably was an asset, for increased adrenalin in response to actual fears gave us the energy needed to fight or flee rapidly from the danger. However, today, we are usually not confronted with life and death situations and our responses to imagined fears remain to manifest themselves in other ways.

Much of the early work on the relationship of strong emotions to physiologic changes was done by Cannon.[49] His interest was primarily in the visceral aspects of emotional expression and the excitement of the sympathetic division of the autonomic nervous system. From his experiments he described the fight or flight reaction in which the body is mobilized through action of the sympathetic nervous system to run from danger or to stand and fight. The emotion involved was either fear or rage, and the physiologic response was as an increase in the secretion of adrenalin, which prepared the body for action.

The results from current research seem to indicate that fear and rage do not produce the same physiologic response, but rather two related responses. Fear tends to release adrenalin, and anger releases noradrenalin. Pelletier says, "There is a discernible difference between proportions of adrenalin and noradrenalin released from one stress response to another. The reason why adrenalin is released in one instance and noradrenalin in another are not clearly understood, but many researchers tend to regard adrenalin as the 'fear hormone' and noradrenalin as the 'anger hormone'."[50]

Other data on the physiologic response to strong emotions come from studies by Wolff.[51] He studied a man who had previously had a gastrostomy performed for feeding purposes because of an occlusion of the esophagus, which followed the drinking of scalding clam chowder. The man was studied for extended periods of time under varying emotional states. The effects of these states upon his gastric activity were noted and reported. When he was fearful or sad there was pallor of the gastric mucosa and an inhibition of muscular contractures and gastric secretions. When he exhibited emotional conflict causing anxiety, hostility, or resentment, there was an engorgement of the gastric mucosa with accompanying hypermotility, hyperemia, and an increase in gastric acid secretions. If the conflict continued for a long period of time physiologic reactions included hemorrhage, lesions, and eventually ulcer formation.

It is now felt that the degree of physiologic response to stress factors is individually determined based upon our genetic equipment and experiences. Hinkle showed that over time a proportionately small number of subjects had a majority of illness conditions, even though they may not have had a great number of objectively determined stress experiences.[52] They perceived their lives as more demanding, depriving, threatening, and conflict producing than their contemporaries. Likewise, Wolff proposed the nonspecific theory of protective adaptive response.[53] He felt that disease could be the end result of protective reactions which in the past had been useful to the organism when faced with symbolic threats. These physiologic reactions, which were protective in nature, became conditioned responses to various psychological stimuli. In addition, the responses themselves could take on symbolic meaning, such as shutting out or rejecting painful situations. For example, the speaker we referred to earlier may develop vague physical discomfort related to his anticipated appearance in public and, thus, excuse himself from the situation because of illness. Individuals, according to Wolff's theory, respond to different stresses in ways that are consistent for them. These responses are based on their genetic equipment and the results of prior conditioning. Wolff stresses the importance of the way individuals perceive situations in which they participate rather than the way an objective observer might perceive them. Stress, and man's adaptation to it, is an important aspect of health and illness and will be elaborated upon in Chapter 10.

Further evidence for the relationship between emotional states and physical distress comes from studies by George Engel and associates at The University of Rochester.[54] This group found that the great majority of patients hospitalized for physical illnesses had experienced a psychological disturbance a short time before becoming ill. Rather than expressing anxiety, fear, or anger, which are usually associated with illness, their group presented feelings of helplessness or hopelessness. These feelings were usually engendered by the loss, or the threat of loss, of someone or something close to the person which was present prior to the onset of the illnesses. The illnesses ranged from cancer, rheumatoid arthritis, ulcerative colitis, cardiovascular disease, diabetes, mental illness to diseases of the nervous system.

It was pointed out that another type of vulnerability was needed to precipitate illness, in addition to the emotional reaction. It could have been a virus, an inherited biochemical defect, or some other biologic predisposition, either inherited or acquired.

When Dr. Schmale looked at the personality characteristics of the various groups that had experienced helplessness or hopelessness prior to physical illness, he found only one individual who had first responded with anger and fear, and then with helplessness.[55] The individuals who experienced hopelessness usually gave a history of long-standing hyperactivity and selfless devotion and a lack of confidence, as compared to those that became angry or fearful. The feelings of hopelessness were often preceded by feelings of guilt and shame.

Further evidence for the relationship of emotional factors to illness were produced with animal studies. A number of studies concluded that both emotional and biologic factors (viruses) were needed to produce an undesirable effect in animals. These findings are consistent with the concept of multiple causation in the etiology of disease processes (see Chap. 9).

At the far end of the continuum of psychological adaptation and maladaptation are the psychoses. These usually involve a gross derangement of mental processes and the inability to evaluate external reality correctly. Again the differentiation between what society considers normal, or abnormal, is probably dependent upon the severity and duration of these processes. For example, in a crisis situation tensions may build to a point that individuals are so focused upon the feelings involved that they are unable to identify the initiating problem. Such situations usually resolve themselves within a 4- to 6-week period, or sooner with assistance, with no drastic change in the underlying personality structure.

In long-term situations, various psychological maladaptations have been identified. The most serious from the standpoint of frequency, duration, and degree of impairment of function are the **schizophrenias,** in which there is a divorcing of the emotional and cognitive processes. The emotional state often seems inappropriate to the thought processes and the situation in which the person is involved. There is often a profound psychological withdrawal from others and distortions of the thought processes. Although we talk about humans as open systems exchanging with their environment, the schizophrenic tends toward a closed system in the psychosocial area of behavior.

Other psychological maladaptations have been labeled as manic-depressive psychoses, chronic brain syndrome, and so forth. These vary with age and social class, and may or may not be related to alterations in the tissue of the brain. In either instance, prevention is possible if intervention is begun early enough. For example, Lemkau distinguishes between psychiatric illnesses from brain damage, and those caused primarily by malfunction of an intact brain.[56] He says, however, that they are not entirely separate. For example, general paresis is caused by destruction of the brain cells, but it usually does not occur unless individuals expose themselves to infection (syphilis), which is usually not without their knowledge. Thus, the brain damage is related to a decision made by the patient.

The concept of the natural history of disease processes and intervention, before man and disease agents are brought together, is important in the prevention of illness and is discussed in Chapter 9.

Although we have said that society considers psychoses to be maladaptive behavior, it is possible that most of these are adaptive for the individual that is faced with a difficult environment. For example, Jackson proposes the **double bind theory** (whereby an individual receives two contradictory messages which must be responded to) as causal in the development of schizophrenia.[57] He believes that communication patterns within a family are somewhat fixed, and these patterns, as well as the behaviors associated with them, can be observed. Communication occurs on multiple levels in all families, but this is particularly so in the schizophrenic family. Jackson says that we should look at the communication patterns, rather than the specific traumatic experiences, when studying the etiology of schizophrenia. The child learns the mental habits (adaptation), which are exemplified in schizophrenic communication, from certain sequential patterns in parents. Or, to put it another way, he says, "the child must live in a universe where the sequence of events are such that his unconventional communication habits will in some sense be appropriate."

Sequences necessary to produce schizophrenia are hypothesized in the double-bind theory as follows: (1) When the individual is involved in an intense relationship—one in which he feels it is vital to discriminate what sort of message is being communicated so that he may respond appropriately; (2) the individual is caught in a situation in which the other person in the relationship is expressing two sets of messages whereby one contradicts the other (verbal–nonverbal, and so forth);

(3) the individual is unable to comment on the messages being expressed to determine which message is valid; and (4) finally the complex set of ingredients is no longer necessary, for the person has learned to perceive his universe in double-bind patterns; that is, he may give incongruent messages, or respond to any and all messages as if they were incongruent.

Another theory for the cause of schizophrenia was proposed by Wynne.[58] Wynne assumes that (1) Movement into relationships with other human beings is a fundamental need of human existence (man is object related), and (2) every human being strives consciously and unconsciously during a lifetime to develop a sense of personal identity.

Wynne believes that the balance between these two needs diferentiates normal from schizophrenic families, and he describes three forms of relatedness: mutuality, nonmutuality, and pseudomutuality. He found that pseudomutuality prevails in schizophrenic families where the family is absorbed in fitting together at the expense of individual family members. Characteristics of these types of families include, rigid role structures, a lack of spontaneity, novelty, and humor, and anxiety about potential deviations from roles.

Both theories seem to point toward adaptation of an individual, or individuals, to a family (suprasystem) that is out of balance. It seems likely that genetic factors may add to ways of adapting to the family environment, and, thus, account for one member being identified as the patient, although, it is becoming increasingly evident that the identified patient is actually indicative of a sick family (entropic). A great deal of theory has evolved around the sick family and forms the basis of family therapy. An assessment of family communication patterns, role structure, and interpersonal relationships is important in community health nursing.

From the foregoing, it is clear that strong emotional reactions relative to environmental energies may lead to physical, mental, and emotional maladaptations. For some individuals, a way to protect themselves from maladaptation is through spiritual development.

In fact, in my opinion spiritual energies can be considered a part of psychosocial exchanges. According to the Bible, Jesus said, "The kingdom of heaven is within," and many groups interpret this to mean the spirit of God is within the physical body.[29] Many people believe that they can attune themselves to God by looking within through meditation and introspection, and by looking without for God in others. The practice of meditation and the demonstration of spiritual attributes, such as, faith, love, and patience in human exchanges can help us develop a better mental attitude toward the physical and social environment, so that both our perceptions of and reactions to situations can change. When negative emotions are removed, there is an increased balance in the endocrine system, and the individual is less prone to lose energy from the system, and, therefore, to illness. Sechrist, using Cayce's data, has related this balance in the endocrine system to attunement with God, and has explained a theory of spiritual development through the endocrine system.[60] In essence, humans, through meditation, demonstration of spiritual attributes, a set of spiritual beliefs, can change their mental attitude, which affects their physical condition (internal environment), which alters their perception of the external environment and the behavior with others (external).

This, in turn, probably has an effect on others in the environment if the studies (quoted earlier) on the influence of negative and positive emotions on plants and other living things are correct.

Love, which is an important component of psychosocial exchanges, is a force that is a part of our affective state and can be considered a spiritual energy. According to the Bible, Christ says, "Thou shalt love the Lord thy God with all thy heart . . . and thy neighbor as thyself."[61] Reference is made to love of a high order, or a perfect love, which is discussed further in the Bible:[62]

> Love is very patient and kind, never jealous or envious, never boastful or proud, never naughty or selfish or rude. Love does not demand its own way. It is not irritable or touchy. It does not hold grudges and will hardly ever notice when others do it wrong. It is never glad about injustice, but rejoices whenever truth wins out.

Maslow sees love as so important to humans that he places it high on his hierarchy of human needs.[63] He says, "When the physiological and safety needs are met, needs for love, affection and belonging emerge. Now the person . . . will hunger for affectionate relations with people in general. . . . He will want to attain such a place more than anything else in the world and maybe even forget that once, when he was hungry, he sneered at love as unreal or unnecessary or unimportant." Likewise, Montague says, "There is good evidence which leads us to believe that not only does a baby want to be loved, but also that it wants love, that all its drives are oriented in the direction of receiving and giving love, and that if it doesn't receive love it is unable to give it—as a child or as an adult."[64]

Smith says, "Every person, regardless of race, sex, culture, or age, has a need to love and to be loved. . . . love has been identified as a basic human need."[65]

The effects of deprivation of love on the developing child have been well-documented by Bowlby.[66] His basic findings show that the deprivation of love led to retarded physical, mental, and emotional development, and often in severe cases it led to the death of the child. The long-range effect of this deprivation was an emotional distance from all humans.

On the other hand, excessive love, which is usually of a selfish, possessive nature, can be damaging to all involved. For example, the selfish love of a mother may lead her to take over for her children, when they are faced with developmental tasks and need to grow (negentropy). This deprives them of the opportunities to become more independent, which may help the mother maintain balance temporarily, but will eventually cause unhealthy consequences from harboring dependency, under the guise of love.

Smith has added to the literature by discussing the components of love. Her concepts relate closely to the definition given earlier.[67]

In addition to psychological energies we also need social energies. Children who lack such energies in early life are unable later to respond to social training. For instance, there are cases on record of children who were lost in infancy and raised by animals (feral children), and exhibited no human social characteristics when brought back to civilization. Some were taught to walk and use their hands, and to say a few words, but there is no case on record of any of these children developing into normal human beings. We can ask whether this is a case of nature–nurture; that is, is it a genetic factor that prevents the learning, rather than the social environment, but it seems more likely that there are critical periods in our life, when certain stimuli must be present if a characteristic trait, behavior, or condition is to develop.

The most noted case on record is that of the feral female child, named Kamala. Although her body was human and she apparently had normal intellectual capacity, she did not have an opportunity to learn human ways. She adapted to her environment by learning the behaviors of the wolves, among whom she lived for 8 years.

She was found by the Reverend J. A. L. Singh in northwest India, when she was about 8 years old. She and another girl about one and one-half years younger were removed from the jungle to Singh's orphanage. The younger girl lived only ten months after her transfer to the orphanage, but Kamala lived about 8 more years. She was slow to adapt to human ways; for example, it was 15 months before she could support herself alone on her knees, and it took 44 months before she could stand on her feet. She never learned to run in an upright position. Initially, she ate her food as a dog would without the use of her hands, and milk was lapped up with her tongue.

Each of us, then, adapts to the particular environment we are socialized into. This process makes an Eskimo baby into an Eskimo and an American baby into an American. However, differences will be found in America because of the differing social-cultural groups that were mentioned earlier. It is little wonder that lower-class children who lack middle-class experiences appear mildly retarded when measured by middle-class intelligence scales. This finding has provided a basis for Head Start programs.

The need for social energies is so important that the concept of "significant others" is found repeatedly in the literature. In addition, because of this need for others, humans are willing to mold their behavior to the expectations of others.

CHANGE IN A PART AFFECTS THE WHOLE INDIVIDUAL

Many of the exchanges between humans and their environment and their adaptation to these changes have been presented. In several examples of change adaptation, changes in interrelated parts of the whole individual were discussed. We will now look more closely at how the parts affect the whole human system.

Exchange Act. Although many of the exchanges between humans and their environment are presented categorically (chemical, biologic, physical, and psychosocial), these exchanges (in total) make up the environment of individuals and impinge upon individuals at all times in varying degrees. Likewise, although the physiologic, psychologic, and mental reactions and adaptations to these energies are presented separately, these reactions occur as a totality and affect the total human being.

Humans are Total Beings. Whitehead in referring to the totality of humans says, ". . . the living organ of experience is the living body as a whole. . . . We cannot determine with what molecules the brain begins and the rest of the body ends. Further we cannot tell with what molecules the body ends and the external world begins. The truth is that the brain is continuous with the body, and the body continuous with the rest of the natural world."[68] Likewise, Dunn says, ". . . a mind is not an entity, a separate thing which inhabits our skull. It is, rather, a complex of activities performed by the brain and the body. . . . My definition would be that it (the mind) is the ability-complex of man which enables him to use his inner world for the purposes of solving the problems of every day living. . . . Man takes the sum total of the information which comes to him through his sense organs from the outer world; stores, integrates, and tries it out by various experiences; modifies and continuously reorganizes it as information available to him from his inner world. The total complex resulting from this process is the mind."[69]

We are so accustomed to thinking of humans as a composite of body, mind, and spirit that it is difficult to conceive of them as a whole being interacting with a whole environment. Specialization and increased knowledge of the body has led to compartmentalization both in the educational process and in the working world. In addition, our methodology for assessing humans and their health has evolved from specialty areas, and, thus, views them in parts.

At this time, some groups are attempting to integrate the parts and view humans as a whole. The concept of interrelated parts recognizes a whole system, which may be composed of subsystems, which are interdependent, so that a change in one part affects all the other parts. With a change in a part, energy is needed (entropy) for the other parts to adapt to the change, and this may affect the energy level of the total system, as it reaches a new balance. This balance, in turn, will affect the environment with which the individual exchanges; that is, if individuals worry about their job (emotional subsystem) they react totally at a lower level of energy. This negative emotion speeds up metabolic processes and alters the internal environment. As a result, there is a lack of vigor, food is distasteful, thinking is unclear, and a variety of other changes occur related to the lowering of the total energy level. Also, interactions with the environment probably also change. Withdrawal into work may take place or a seeking of approval from friends. Inadequate feelings may be projected onto others, using whatever defense mechanisms will help maintain a balance in the light of the altered energy level.

There is a great deal of evidence in the literature to substantiate the concept of subsystem alteration affecting the whole person. We know that when we are physically ill, we have difficulty thinking and we become more sensitive emotionally because of our lowered energy level. At these times, the body needs an alteration in external energies, so that the internal energies of the individual can regain a balance. Usually there is an increased need for psychosocial support, and physical care, so that the body can rest and heal itself. There may be a need for decreased environmental stimuli to facilitate this process, and, at times, increased chemical exchanges in the form of drugs, special diets, and oxygen may be initiated. This need for a decreased amount of energy expenditure during illness is so well-documented that Parsons has conceptualized the role of the sick.[70] The sick role includes dimensions, such as, dependency, exemption from usual activities, and so forth, and although these dimensions apply to the physical, they are equally appropriate to mental and emotional disorders of the whole persons. In addition, studies on the effects of anxiety have shown a total response by humans. When anxiety is too high emotions and mental processes are affected as a result of physiologic changes, and a new balance is established. In a preceeding section on adaptation, we discussed many examples of human adaptation as total beings. In addition to physiologic changes, we pointed out how humans use their mind to facilitate adaptation and how the emotions may assist, or hamper, such adaptation (*e.g.*, when humans are exposed to high temperatures, their physiologic mechanisms assist them in maintaining body temperature, but in addition, they use their minds to assist in this process of trying to remain within a range of adaptability). We also pointed out how emotions could assist or hamper this process.

We have all experienced periods when we felt in excellent health, where our bodies, minds and spirits are functioning at a high order, and we relate at a higher level with our environment. Dunn, Maslow, and others, have named these periods **peak experiences,** and have attempted to describe and conceptualize them.[71,72] It seems likely that if humans wish to move to a higher level of functioning, they must work on the parts of the total system concurrently; that is, they must pay attention to the physical, mental, and emotional subsystems in their day-to-day life. By moving to a higher level of energy, humans are better able to withstand impinging environmental energies and are thus better able to adapt.

Many of the failures in the health sciences are related to our inability to treat humans as total beings, when they are suffering from maladaptations. Although we accept the theory of multicausation in disease processes (*i.e.*, an imbalance in the energies in the human environment [physical, biologic, social, chemical], and within humans [physical, mental, spiritual]), leading to a breakdown in adaptive ability, we do not apply this concept once a disease process is initiated. Many in the health professions believe a diseased part can be removed, or treated with drugs (chemical energy), without dealing with the total person. This in combination with nursing measures, such as, emotional support, physical care, and so forth, may allow the body to heal itself and regain a degree of balance, but further breakdowns are possible once individuals return to their usual environment, because initial patterns (which were instrumental in the maladaptation) have been left unchanged. For example, if attitudes, emotions, and thoughts were instrumental in initiating the disease process, they should also be assessed and efforts made to help the individual change the resulting behavior.

The literature on spiritual concepts and healing seem to have moved further ahead in conceptualizing treatment for the whole man, than has the scientific literature. One important concept, from the Cayce reading, is the idea that, Spirit is the Essence, Mind the Builder, and Physical the Result.[73] If we think that diet, exercise, rest, and the other aspects of a balanced physical body are important, we will carry out an appropriate program in our lives, which will express these thoughts. If we understand and express spiritual attributes of love, patience, faith, and forgiveness, and develop the appropriate mental attitude toward ourselves, and others, our behaviors will manifest this, and our emotions and mental apparatus remain in balance. If on the other hand, our thoughts about ourselves and others are negative, and we neglect our bodies, we may establish a balance that does not allow us to remain adapted, and we experience illness. Illness may give us an opportunity to reevaluate our goals in life and our methods for reaching these goals, and thus, point us in the more healthy direction.

Because we have become so specialized, and tend to go into depth in one area of human behavior, our research and diagnostic tools for looking at sickness and health reflect this narrowness. Consequently, although theories of humans as total beings are evolving, the methodology for evaluating our health status has lagged behind, and we are forced to evaluate or view humans and their environment in parts, rather than as a totality. For example, the doctor may look at a chest x-ray film, palpate the liver, listen to chest sounds, and so forth, and the nurse may take the patient's temperature, blood pressure, and check the urine for sugar. The social worker may evaluate the social history and the psychologist the patient's psychological status. These parts give some indication of the functioning of the whole. In the community, the community health nurse may obtain a health and nutritional history, observe living and sleeping arrangements in the home, observe sanitary conditions and practices, observe family relationships, and so forth. Although this methodology allows us to observe and evaluate the parts of human behavior and the environment, these parts fit together to form a whole, where many factors lead to disease processes (multicausal theory of disease processes as a result of maladaptation). The multicausation theory allows us to interact to put humans in a favorable balance of health as a result of a theoretical base. In other words, the concept of multifactor causation in disease processes, our knowledge of various processes (effect of strong emotions on the body and mind, the effect of high numbers of bacteria in a weakened body), and our observational and interviewing skills, with families, allow us to predict to some degree the effect on humans if certain patterns are left unchanged.

As we continue to conceptualize man as a total being and move away from specialization to generalization, it seems likely that more methodology for viewing the total man may evolve. There have been some beginning developments in this direction in Russia. Machines, such as the Kurlin machine, which can photograph an energy field around the body so that physical, mental, and emotional problems can be identified before they manifest themselves, may eventually allow for preventive intervention of energies that affect the human being. Likewise, efforts to change energy-flows within man by using acupuncture techniques may become effective as treatment of whole man.

Humans Interact with a Total Environment. Various energies in the environment were previously singled out for discussion. Although these were presented separately for clarification (*e.g.*, biologic, chemical, physical and psychosocial energies), these and other energies *in toto* make up our environment. We are not exposed to energies singly but *in toto,* and multiple adaptive processes on our part are occurring simultaneously. It is interesting to consider a few of the energies impinging upon us in a single day as we lose or gain energy in our efforts to adapt. We may awaken in the morning and rush through a cup of coffee (which gives us no energy), or we may eat a leisurely well-balanced breakfast, which contributes to our energy intake. In the first instance, we may actually lose more energy from the rushing around, which increases metabolic processes, and causes a proportional increase in energy output. After preparing for work, we may begin our drive to the office moving from an air-conditioned home to a warm outdoors and back into an air-conditioned car calling into play other energy exchanges. During our drive, we are confronted with heavy traffic, which initiates a fear of being late and losing our job, or else we rest comfortably in the knowledge that we have allowed time for such occurrences. Again we lose energy from the increased metabolic processes resulting from adrenalin, or we maintain a normal energy exchange from the positive assurance of adequate time. If a child darts in front of the car, there is a total response that lowers our energy level. Finally, we move from the air-conditioned car into the warm outdoors and back into the air-conditioned office calling into play adaptive heat-exchange mechanisms with shifts in energy levels. We may be greeted by angry co-workers who call forth negative feelings, which decreases our energy and calls into play psychological defenses that tend to reestablish our balance, or we may be greeted by congenial co-workers who express concern and thus increase our energy level. We may influence our energy level by enjoying our work, exercising our minds and feeling productive, or we may be pressured and annoyed. At lunch, we may be exposed to chemical energies, which may be adequate or inadequate for the afternoon work, and thus may increase or decrease the internal energy level. We return to the office and may worry about completing work further losing energy. Again psychological defenses may come to our rescue and we may say "Oh well, no one could do that much in one day." We return home at night over the same road with some of the same problems as discussed earlier, but, in addition, carrying some of the problems of the day. These are just a few of the exchanges between average middle class individuals and their environment, which affect the energy level of the human system.

In most instances, we are able through physiologic adaptive maneuvers, psychological defenses, and learned patterns of behavior to maintain a degree of balance, although some of these patterns may be conducive to later periods of maladaptation if we are confronted with increased environmental energies (frequency, duration, or severity) that pose a strain on our characteristic patterns of response. This is discussed further in Chapter 10, which incorporates crisis.

ENTROPY AND NEGENTROPY OF INDIVIDUALS

ENTROPY

In the individual, as in any open system, entropy is always present because the parts of the system (circulatory, nervous, respiratory) must continually adjust to the input of energy as energy is lost in the process of transformation and subsequent feedback. In each of the exchanges discussed earlier (food, oxygen, psychosocial), some energy is lost and unavailable for work because of the transformation of the energy input within the system (see Braden for a discussion of this process).[74] This loss of energy and tendency toward disorganization (entropy) is not detrimental to a system in which the parts are functioning efficiently to maintain the whole, because there is always enough energy to sustain the individual beyond the disorganization, to meet the needs of the system (adaptation), and to move to a higher organization and order (negentropy). For example, even though energy is lost (entropy) in the process of food digestion, there is still adequate energy to meet the needs of the cells and tissues, which was discussed earlier under the process of adaptation. Growth, or negentropy, is a result of an increase in the building-up forces within the individual over the breaking-down forces (entropy). In other words, entropy results from an increase in breaking-down forces over the building-up forces. Growth is stationary (temporary equilibrium) when the two forces are equal.

Entropic processes may result from a breakdown of a part of the system that affects other parts and the system is no longer able to work effectively to meet the goals and purposes of the system. This may result from excesses and deprivations in the exchange between the individual and the environment, and if continued over a long period of time leads to changes in the organized, kinetic, or potential, energy of the individual. At such times the individual is faced with a crisis (physiologic, psychological) and usually needs outside assistance to regain balance. These excesses and deprivations as they affect the individual were discussed earlier under adaptation. An example of an entropic process is food deprivation whereby the body's carbohydrates are used up within 24 to 48 hours. This is followed by depletion of the body's fat and finally by the depletion of protein. This entropic process, if continued, will lead to death of the individual. Many entropic processes can be identified in individuals with whom we work. Disease processes such as cancer, cardiovascular disease, allergies, arthritis, emphysema, and mental illness would all constitute entropic processes in the individual. In addition, we can identify potential entropic processes as a result of our knowledge of the natural history of diseases and our knowledge of the range of adaptability of individuals. For example, cigarette smoking, inadequate food intake, exposure to excessive heat and sound in industry, and contaminated food, water, and air are all potential areas to cause entropic processes in individuals. Any of these, if prolonged, can lead to a breakdown of a part, which will affect the individual as a whole. Application of the nursing processes (Chaps. 6 and 7), and knowledge of the dynamics of the individual and the environment (Chap. 9) form a basis for determining whether or not the nurse should intervene. When the nurse does intervene, the interventions are aimed at counteracting the entropic forces to bring about a degree of equilibrium, or to restore negentropy. Putt discusses many nursing measures that will counteract entropic processes.[75] For example, teaching deep breathing will increase the oxygen–carbon dioxide exchange (negentropy) in an emphysemic patient (entropic) and move him toward equilibrium. Teaching a balanced diet to a person whose diet is inadequate will remove the potential for entropic processes. However, when we are working with preventive care (potential entropic processes) we must be aware of the reason for the behavior observed (see Nursing Process, Chap. 6), and our philosophy of community health nursing (Chap. 5). For example, if an individual consumes an inadequate diet we identify the reason for the behavior or the need it meets (Chap. 6). Otherwise, we may disrupt the temporary balance by attempting to implement change before the person is ready. This may lead to other entropic processes. For instance, if we talk with a client about quitting smoking and the client complies because of a desire for reward or to avoid punishment (Chap. 6), the client may quit but begin overeating to satisfy an unresolved need and to maintain a temporary balance. This behavior can also lead to entropic processes. In addition, the nurse's behavior would be inconsistent with our philosophy which identifies actual and potential health problems, points out alternatives and consequences of behavior, but leaves the decision for change up to the client (see Chap. 5)

In addition to a failure in an individual's subsystem affecting the whole system leading to entropic processes, the superordinate system may also facilitate entropy. Earlier we talked about the double-bind theory and the family that is so concerned with cohesiveness that it ignores the identities of its individual members. Such families do not allow members to grow into increasingly ordered and complex individuals, which may eventually cause disordered behavior (entropy) in one, or more, of its members. In addition, the ability to love, to develop self-esteem, to trust, to feel good about ourselves (self-concept), and various other growth processes, are developed within the family. Failure of the family to meet these needs leads to entropic processes such as poor self-concept, low self-esteem, emotional deprivation, and so forth. For example, a poor self-concept and low self-esteem often prevent individuals from entering into important roles and relationships, which would facilitate their growth. When two such people come together and marry, they form the core of another sick family.

NEGENTROPY

When individuals are not demonstrating entropic processes, or a temporary steady state (entropic processes balanced with negentropic processes), they are evolving toward increased order and organization (negentropy). Individuals grow from infancy to adulthood physically, mentally, and emotionally. The adult has a greater body mass, communication, learning, and other skills that the child does not have, because of negentropy. Sutterley discusses many of these negentropic processes.[76] Because there are established norms for groups in relation to these negentropic processes, we can identify how individuals are or should be progressing. For example, the 12-month-old child triples his birth weight, walks with support of one hand and reverts to creeping when support is not available, can grasp two small objects at the same time, pick up minute objects, and so forth. Several guides for assessing the child's level of development are available. The one most frequently used in local health departments is the Denver Developmental Screening Test.[77] In addition, Piaget has described stages of psychosocial development.[78,79] Sheehy has also discussed the development of individuals throughout their lifetime.[80] These guides and tools are useful in the nurse's assessment to determine if the patient is within an acceptable range regarding negentropic processes.

Humans and Their Environment are Evolving in One Direction. Both humans and their environment are continually changing and evolving—neither are static forms of energy. Humans grow through the process of cell anabolism and catabolism from infancy to adulthood. Such growth is inherent in the nature of the cells, and each specialized cell is made up of molecular patterns that are coded for exact replication by hereditary factors. All living forms are made up of these molecular patterns of energy ensuring an ordered and continued pattern of growth. From birth to death, human sequential stages of development (birth, infancy, adolescence, adulthood, and old age) have been generalized and categorized for consistency. Although we have standards for physical, intellectual, and psychological development that apply to groups, these standards may vary with time and place because of evolving environmental energies (natural and man-made) and humans themselves (genetically, experientially). Growth is dependent upon this exchange of energy and Guyton says that cells can survive and reproduce, provided they are surrounded with fluids containing nutrients.[81] Oxygen and food, then, as well as the other energies we discussed earlier are necessary for the growth and continued evolvement of humans.

During the process of growth, humans are exposed to various degrees of environmental energies, which are also changing because of natural and man-made transformations of energy. During this process, we are exposed to various energies that influence internal processes (physical, psychological, spiritual). Some of these environmental challenges are within a usual range of adaptation and are thus responded to in a somewhat automatic fashion. Others may be beyond the usual range of adaptation creating more stress leading to conscious ways of coping and a new level of balance. During these periods, humans may learn new information, new coping skills, and new attitudes and feelings that leave them a different person than before.

In a general sense, human growth and evolution can be thought of as on an energy continuum where more and more energy is available, as humans, over time, become organized into a greater energy system through the growth process (physically, intellectually, spiritually, influencing behavior). As humans grow, they take in more energy in the form of food, heat, information, and so forth, and they develop into more complex beings at a time when they are moving into situations requiring greater reserves of physical, psychological, and spiritual energies. Eventually there is a decreased intake of some energies, which coincides with a decline in performance. As the life cycle progresses, more and more energy restores what is worn away by attrition, until the body, as an organized structure, breaks down and eventually dies.

Although humans are progressing in a forward manner maturing physically, mentally, and spiritually as a result of their exchange with their environment, some behaviors and adaptations seem to have a cyclic nature, rather than a straightforward movement. This is most clearly seen in biorhythmic functions and in learned patterns of response (both intellectual and emotional) to environmental energies, in our attempt to maintain balance. However, since the environment too is changing and evolving, these response patterns cannot continue indefinitely in a cyclic fashion, but must eventually move to another level. For example, we may automatically respond to minor stresses by worrying and then rationalizing and projecting. This pattern of response may help us maintain a balance for awhile, but as the environment changes and we are faced with increased amounts of stress this response pattern increases and may lead to changes in our organized energy (ulcers); then, we must learn new methods of adapting to stress.

Evolving Environment. Our environment is also evolving in a forward direction primarily because of our interventions and our attempts at manipulating and transforming energy for our use. We have moved from an agricultural society where we were fairly self-sufficient to an industrial society where specialization and interdependence flourish. During this process, humans collectively used their minds to improve the standard of living by transforming energy into forms for human use. The horse-drawn carriages were replaced with automobiles, buses, and airplanes. And now that we are moving into the space age, there is the potential for interplanetary travel. We have replaced the woodburning stove with electric and gas heat, which can be adjusted by the movement of a switch. During the summer months we now turn on the air conditioner, and reading and physical work have been replaced with television, movies, and the radio. This list of energy transformations for our use and comfort could go on indefinitely. These changes in our lives have had a profound effect on our health and behavior. Energy excesses and more leisure time as a result of these timesavers have created, or increased, such problems as pollution, crime, mental, and chronic illnesses, to name a few.

In terms of energy output, it seems that humans collectively have gone through three periods of development over time and although some individuals may have maintained a balance of mental, spiritual, and physical energy output, most humans stress one kind of energy more than the others. During our agricultural period of evolution the physical was overstressed because of the need to grow food, provide shelter, and other physical needs. For most people there was probably little time or access to materials to stimulate the mind and the spirit. With industrialization, specialization, and mass production came more free time and social changes in the form of laws that began to focus our energies on mental activities. For example, laws such as compulsory education, prohibition against child labor, state and federal expenditures for education, made education available and mandatory. Now that we have moved beyond the necessity for overstressing the physical and intellectual to meet our needs, we seem to be entering a period where there is a major thrust, especially among young people, to find meaning in life and to develop spiritual concepts.

This third focus of energies has led to experimenting with drugs among some, to the growth of courses on meditation, offered on university campuses and elsewhere, and to a seeking of enlightenment in many other ways, rather than an emphasis on material possessions and mental acquisitions. It seems as if a larger group of people is moving toward a balance of mental, spiritual, and physical activities than has previously been the case. We could almost compare these changes in society with Maslow's Hierarchy of Needs for individuals.[82] This hierarchy lists the needs that motivate individuals as they move up the hierarchy. When one need is met, it no longer motivates the person. The first needs are in the physical area, which can be likened to society during the agricultural period. Once these basic needs are met, an individual (or society) begins to focus on needs for security, social contact, and status, in that order. Maslow's last need is for self-fulfillment and this relates to the search for meaning in life that is the concern of our current generation.

Many changes within society have brought about this refocusing. In general, it can be said that all human efforts have been geared toward increasing or conserving energy. Technology brought about a variety of home appliances that were within the economic reach of large segments of the population. Such things as air conditioners, improved methods of heating, and electric lights, improved methods of farming and food distribution; dishwashers and man-made gadgets have decreased the amount of energy output in meeting our physical needs. At the same time, improved methods of transportation and roads, refrigeration, and so forth, have allowed for a greater food supply (energy) among larger segments of the population. Technology has also allowed humans to move from place to place with a minimal amount of energy expenditure. Labor unions have evolved for the same purposes, that is, to protect the rights and energy of the workers. Likewise, the social and health services have evolved to increase and conserve the energy of populations. For example, many of the teaching functions of nurses and social workers are geared toward helping humans improve their knowledge and, thus, helps them adapt better to their changing environment (knowledge of preventive measures, coping skills). At other times, when humans are at a low level of energy, such as, coping with a physical or psychological crisis, these services may provide the support until individuals return to their usual level of functioning.

At the same time, as these efforts to increase and conserve human energy have been going on, there have been by-products, or unexpendable energy, from these transformations, which have been detrimental to the group. Such factors as water and air pollution, drugs, boredom, and mental illnesses, are among the many in present-day society.

As with humans, many of the environmental forces seem to have a cyclic pattern. This is most evident in the daily cycle of light and dark, the seasons, and so forth.

Evolving Humans Adapt to an Evolving Environment. At any point in time, humans are the result of their genetic base and their environmental experiences. During some periods of growth, we adapt easily to environmental energies because they are within our range of adaptability. At other times, energies are beyond our adaptative abilities (physiologic, intellectual, and emotional) and the excesses or deprivations have led to entropy with reversible, or irreversible, changes in our organized energy. Following readaptation, our balance is at a different level because of physiologic, intellectual, or emotional changes, including, new knowledge, attitudes, and skills. For example, lack of sensory stimulation in early life may have created a breakdown in the adaptive mechanism of the child creating irreversible damage to the eyes, or thinking processes, and readaptation would occur on a lower intellectual level, or without full functioning of the eyes. This alters total behavior; that is, the child is less able to grasp mental concepts that assist in adaptation. Likewise, the child may have experienced maternal deprivation and lack of love in early life. This imbalance could lead to physical-psychological damage, which would influence later behavior. Readjustment, then, is at a lower level.

Exposure to energies that create entropy may also leave the body at a higher level following readjustment. For example, if we have an illness such as mumps, we develop an immunity to further illnesses of this sort. Dubos says,

> Acquired immunity, whatever its mechanism, is a sort of biological learning which makes the body better prepared to meet a danger already encountered in the past. . . . Biological learning can range all the way from the production of antibodies detectable by chemical techniques in the serum of an im-

> muned individual, to the wisdom of the world, and to the social knowledge which schools and books try to convey by describing the various aspects of human experiences.[83]

Then, in addition to changes taking place in the body as a result of illness, we may have learned new knowledge of caring for ourselves, who to turn to when ill (community resources), and ways of preventing further illness. Also, depending upon how we are treated during this dependency period, we develop new attitudes and values. Humans, then, respond as a total being and our future behavior is changed accordingly. In relation to this last point, Byrne and Thompson see man as a whole individual reacting to internal and external environments, while meeting basic needs.[84]

In summary, human reactions to energies impinging upon them at any point in time are based upon genetic equipment and previous experiences. This is a total reaction of body, mind, and spirit, which remain in balance, or do not, depending upon the physical condition of the body, use of previous knowledge, values, attitudes, emotional responses, and so forth. One means of helping humans regain balance when faced with environmental stress (physical–psychosocial), which was proposed by Dunn, is to place people in a protected environment (hospital or other care facility), where stress is reduced. Many other methods of building up humans to reduce the chances of entropy, when faced with environmental stresses, will be discussed in Chapters 6 and 7. These include activities, such as, establishing helping relationships and assisting families in changing attitudes and values in health; helping children in schools or family members to solve problems and thereby prepare them for problem solving during later crisis situations; helping to increase knowledge about care of the ill, ways of preventing illness, and community resources; and immunizations that give immunity to disease. All preventive and nursing-care services should be offered in a way that families can accept them and thereby increase their ability to maintain balance when faced later with environmental stress.

FEEDBACK IN INDIVIDUALS

Feedback in humans facilitates self-regulatory processes and, as mentioned before, is the process where some output from the system is fed back into the system as input.

Under the concept of adaptation, we talked about some kinds of **negative feedback**—that is, the body's attempt to maintain a steady state consistent with the individual's goal of remaining in balance, in view of changing internal and external exchanges. We also indicated that, at times, if the individual goes outside the range of adaptability in exchanges, the result is crisis (entropy).

The other aspect of feedback for individuals involves **positive feedback,** which amplifies deviations away from the steady state and facilitates learning and growth (negentropy). These occur as the system grows in multiple areas as discussed under the concept of negentropy. For example, the child moves from the stage of trust–mistrust to the stage of autonomy as outlined by Erikson or through the various physical developmental stages identified on the Denver Developmental Test.[85,86] During these transition stages there is a need for a change in the energy exchanges if children are to meet their goals of maintaining balance and growing more complex (negentropy). For instance, there may be a need for an increase in chemical exchanges (food) and a decrease in the need for outside resources as children use their own resources more (e.g., walking; does not need to be carried), and an increase in the need for psychosocial energy (in the form of encouragement), and in information, as the parent tells the child how to master the new task.

This change will necessiate a change in both the subsystems and in the whole system, as well as the suprasystem. For example, before children can walk, their bone and muscular structure, brain, and so forth, must be developed to the point that they can receive and transmit signals from the brain to the body to maintain an upright position. In addition, parents, and others, in the social environment must allow children to experiment and move to this new level of development rather than continue to carry out an old pattern of carrying the child if the child is to move successfully into a new stage (negentropy). This applies to all patterns of growth; that is, the body must be ready in total, and the social environment must change, to facilitate growth as we move away from a steady state in areas, such as, physical, psychosocial and sexual development. Otherwise, these processes of growth may be stifled through excesses and deprivations of exchanges and we move toward entropy.

The process whereby these growth periods occur or whereby we move away from a steady state seem to follow a pattern. At any point in time, we have patterned behaviors to which others in our environment adapt temporarily. For example, as very young children crawl, parents or siblings may carry or wait on them. When the body as a whole is ready to move away from this temporary steady state, the system receives mismatched information between its behavior (crawling) and its internal standard or internal criteria. The internal goal then forces a change in the patterned behavior (walking, instead of creeping). The child's system experiences increased tension and conflict until a new patterned behavior is reached, which is consistent with the new goal or a decision is made to give up the goal.

As children get older various learned maneuvers are tried in an attempt to move to new stages of development when faced with opposition from the family or others in the social environment. These maneuvers include, bargaining, coaxing, threatening, and others, which are elaborated upon in the next chapter. Following the transition to a new stage there is again a temporary steady state until a new growth spurt (physical, psychosocial) occurs, and a new goal, necessitating a change in both the subordinate and superordinate system to which the individual is closely tied.

As indicated in the last chapter, some of the changes away from a steady state (positive feedback) in an individual may be disastrous for the system. If an individual decides that stealing is a way of living life, this person may move away from a steady state of instilled values of honesty and integrity (internal standard) to this new steady state. The mismatch of information causes an incongruence between internal standards of conduct and the new behavior, which creates tension and conflict. If there is peer support (*e.g.*, "It's OK to steal—the world owes us a living"), and the person can replace the internal values with this new behavior, there will be continued movement toward this new behavior. Perhaps the behavior is tried a few times and the person gets away with it, the behavior is reinforced and it becomes a new steady state.

EQUIFINALITY IN INDIVIDUALS

Each individual has goals and a particular way of reaching these goals based upon current and past experiences. Some individuals may need money for basic necessities and turn to the community for assistance. This may result from an awareness of community resources, internal values that stealing is wrong, but using community resources, which are tax supported, is all right. In addition, the current needs are such that they can meet their basic needs with community assistance. Other individuals may decide stealing is the only way to meet their needs and goals.

A consistent goal for all individuals is to maintain their self-regulatory processes throughout their life span. However, as indicated earlier, we all learn different ways to maintain balance in view of changing internal and external needs and based upon our background, and, thus, may go outside our adaptive abilities where the self-regulatory processes break down. In addition, as we grow and develop through the process of negentropy, our goals will change.

A FOCAL POINT FOR COMMUNITY HEALTH NURSES

Community health nurses must focus on individuals as holistic systems, that is, systems whose behavior reflects the interaction of the subordinate (organ) system and superordinate (family) system. An assessment of the behavior of the individual in relation to all exchanges, including the family, is a necessary part of the nursing process. This behavior should then be compared with acceptable standards for the particular age, sex, and activity level. For example, are the body parts of a 6-month-old ready for toilet training in a family that is pressuring for this change? And what is the actual and potential effect on the child? We know from standards of growth and development (negentropy) that children of 6 months are not ready for this change and may react by frustration and rebellion (feedback process). Has the pressure by the family and the rebellion by the child led to a deprivation of psychosocial energy for the child? This assessment should lead to interventions that are in keeping with the child's level of development and the families peace of mind. Thus, we must use our knowledge of readiness of body parts for growth (negentropy) and readiness for new goals, as well as family dynamics, as a basis for deciding how to intervene effectively to allow individuals to move to new steady states (negentropy).

Often we can help families adapt to change in members by providing anticipatory guidance, that is, by telling them beforehand what to expect in individual members before they reach certain stages of change. For example, if we tell families with 1-year-olds that 2-year-olds become negative, reduce their food intake, and are ready for bowel training based upon the growth and development of body parts (negentropy), they are prepared for these behaviors and perhaps avoid unnecessary difficulties.

Community health nurses should also have a good understanding of the changing needs of individuals for exchanges at various stages of development (negentropy), and the range of adaptability of these exchanges. This knowledge can be compared with the assessed behavior in individuals to determine how nurses can best help individuals maintain their goal of self-regulation.

Some goals (equifinality) of individuals are unconscious, whereas others are conscious and change over time. Unconscious goals include, the goal of self-preservation and the maintenance of balance (steady state and negentropy). Although these unconscious goals are out of our awareness, individual behavior regarding exchanges may facilitate or hamper the goals. Conscious goals change over time and should be assessed by community health nurses, as a basis for planning. For example, if a family goal is to maintain a good home in a good neighborhood and this goal is straining the budget, nurses must be aware of this goal in planning. Rather than referring the family or individual to low-cost housing, nurses may more appropriately work with other aspects of the budget, such as, recreation, transportation, or any unnecessary items to see where the strain can be reduced without sacrificing needs. Thus, an assessment of individual goals and joint planning by the nurse and individual are important.

At times community health nurses may intervene at a point to prevent entropic processes or to facilitate negentropic processes and meet the goal of self-regulation. For example, there may be an inadequate diet consumed by the individual, or there may be chain smoking that interferes with the oxygen-carbon dioxide cycle. If nurses teach proper diet and ways to reduce smoking, and the individual makes changes in a positive direction, the intervention has prevented entropic processes. Or, if nurses intervene on behalf of a child who is unloved and help encourage an adequate supply of this psychosocial energy by the mother or any significant others, they are facilitating negentropy for the child. These examples involve primary-prevention interventions, which are discussed in Chapter 9.

At other times, community health nurses may intervene to counteract entropic processes. These interventions may occur at the secondary or tertiary levels of prevention, depending upon the location of the individual on the health continuum. For example, community health nurses may identify individuals who have beginning signs of emphysema (entropy), and in addition to carrying out other prescribed treatment, might teach deep breathing to the person (negentropy). Because the illness was identified at the early stages, secondary-prevention interventions are useful. At a later stage in the illness, such teaching might not be effective and the individual may be moved to a hospital where machines and personnel would assist the patients breathing and, at the same time, reduce the demands upon the lungs by reduced physical activity.

REFERENCES

1. Jones K, et al: Dimensions III: A Changing Concept of Health, p 441. San Francisco, Ganfield, 1976
2. Dubos R: Man Adapting, pp 55–57. New Haven, Yale University, 1967 (Reproduced with permission)
3. Guyton A: Textbook of Medical Physiology, pp 956–961. Philadelphia, W B Saunders, 1976
4. Dubos R, Man Adapting, p 55 (Reproduced with permission)
5. Dubos R: So Human An Animal, p 73. New York, Charles Schribner's, 1968
6. Luce G: Biological Rhythms in Human and Animal Physiology. New York, Dover Publications, 1971
7. Guyton A, op cit, pp 826–837
8. CBS News Television Report from Temple Buell College Denver, Oct 16, 1970
9. Baetzer A: Radiation. In Sartwell P (ed): Preventive

Medicine and Public Health, pp 847–858. New York, Appleton-Century-Crofts, 1973
10. Dubos R: Man Adapting, p 22. New Haven, Yale University, 1967 (Reproduced with permission)
11. Ibid
12. Dubos R, Man Adapting, pp 135–136 (Reproduced with permission)
13. Koos E: The Health of Regionville. New York, Columbia University, 1961
14. White J: Plants, polygraphs and paraphysics. In White J (ed): Frontiers of Consciousness. New York, Julian, 1974
15. Vogel M: May-plant communication. In White J (ed): Psychic Explorations, p 289. New York, Edgar D Mitchell and Associates, 1974
16. Ostrander S, Schroeder L: Psychic Discoveries Behind the Iron Curtain, p 32–35. New Jersey, Prentice-Hall, 1971
17. White J, op cit
18. Ostrander S, Schroeder L, op cit
19. Ibid
20. Ibid
21. Ibid
22. Bredemeier HC: Social systems integration and adaptation. (Unpublished) Cited by Shirley A Smoyak: Toward understanding nursing situations: A transactional paradigm. Nurs Res 18:407, Sept–Oct, 1969
23. Sutterley D, Donnelly G: Perspectives in Human Development. Philadelphia, J B Lippincott, 1973
24. Beland I: Clinical Nursing: Pathophysiological and Psychosocial Approaches. New York, Macmillan, 1975
25. Jones K, et al: Dimensions III: A Changing Concept of Health, p 175. San Francisco, Ganfield, 1976
26. Birch HG: Malnutrition, learning and intelligence. Am J Public Health 62, No. 6:773–784 June 1972
27. Guyton A, op cit, pp 589–590
28. Guyton A, op cit, p 600
29. Baetzer A, op cit
30. Beland I, op cit
31. Levine, Myra. Introduction to Clinical Nursing. Philadelphia, F A Davis, 1973
32. Dubos, R, Mirage of Health. New York, Harper & Row, 1971
33. Guyton A, op cit, p 966
34. Dubos R, Man Adapting, p 56 (Reproduced with permission)
35. Baetzer A, op cit, p 837
36. Dubos R, Man Adapting, p 57 (Reproduced with permission)
37. Baetzer A: op cit, p 838
38. Dubos R, Man Adapting, pp 50–51
39. Ibid
40. Ibid
41. Thommen G: Biorthythm: Is This Your Day? New York, Award Books, 1969
42. Baetzer A, op cit, p 864
43. Dubos R, Man Adapting p 25 (Reproduced with permission)
44. Ibid (Reproduced with permission)
45. Ibid, p 22 (Reproduced with permission)
46. Ibid, p 51 (Reproduced with permission)
47. Baetzer A, op cit, p 854
48. Freud A: Aggression in relation to emotional development. The Annual 3, No. 4, 1949
49. Cannon WB: The Wisdom of the Body. New York W W Norton, 1939
50. Pelletier K: Mind as Healer, Mind as Slayer, p 62. New York, Delta, 1977
51. Wolff HG, Wolf S, Goodell H (eds): Stress and Disease, 2nd ed. Springfield, C C Thomas, 1968
52. Hinkle LE, et al: The effect of exposure to cultural changes, social changes and changes in interpersonal relationships on health. In Dohrenwend BS, Dohrenwend BP (eds): Stressful Life Events: Their Nature and Effect. New York, Wiley, 1974
53. Wolff HG: Stress and Disease
54. Engle G, et al: Psychological factors in organic disease. Mental Health Program Reports, pp 1–23. Bethesda, NIMH, Feb 1967
55. Ibid
56. Lemkau P: Basic Issues in Psychiatry. Springfield, Charles C Thomas, 1959
57. Jackson D: Communication, Family, and Marriage. Human Communication Series, Vol 1. Palo Alto, Science and Behavioral Books, 1968
58. Wynn, L, et al: Pseudomutuality in the family relations of schizophrenics. Psychiatry 21: 205–220, May 1958
59. The Living Bible, p 825. Wheaton, Tyndale House, 1973
60. Sechrist E: Meditation, Gateway to Light. Virginia Beach, ARE Press, 1972
61. The Living Bible, p 793
62. The Living Bible, p 925
63. Maslow AH: Motivation and Personality. New York, Harper & Row, 1954
64. Montague A: The Practice of Love, p 6. Englewood Cliffs, Prentice-Hall, 1975
65. Smith K: The need to love and be loved. In Yura H, Walsh M (eds): Human Needs and the Nursing Process, pp 171–212. New York, Appleton-Century-Crofts, 1978
66. Bowlby J: Maternal Care and Mental Health. Geneva, World Health Organization, 1952
67. Smith K, op cit
68. Whitehead AN: Adventures in Ideas. New American Library of World Ideas, 1964

69. Dunn H: High Level Wellness, pp 79–81. Arlington, R W Beatty, 1961
70. Parsons T: The Social System. Glencoe, The Free Press of Glencoe, 1951
71. Dunn Halbert: What high level wellness means. Can J Public Health 50:11 1959
72. Maslow A, op cit
73. Cayce E: Psychic Readings Housed at Association For Research and Enlightenment, Virginia Beach, Virginia
74. Braden C, Hebran N: Community Health: A Systems Approach. New York, Appleton-Century-Crofts, 1976
75. Putt A: General Systems Theory Applied to Nursing. Boston, Little Brown, 1978
76. Sutterley D, Donnelly G, op cit
77. Frankenberg WK, Dodds JB: The Denver Developmental Screening Test. J Pediatr 71:181, 1967
78. Piaget J: Introduction to the Language and Thought of the Child. New York, Harcourt, 1926
79. Erikson E: Identity and the life cycle. Psychological Issues. New York, International University, 1959
80. Sheehy G: Passages. New York, Bantam, 1977
81. Guyton A: Textbook of Medical Physiology, p 12. Philadelphia, W B Saunders, 1976
82. Maslow A: op cit
83. Dubos R: Mirage of Health (Reproduced with permission)
84. Byrne M, Thompson L: Key Concepts for the Study and Practice of Nursing. St Louis, C V Mosby, 1972
85. Erikson Eric, op cit
86. Frankenberg WK, Dodds JB, op cit

3

The Family as a System

In this chapter, systems theory is related to the family, which is a major focus of attention for community health nursing. The family is so important that it is recognized in every society. Despite the fact that there are more than 4000 human societies, Benson says, "The family, as a social institution has existed from the beginning of time in every corner of the world. It is the most stable, enduring, and universal cultural form."[1]

CONCEPT OF THE FAMILY

DISCIPLINARY ATTEMPTS

There have been many attempts to define and conceptualize the family, by various disciplines. Each discipline has its own point of view, or frame of reference, for viewing the family and its attempt reflects its particular framework. Biologists are concerned with the biologic functions of the family, and focus on the perpetuation of the species, the union of male and female to produce offspring, and the effects on the offspring of biologic variations (genetic patterns) in parents. They tend to define the family from a biologic point of view. For example, Freeman quotes Farber who describes the family as, ". . . a collective enterprise based on relationships defined by birth and marriage . . . a kinship organization mobilized to endure."[2]

Psychologists and psychiatrists have been concerned primarily with family relationships and the prevention of mental illnesses resulting from these relationships. They have also looked at individual personality development, and how individuals see themselves as individuals and in relation to their families. At times they have also looked at subgroups of the family, such as marital relationships from a psychodynamic point of view. For example, Murray and Zentner say that, "many experts agree that the family is the basic unit of growth, experience, and adaptation . . . it is also a basic unit of health and illness."[3]

Economists have been concerned with how the family works together to meet their material needs, and sociologists have looked at how the family as a group functions socially, using the theory of group process and dynamics. Sociologists have also looked at how the family as a group relates to the larger society.

Unfortunately, there is no one concept of the family that is useful to community health nursing, despite current attempts at multidisciplinary research. Some of the sociologic studies consider only biologic theories of families, and they discount unwed mothers and single people in a family. Farber's definition (quoted earlier) is such a concept. Sociologists also use the biologic basis of the family when they talk about the family of orientation or procreation. Other difficulties with sociologic concepts of the family result from a lack of dynamics in concepts accounting for shifts in family structure and function, during phases of the life cycle.

Likewise, some psychologists limit their concepts of family to the biologic family (two parents and offspring) or to certain racial or social-class groups, and these concepts cannot be generalized to all families. In other instances, psychologists may focus only on internal relationships of families, as though they were closed systems uninfluenced by the larger society.

Some recent attempts to define and conceptualize the family, using systems theory, have been more appropriate for community health nursing because of the focus on internal and external relationships and dynamics. For example, Sussman looks at selected internal and external relationships of the family and identifies traditional and emerging categories of family structure.[4] Rae defines the family as "an integrated system of interdependent structure and functions, is constituted of relationships, and consists of people who must learn to live together."[5] Leininger says, "a social system may be viewed as a network of persons who regularly interact with one another and manifest signs of being interdependent and interrelated in order to achieve common institutional goals."[6]

Although we can learn a great deal, then, from the literature about internal family relationships, about normal family functioning, and about how certain types of families relate to the broader community, there is no one concept that will encompass all levels of concern in community health nursing. For example, focusing only on internal family relationships would disqualify the influence of the broader society on these relationships, or applying concepts of families derived from middle-class studies might not be pertinent to lower-class families. Likewise, tuberculosis casefinding by the nurse, using a family definition of father, mother, and offspring, in a household where extended-family members or other unrelated individuals also live, would be inadequate casefinding. It is also obvious that we cannot use only one disciplinary focus when we are concerned about health patterns and behaviors in the family. We may be concerned about reproductive patterns in a family, but we are equally concerned with internal relationships, economic factors, and a variety of other conditions, and factors, which may influence health. Likewise, authors such as Koos indicate, for example, that the health behavior of one social class differs significantly from another.[7] However, systems theory provides the framework onto which these concepts can be attached.

FAMILY DEFINED FOR COMMUNITY HEALTH NURSING

Because the family as defined in the literature often refers to a biologic family, a broader definition is needed in community health nursing, as indicated previously. One useful definition is that the **family** is "a primary group of people living in a household in consistent proximity and intimate relationships." Using this definition of family, the nurse can include various patterns of family groups found in the community, such as the normal biologic family of procreation, the family of procreation that incorporates one or more members of the extended family (family of orientation), the single parent and offspring, a communal family that is together because of common interests and goals, or a homosexual couple. Under each of these family patterns there is a distribution of privileges and demands, encompassed in interdependent roles, that may change as the family moves through time, and the family relates to a broader society, which may move them toward or away from health. Thus, this definition views the family as a system.

FAMILY'S PLACE IN THE HIERARCHY

In the hierarchy presented in Chapter 1, the family is located between the individual and the community. The subordinate system of the family is the individual and the superordinate system is the community. In order to adequately understand the family and to assist its members in health matters, we must look not only at the family as a unit, but also at the individual members and community and how they influence the family's behavior and health.

BOUNDARY OF THE FAMILY

There is a greater concentration of energy within the family than there is between the family and those outside the family system; thus, the family has a boundary. This greater concentration of energy is seen in the more intimate relationships and the interdependent functions within the family. For example, although these functions are changing, mothers have traditionally cleaned, washed clothes, cooked, shopped for food, supported children emotionally, and so forth; whereas, the father has provided the economic base for the family, kept the car in working order, and maintained the exterior of the house. As children were added to families and grew to the point where they could assume more independent functions, they were assigned tasks, such as, taking garbage outside, washing dishes, cutting the grass, and so forth, depending upon the age and sex of the child and the attitudes and values of the parents. Whatever the pattern of family functioning (who does what), the family remained interdependent because these functions in total were needed to meet the goals of the family as a unit.

In addition, families are more emotionally interdependent with each other than they are with members outside the family unit (in the community). A family member can more easily take their hurts and anxieties to another family member, who will provide the necessary support and reassurance, than they can to a friend in the community.

The family's boundary serves as a filter for screening exchanges of elements, energy, and mass between the family and community and can expand or contract to increase or decrease this exchange. The family has various needs for energy and information exchanged with the community at different points during its life cycle (see negentropic section in this chapter), depending upon its location in the life cycle, its physical status, its preventive and curative resources, and so forth. For example, the family with preschool children may need exchanges with the well-child conference for preventive services, but it does not need exchanges with the school subsystem of the community. On the other hand, the family with school-age children needs the school exchange, but does not exchange with the well-child conference.

In addition, families at the same point in the family life cycle may vary in their exchanges or they may filter different exchanges, because of their attitudes, values, and purposes. For example, one family may readily admit the community health nurse to their home because they see a need for the service that is consistent with their goals, whereas another may not. Or a family may vary its feelings over time because of their changed perceptions or needs. For instance, as a community health nurse in California, I was denied access to the home of one prenatal mother in my case load (by the mother herself). Thus, no exchange between the family and myself as a part of the community subsystem of health took place. Because there was no interchange, it was unknown whether this contracting of the family's boundary was a result of attitudes, values, lack of time, or a lack of a perceived need for the exchange. However, after the child was born a defect was identified for which the family contacted me to discuss the Crippled Childrens' Program of the health department which provides corrective medical services for the child.

The screening of energy and information across the boundary of the family allows its members to maintain a degree of balance in terms of changing internal and external demands upon the system. Examples of expanding the boundary of a family include increased input from the legal system of the community when there are legal problems in the family, such as a pending divorce or adoption, or increased health services given to the family when there is an illness or an addition (new member) to the family structure. On the other hand, the family may contract its boundary.

Many of the expanding and contracting functions of the boundary of the family result from the family's perception of the exchanges and its particular short- or long-term goals. This, in turn, may be a result of family knowledge, attitudes, and values based upon experiences and the current situation of the family, but all are attempts by the family to maintain its homeodynamic balance by preventing overload or underload. However, these attempts may meet with failure in the long-range view.

STRUCTURE OF THE FAMILY

The family is made up of individual members who have their own distinctive biologic, psychological, social, and cultural needs and expectations. Members also have their own circadian patterns and needs for independence. However, these individual qualities are blurred as they merge with the family, which then takes on its own identity. Thus, although the family is made up of individual members, these members are interrelated and interdependent in a way similar to the organ subsystems of the individual as a system, and the family is the interacting unit.

Although all families are comprised of the individual members who are interrelated and interdependent, the structure can take various forms, which is consistent with the definition presented earlier. The most common structure of a family, the nuclear family, is composed of an adult male and female who are married with children. Many variations of this structure are possible. There is the family of two married adults without children, a remarried nuclear family, and the single-parent family. In addition, there are communal families, homosexual families, and couples living together but not married. In each of these structures there will be a division of labor and a sharing and caring relationship or an interdependence physically and emotionally to meet family needs.

Sussman in 1972, estimated the U. S. population to be composed of the following family types.[8]

FAMILY TYPE	PERCENT
Nuclear family	44
Married adults without children	15
Remarried adults (nuclear)	15
Single parent	13
Experimental family	8
Other traditional (3 generations)	5

Thus, he viewed about 79% of all families as being essentially nuclear. With further changes in cultural values, this percentage may be smaller as the number of experimental and nontraditional families (*e.g.*, unmarried adults sharing a residence) increases. These might include homosexual families, communal groups of individuals or couples living together, with or without sexual sharing, and male-female unmarried couples.

Most single-parent households are made up of a woman and her offspring. According to Burden, 90% of the single-parent households in the U. S. are headed by women, and over 9 million children under the age of 18 live in single-parent families.[10] Of these, 2.2 million children are under the age of 6 and constitute 10% of all children in the under-6 age category. Single-parent households are also high among low-income families. Forty-five percent of all children under the age of 6 from families in the poverty group live in single-parent households.

A particular family's structure may change over time because of factors such as the addition of children through adoption or birth, the loss of children through marriage or leaving for college, or through death or a long-term illness and the institutionalization of the sick member. As the structure of a family changes, the dynamics also change. A family may adapt easily or poorly to these changes.

Anderson and Carter identify four structural characteristics of families: organization, boundary, differentiation and specialization, and territoriality.[11]

Family **organization** is identified by a high degree of interrelatedness and interdependence. Its effectiveness is dependent upon the degree to which its goals are fulfilled—the goals of its members and of society. Securing and conserving energy from both internal and external sources through organization is necessary for the family to achieve these goals.

A second characteristic, **boundary,** from a structural point of view refers to the intense and frequent interactions among the components (*i.e.*, the members). "It is within the interactional boundaries of the family that the members participate in a particularly close network of feelings, both positive and negative, with a minimal sense of needing to put up a front."[12]

Another structural characteristic, according to Anderson and Carter, is **differentiation** and **specialization.** Differentiation and specialization are seen in the role allocations used to meet goals. One member may be the breadwinner, another may care for the house, prepare meals, wash clothing, and so forth. This concept is discussed in more depth later in this chapter.

The last characteristic of family structure is its **territoriality.** Members have a sense of place and belonging because of the closeness to other members. In addition, the family occupies a physical territory—the apartment or house at a certain place with a certain address.

Thus, another aspect of family structure is the roles and associated behaviors within a family that function interdependently to meet family goals. The roles and associated behaviors of members that function together are similar to the interrelated organ systems of individuals who are one step lower in the system's hierarchy.

PROCESSES IN FAMILIES

EXCHANGES WITH THE ENVIRONMENT

The family exchanges energy and information with its environment throughout its life cycle. Some of the exchanges between the family and the environment or community are the same as outlined in Chapter 2 and are not necessarily repeated here in that form. Other exchanges between the family and community follow.

Economic Subsystem. One exchange between the family and community is with the economic subsystem. One or more family members provide goods or services to the community (output) in exchange for money (input), which is then used to pay (output) for family needs to meet the family's goals of food, shelter, recreation, and health care (input) necessary to meet the self-regulatory processes of individual family members and the family as a unit. In addition, families pay taxes (output) that provide other services to the family (input), such as, mail delivery, garbage pickup, community health and social services, and public education.

Education Subsystem. The family also exchanges with the education subsystem of the community. Children attend the schools and learn ways of coping with the environment (input), and adults may attend college. For this input, families pay tuition to private institutions at the elementary and secondary school level or they pay taxes for public institutions at the elementary and secondary level of education. For adult education (input), they may also pay tuition at various rates at both public and private institutions (output).

In addition, there are many less formal exchanges between the family and the education subsystem of the community. The family pays taxes or a fee to support community nursing services (output) and, in return, receives education for health matters (input), as part of the nursing care, when needed. The family may also use the public library, neighbors, and other professional and nonprofessional sources for information. A simple diagram of these exchanges follows in Figure 3–1. (In reality these exchanges are much more elaborate.) In Figure 3–1, the individuals in the family system learn concepts and ways of coping with the environment (input) from teachers in schools, from neighbors and other informal contacts, from reading, from the mass media and from health care and other professional personnel, such as, lawyers, social service or recreational personnel, as appropriate to the particular family. Output from the family is in the form of work (job), school, community organizations, or with neighbors and other informal groups. Because the input varies from family to family depending upon their goals, the output will also vary. Thus, members of one family may obtain a medical education and provide output in the form of medical treatment in private practice, whereas members of another family may quit secondary school and provide output in the form of factory work. Likewise, the goals and skills (input) of members of one family may be more conducive to community organizational work, than those of another family. In return for this output, the members receive compensation in the form of money to meet basic physiologic needs and may or may not receive satisfaction and recognition from their job, which influences self-esteem. This feedback is fed into the system and influences further output.

Health Subsystem. At different times throughout the life span of the family there may be various exchanges with the health system. At the beginning of the family life cycle, the couple about to be married is required to have a blood test (input), for

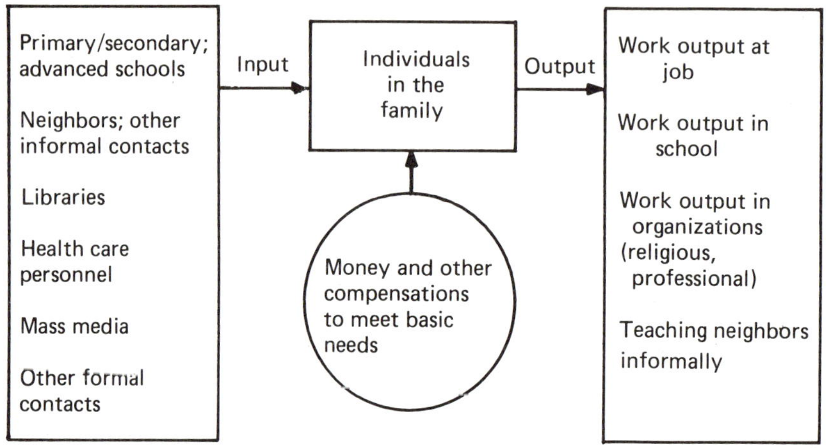

Figure 3–1
Family-educational subsystem exchanges.

which they pay a fee (output). When the couple moves into the childbearing years, they again interact with the health subsystem of the community for prenatal care, labor and delivery and newborn follow up (input), for which they pay a fee or taxes (output). Families may also receive community health nursing services (input) during this process. Throughout the rest of its life cycle the family may exchange with the health system for preventive services such as immunizations, health teaching, and supervision in various areas (care of the newborn, accident prevention, adequate diet, growth and development including anticipatory guidance, sex education, the effects of alcohol and tobacco, and so forth). They may also exchange with community health nurses when there is a need for casefinding and early health care (unsupervised prenatal mothers, abused children, a case of tuberculosis, venereal disease or other communicable diseases), or when there is a need for bedside care in the home. Home care is most likely to occur in the later years of the life cycle and may be provided by either the community health nurse from an official agency (tax supported) or from the voluntary nursing service (fee for services), or from a combined agency.

Other exchanges between the family and health subsystem of the community take place in the dentist's office for preventive or restorative dental care, in the doctor's office for preventive or curative care or in the pharmacy (prescribed drugs for an illness). It may also take place in surgical supply stores where special appliances are provided (leg braces, crutches). Many exchanges between family members and health subsystems also take place in schools, industrial, or other work organizations and hospitals.

Social-Service Subsystem. Families in a community may also exchange with the social-service subsystem, which was formerly known as the welfare subsystem. Some families continually exchange with this system because circumstances have prevented growth and development (negentropy) in the area of productivity, and these families remain chronically dependent. Or there may be an exchange with this subsystem because of an accident or disease process having long-term effects (entropy) on the breadwinner in the family with no one else to take over this role.

Some families exchange with this subsystem temporarily or periodically because of temporary illness or temporary unemployment of the family breadwinner. Since social-service programs are tax supported, taxes make up part of the family's output. During times of need, families may receive money, food stamps, and other necessary basic items (input) that, in turn, are paid out to other sybsystems of the community (output) to meet the families' basic needs and goals.

Sociocultural Subsystem. Families also exchange with the sociocultural subsystem of the community. Societal expectations of families influence and are influenced by family functioning through this exchange. Patterns of child-rearing, marital interaction, family-member functioning, and so forth are influenced by this exchange. For example, in the past most women in a family were cast in a homemaker role. This role has changed and many now work in the community. In addition, there were many rigid husband and wife roles as to who cooked, who cleaned, who provided the basic financial support, who nurtured, and so forth. Many of these rigidly defined roles are changing as a result of this two-way interaction.

Likewise, society is becoming more tolerant of new and emerging types of family structure as a result of this exchange. For example, so called nontraditional family types, such as, the communal family, homosexual family, or unmarried adults of opposite sex living together have emerged and in some cases are supported or maintained by changes in other subsystems, such as the legal system. Such societal changes, which allow families to change and grow as a result of this exchange, indicate negentropic processes at the community level.

Legal Subsystem. Families may also exchange with the legal subsystem at various points throughout their life cycle. An initial contact may be made for a marriage license in which a fee (output) is provided for this service (input). There may also be exchanges for birth certificates, divorces, wills, or legal problems involving other individuals or organizations.

Recreation Subsystem. The family has many exchanges with the recreation subsystem of the community. Its members may exchange money (output) for relaxation and entertainment (input) at the movies, theater, opera, ballet, symphony, at lectures, and so forth. Or they may enjoy a leisurely afternoon at the community park, playground, at bandstand performances, or at other planned social-recreational functions (input), which are tax supported (output).

Interrelated Exchanges. Although some of the family–community exchanges have been separated into economic, educational, and political categories, these exchanges in reality cannot be separated and there are considerable overlaps within categories. For example, the family does exchange with the economic or educational subsystem of the community but these may also serve as a social exchange, that is, work and school are sources of continuing contact with other humans, and friendships and social contacts may result from these exchanges. In addition, one may learn from these exchanges and, thus, education may become a part of the economic–social exchange.

These exchanges will vary throughout the family's life cycle depending upon their needs and goals, their knowledge, attitudes and skills, and their ability to apply resources. For instance, if a member of the family is ill at home and family members have the resources (physical, intellectual, psychological), they may not need to exchange with the health system. If another family has an ill member and has the physical and psychological resources to provide the care but lack the knowledge and skills, they may have limited contact with the health subsystem (community health nurse), which will provide the necessary education. Yet another family may lack the physical and psychological resources to care for the ill member and require skilled nursing care in the home or may need other community resources.

Or a family may have an ill member who is the breadwinner and they may use a different means to reach the goal (equifinality) of providing for food, shelter, and other basic necessities. Depending upon their decisions about reaching this goal, they may have various exchanges with the community. One family may have a member who has knowledge, skills, and attitudes that are in demand in the job market and decide to let this member take the place of the previous breadwinner. Thus, there will be no exchange with the social-service subsystem, but there will be an exchange with the economic subsystem. Another family may lack any members who have skills in demand by the job market and have to turn to social service for assistance. Thus, they do not exchange with the economic subsystem for work output, but receive money (input) from social services, which is paid out (output) to provide for the basic necessities (input).

In community health nursing we are always aware of the need for individuals and families to grow and to become increasingly more complex and organized (negentropy). Thus, community health nurses are always assisting families by teaching them new knowledge and skills and by fostering positive attitudes that help individuals remain independent or become more interdependent. For example, if there is an ill member in the family where there are other members who are capable of caring for the individual, nurses teach prevention of further illness, how to care for the ill member, explain community resources, and so forth, depending upon their assessment. This would assist the family in remaining as independent as possible. In the process, the family has learned new knowledge and skills and has hopefully developed positive attitudes that will benefit them in the future. Or, a nurse might support an individual family member's efforts to work part-time while receiving an education, rather than apply for social-service funds. This would decrease the individual's exchange with the social-service subsystem and increase exchange with the education and economic subsystems, which would help the individual to maintain a degree of independence and interdependence. At the same time, it would help the individual learn new knowledge and skills that would ensure interdependence.

Category of Exchanges. There are various ways to categorize these multiple exchanges between the family and community. One way that is useful to community health nurses involves using the concepts of health, autonomy, and resources.

In community health nursing we continually look at the exchanges between the family and community. From a health point of view, we can consider these exchanges in terms of health problems, autonomy, and resources. If there is an epidemic or harmful pollution in the larger community, families may be affected by this exchange and thus should be assisted in obtaining immunizations, information, and whatever other health-preventive measures are indicated. Likewise, if a communicable disease occurs in a family, we are concerned about the community, and in addition to helping families adjust their roles, to learn preventive measures, and so forth, we are also interested in casefinding among the other family members and in isolating other cases to protect the community.

Or, community health nurses may be interested in the family's diet (input) as it affects their health, for an inadequate diet may eventually lead to the need for free health care and this indirectly affects the tax structure of the community. Likewise, leaving garbage beside the house in uncovered containers (output), which attracts rats and affects the community (neighborhood), would be a concern for community health nursing.

Families have various resources (physical, intellectual, psychological, financial) that have developed over time. When families lack the resources to meet their needs and goals, they may turn to the community for these resources. For example, when a family needs financial assistance they may turn to social services or other financial assistance programs in the community. If health care is needed, they may turn to the health subsystem. As families grow (negentropy), the need for outside resources changes because of changes in internal resources. For example, when a second child is added to a family, the members usually have more knowledge and skills for dealing with the new member from interactions with the previous child.

An example of relating family resources to community resources is the family who lacks the physical and intellectual resources to care for a sick member. Here we would look to the community to provide care, and we would arrange for assistance through a program of care at home, in the hospital, or in a nursing home. If we think of resources in the broader sense to include the knowledge and skills of the family members, feelings, attitudes, and finances, then other examples will come to mind.

Likewise, community and family autonomy (see Philosophy, Chap. 5) are interrelated and the community health nurse continually relates one to the other in her assessment of the family. For example, if compulsory vaccination for all children is initiated on a community level, the family must give up their freedom of choice in this area for the self-preservation needs of the group. Thus, some families who have religious beliefs that are opposed to blood transfusions or immunizations must comply with this exchange with the health subsystem even though it may create a temporary imbalance because of the discrepancy between their religious beliefs (internal standard) and the behavior required by the health subsystem (see Feedback Concept in this chapter for the process for resolving this conflict in families). On the other hand, the community health nurse may assess the need for family planning in a particular family but, in this instance, can only point out the possible consequences of not practicing family planning to this family. The decision to use or not to use this resource is left to the family because their autonomy supersedes community autonomy, at this point in time. Currently we are seeing a loss of individual autonomy to the community because of the energy crisis. These relationships, or exchanges, may likewise move families toward or away from health.

In community health nursing, we continually view the exchanges between a family and community in an effort to move the family toward a higher level of health. The nursing process is a method for viewing and intervening in these processes, if needed.

Social Changes Influence Family Exchanges. Many of the exchanges between the family and the community have changed over time because of societal changes. Education, health, welfare, food processing, and many other tasks performed by the family when we were an agricultural nation have been taken over by the community. With increased specialization and the complexities of an industrial society, the individual members are exposed to many more stresses than were previously there. Thus, dependence on the family for affection, satisfaction of emotional needs, and the relief of pressure has increased.

Although fewer tasks are performed by the family, several authors have identified family functions at this point in our development as a nation. Sussman says the main tasks of the family are (1) the socialization of children, (2) to enhance the competencies of family members to cope with the demands of organizations in which they function, (3) to utilize organizations, (4) to provide an environment in which identities and affectional responses can develop, and (5) to create a mentally healing and satisfying environment intrinsic to the well-being of a family.[13]

Leitch says that the American family currently has seven functions including (1) mediation between the individual family members and society, (2) socialization of its members, (3) conferring status such as ethnicity and social class, which is the foundation of aspirations, traditions, rights, group identification, and educational possibility, (4) care and affection, (5) legality or providing a name for members and support and care, (6) reproduction, and (7) a sense of self-hood or belonging and separateness.[14]

Thus, although the family has given over many functions to society, which increases the exchanges with the community, the members maintain functions that bind the group together as a system. If families are to maintain themselves as families, they must meet some or all of these functions and the particular functions depend upon whether the family is a biologic traditional family or one of the emerging family structures identified earlier. Some functions such as care and affection, a sense of belonging, and a satisfying environment are necessary for all families, whereas, other functions pertain only to the traditionally defined family.

Families Obtain, Retain, Contain, and Dispose. Bredemeier's concept of systems adaptation says that systems need to obtain energy, information, and matter, to dispose of energy, information, and matter, and to contain or retain certain energies, information, and matter. This concept is useful in understanding families.[15]

Obtaining refers to the family's input and disposing refers to the family's output as discussed previously. For example, the family may require community health nursing services (input) when a member is sick for which a fee or taxes (output) are paid for this service. Or, family members may provide a service to the community in their jobs or positions (output) for which they receive money (input) to provide for other basic needs (input) that are consistent with their goals. Because of the process of retaining, containing, and transforming, the output from the family system varies from the input.

In addition, families contain certain energies, matter, or information in the environment so that unwanted exchanges cannot cross their boundaries. Much of the containment by families is a result of learned behaviors. For example, according to Koos' study a lower-class family often does not identify the physician as the appropriate resource for dealing with any type of illness, whereas, a middle- or upper-class family will use this resource.[16] Fifty-eight percent of the lower-class respondents in the study indicated they would use a chiropractor for any illness. Therefore, a lower-class family would be less likely to seek out health care from physicians or would contain this exchange outside their boundaries. Likewise, the family may not see immunizations and other preventive services as useful and would not see the need for this aspect of health services (containment). In this way, families may contain certain energies, information, and matter because they do not see their value in meeting goals or because they lack the knowledge of how they can be helpful. For instance, one family may not allow their daughter to bring boyfriends home (containment) because their goal is to remain a close-knit family with a rigid role structure (and behavior to the contrary would create tension and anxiety). This family, which fails to recognize the identities and needs of its members to grow, is moving toward entropy. Another family may deny entry to their home of the community health nurses (containment) because they do not see how they could be of assistance.

Families also retain certain energies, information, and matter from their exchanges with the community. Individual members of families retain from the chemical, physical, biologic, and psychosocial exchanges as discussed in Chapter 2. In addition, the individual members or the family itself retains from the exchanges made with the education, economic, recreation, and other community subsystems. (For example, some families may put money in the bank [retain] to meet a long-term goal of a trip to Europe or for retirement.) All families will retain some knowledge, attitudes, and skills from their interaction with many community subsystems. Families are more likely to retain information that will help them cope with their environment if it is presented in a way that is acceptable to them, has meaning for them, and can be related to their goals.

Obtaining, containing, retaining, and disposing are all processes that families use to help them maintain a degree of balance at any particular time and are based upon their learned behaviors and their particular goals at that time. Many of these behaviors can be compared with established standards to determine if the obtaining, retaining, disposing, and containing are merely meeting a temporary balance, which may be shattered later, or whether the behaviors are in accordance with established standards of family behavior.

COMMUNITY HEALTH NURSING AND FAMILY EXCHANGES

Community health nurses should assess family exchanges with the community and the family's adaptation to these exchanges, as a basis for interventions. Since the output from a system varies from the input, nurses should assess, where possible, both the input and the output, and the retention of input by the family. These exchanges can then be compared with established norms and the family's goals as a basis for planning and implementing a nursing care plan.

Economic Exchange. The nurse should assess the source and total amount of family income. In some families, one or more members may be employed, while in other families, the members may receive funds from social services, social security, or other public assistance programs. It is also important to assess how the family uses this money (output and retention). For instance, do they have a savings account? How much do they spend for housing? Are they interested in and eligible for low-cost housing? How much does the family spend for food? Do they buy in bulk or in small quanties? If the housing is poor because of economics, is it adequate for the safety and the privacy needs of the members? Are there ways in which the nurse can help the family reduce the potential of accidents? Can the home be rearranged to increase privacy for the members? Is this important to them? Also, do they have adequate storage space and refrigeration for food? Is the family's diet adequate in quality and quantity? What are the personal hygiene habits of the food handlers in the home? How much of the income is spent for furnishings and leisure materials such as books, magazines, television, radios, and toys for children? Are the furnishings adequate to meet the family's needs? Does the family have an automobile or do they use public transportation? If they use public transportation, is it accessible? These and other questions should be asked about the economic exchanges between the family and the community.

Education Exchange. Community health nurses should also assess the educational exchanges between the family and the community. What is the educational level of the parents in the family? Do they wish to obtain further education? Have they made any plans for this? Are the children enrolled in public or private schools? What are the aspirations of the parents for their children? Does the family have the educational level to stimulate small children intellectually? Would a Head Start program be appropriate? Does the family have the ability to understand the nurse's instructions about growth and development, community resources, prevention, and anticipatory guidance? Does the family accept the nurse as an educational resource? Where does the family usually turn when they need advice? Do they seek out professionals, neighbors, extended family or friends? What knowledge do they have about health, preventive services and community health nursing services? Do they have any misinformation in these areas? These and other areas of educational exchanges between the family and the community should be assessed, as a basis for planning interventions.

Health Exchange. The family also exchanges with the health subsystem of the community, which should be assessed. Is there a history of illnesses or defects among family members? Are any members currently on medications? Do they take these as prescribed? Do they obtain medications from physicians, or other health personnel, or are they self-prescribed? Do any of the medications counteract and nullify the effects of one another or produce toxic effects? Are the members aware of the symptoms of toxicity? What is their source of medical care? Do the children receive immunizations and other preventive health services? Do the adults have periodic health examinations? Are there accident potentials in the home? Are personal hygiene habits adequate to prevent contamination of food and air? Does the family obtain regular dental care? Do they see the need for prenatal supervision? Are the children well-cared-for physically and emotionally? These and other questions will provide community health nurses with information for the assessment of family health patterns and behaviors from which plans can be developed.

Legal Exchange. The nurse may also question whether or not there are any current exchanges with the legal system that may have an influence on the family's health. For example, has there recently been a death or divorce in the family? Are the members working through these potential crisis situations or are they using defense mechanisms such as denial? Do they have an adequate support system? Are they able to identify the problems creating the pain or are they engrossed in the pain alone to the point that they are unable to focus on the problem and look for way to resolve it? Do they know of community sources that can assist them, or is the nurse able to help them resolve the problem? If there has been a recent divorce in a family with children, what plans have been made for the children? These and other questions about the family's exchange with the legal subsystem of the community should be asked and assessed.

Recreation Exchange. The nurse should also assess the recreational and leisure-time activities of the family. Does the family do things together as a family or do the members each go their own way? Do most of the leisure activities take place at home or in the community? Are parks, playgrounds, and other recreational facilities accessible to the family? Do they have television and reading materials in the home? Do all the members take time for leisure activities and get adequate rest?

Other Exchanges. The exchanges for individuals identified in Chapter 2 also pertain to family members and should be assessed. The reader may review these exchanges in Chapter 2 or refer to the family assessment guide in Chapter 6.

Nursing Interventions. Although community health nurses may give physical care and emotional support to family members, many of their interventions involve working with the learned behaviors of families. If families are having difficulty maintaining their health status with their economic resources (input), nurses may help them budget their money, plan low-cost nutritional meals, locate free or part-pay medical, health, and preventive services, obtain food stamps, locate low-cost housing or whatever other plans will reduce the economic strain and meet the families' goals. Many of these interventions involve teaching about diet, community resources, and the need for health and preventive services and should be based upon the families' goals, their knowledge and their interests. In relation to the families' exchanges with the health subsystem of the community, nurses may also teach the signs and symptoms of illness, prevention, and the treatment of illness, ways to remember taking prescribed medications, sources of public or private medical health and dental care, personal hygiene measures, care of the sick, and ways to reduce accidents in the home, if appropriate.

INTERNAL PROCESSES

Subsystem Change. In the family, the interrelated parts function as a whole and because the parts are interrelated, a change in one part affects all other parts and therefore the whole. These changes can be the result of either internal or external factors.

Internally, the family needs organization to meet its needs and goals. To meet these, it places certain demands upon members and, in exchange, gives them specific privileges and freedoms. The demands and freedoms on members in a family are directed into roles that help the family maintain its functioning as a whole.

The pattern of behavior assigned to a family role must be complementary or fit with the other roles. Thus, it is meaningless to think of the mother-role without thinking of the child-role, or the husband-role without the wife-role. The behavior of all the family roles in total comprise family functioning the same as the behavior of all the subsystems of individuals comprise individual functioning. Roles are culturally determined and labeled, and are, thus, general as well as specifically developed in every family. Culturally, there are the general complementary roles of husband–wife, mother–father, parent–child, and sibling–sibling in nuclear families. Similar complementary roles are developed in nontraditional alterations of the nuclear-family structure, but they may be labeled in other ways. These general, culturally determined roles are present in families, although each family modifies them into its own unique forms. Each family will vary the patterns of behavior associated with the role at any point in time, and the behavior patterns may change over time because of internal and external forces. Behavior-pattern changes in one member will affect the other members.

The traditional wife–mother and husband–father role behaviors were identified earlier. Sociologists usually think of the male role in the family as being instrumental, whereas the female role is expressive. In addition, as children are added to the family and grow and develop, they are also assigned role behaviors that complement the parental roles. Thus, the roles of the family members comprise family functioning. As society changes, many of the traditional roles of family members are fusing and there are more overlaps (*e.g.*, it is more common now for both parents to work). In June, 1979, 47.6% of the wives in the U.S. were working and this group made up 4.9% of the labor force.[17] This is in contrast to 1967 when 37.9% of married females over 14 years of age worked and 1940 when 16.7% of this group worked.[18] With the increased numbers of wives in the work force, husbands may participate in more household functions. Whatever patterns of behavior are assigned to roles by the family, the roles in total should be inclusive enough to carry out the family's functions. However, earlier we discussed exchanges between the family and the community, and as an open system the family may turn to the community for assistance at times when they are unable to meet their own needs.

In addition to these culturally defined roles that families modify to meet their needs, each family develops an overlapping, separate, and specific set of unique roles that may be easy or difficult to spot and label. For example, one member of a family may become the family mediator, whereas another may become the troublemaker. There may be a family clown, a helpless one, a bright one, an independent one, a stupid one, and so forth. These various roles serve a useful purpose in the smooth functioning of the family group as perceived through the member's eyes (overtly or covertly), and members will fit into roles by acting as others expect that they should act. The concept of fitting into the expectations of others has been developed by Cooley and labeled "The Looking Glass Process".[19]

Internal changes affecting a part of the family system, which affects the total system, may include a change in the structure such as the introduction of a new member into the family or the death or movement of a member away from the family; a change in the physiologic condition of a member, such as, pregnancy, adolescence, or illness, which moves an individual from an independent to a dependent role, or a change in a member from movement to a higher level of growth and development (negentropy), which usually moves the individual to a more interdependent role.

When there is a change in the family, there is a need to reshuffle some of the role behaviors and the autonomy of the group. For example, if the breadwinner of the family becomes sick producing a gap in family income, another person must take over this function or perhaps the decision-making role to find another source of income. In addition, members may be called upon to care for the sick individual until recovery. If the mother, for example, takes over this role, the whole family will be affected. She will have less time to perform her usual role behaviors because of the additional role functions (*i.e.*, earning a living for the family and caring for the father). Perhaps, in addition, to less time to meet physical needs of family members, she is somewhat anxious about her new role behaviors and thus less able to meet the psychosocial needs of family members, or she may need to reallocate part of her role behaviors, such as, cooking, cleaning, and washing clothes to another family member. As indicated earlier, if families are unable to meet their needs and goals when change is initiated, they may turn to the community for assistance (family–community exchange). For example, the family might place the sick individual in the hospital where he would receive care, or they might employ part-time nursing care in the home. Or, they may need to turn to the community for financial assistance during this period. Whatever arrangement is made with the family for redistributing family resources, all members will be affected by the change. Community health nurses have an important role in helping families solve problems and identify solutions to the problems presented by the change.

Pregnancy presents an interesting internal change in the family. Findings by Caplan show that the metabolic changes in the woman lead to increased dependency needs psychologically.[20] Thus, she is not only less able to perform her physical functions late in pregnancy, but she has an increased need for psychological support throughout the pregnancy. This requires increased time and consideration for her needs on the part of other family members and will thus require a reshuffling of family roles and autonomy. If the family is unable to meet this need, the woman may turn to the community. However, this solution to the problem will also have ramifications for other family members.

Less obvious changes in a part of the system, which affects the whole system, result from the developmental changes of members of the family as a whole. For example, as the child moves from a completely dependent stage to beginning independence and interdependence (see negentropic process of individual, Chap. 2), the mother and others in the family must also change (stop doing so much for the child and find other things to do with the increased time) to accommodate the child's needs, if both members in the complementary role (mother–child) are to develop in a healthy fashion. Erikson has conceptualized these stages of individual development and they are mentioned in Chapter 2 and are discussed in Chapter 10.[21] Likewise, there is a need to change role behaviors as the family as a group develops. Duvall has identified the behaviors or tasks required by family members at each stage of development as they move from the beginning family, to the childbearing family, to a family with preschoolers, to a family with school-age children and teenagers, and to a contracting family in the middle and late years.[22] These stages of the family life cycle will be enlarged upon later in this chapter when we look at negentropic processes in the family.

ADAPTATION IN FAMILIES

When change occurs in a part of the family, the change will be counteracted by the other parts of the system in an attempt to maintain a homeodynamic balance. In other words, families tend toward a homeodynamic balance or equilibrium. It is characteristic of an open system to counteract disturbances and return to a previous state of balance. Although this is easier to see in an individual who is challenged by internal or external demands for change, the same process occurs in families.

The family will attempt to maintain its steady state or homeodynamic balance by overt and covert rules about family roles, which must be played according to these rules. Any individual deviating outside family norms for roles, causes conflict, and other members try to eliminate the conflict. For example, a son may be prohibited from behaving in a femalelike way, the family clown may not be allowed to show sadness, or the bright one may not be allowed to fail. It has even been found that once the sick role (mentally ill) has been established, the individual in this role is often prevented from getting well until the family as a group receives therapy and moves to another homeodynamic balance.

The amount of deviation permitted within a role and from role to role serves to delineate the homeostatic range that allows the family to maintain a homeodynamic balance, and this range will vary from family to family. For example, some families may tolerate a considerable amount of "bad" or rebellious behavior in their children. Beyond a certain point, they will step in to control this behavior through punishment, reward, and so forth. Other families may tolerate a greater or lesser degree of rebellious behavior. The range of behaviors with regard to any issue is its homeodynamic range.

This range has both advantages and disadvantages in the family. It has the advantage of providing a relatively stable environment for the family members and prevents the creation of a possible state of anarchy and chaos. This stable environment is important for the child's growth and education. On the other hand, it has the possible disadvantage, when the range is extremely constricted or narrow, of preventing the family from allowing each of its members the amount of freedom that is needed to develop in a particular way, and may lead to entropy.

One author, Wynne, has seen this as a major factor in causing schizophrenia, where the family is absorbed in fitting together at the expense of the differentiation of the identities of the persons in the relationships.[23] A balance of these factors of fitting together and personal identity seems necessary for healthy development.

The concept of steady state in a family also operates when there is a need to reshuffle roles and autonomy that is necessitated by a change, such as, a birth, a death, or an illness of a family member. Some families will adapt better than others to these changes because they have a greater range of tolerable behaviors—homeodynamic range—and resources (physical, mental, social) to take over and adjust in an emergency. In fact, some families reshuffle and take over vacated roles so well that there is actually a closing of the ranks. This closing of ranks has been found especially among families where a member has been hospitalized for mental illness, or has been drafted into the army and gone into combat zones. When the individual returns to the family, his role has been taken over by the others and there is no place for him. At the other extreme is the family that is thrown into a crisis by illness, death, or birth and is unable to reshuffle roles. Glasser and Glasser have discussed this phenomenon and it is discussed in Chapter 10.[24] Any of these extremes in roles may lead to entropic processes in a family.

Thus, there is a homeodynamic range that will help the family maintain a balance toward health when faced with internal or external changes. Beyond this range, in either direction (*i.e.*, too constricting or too loose), the family faced with change will not cope in a healthy way. This is similar to disease processes experienced by humans when they move outside the range of adaptability to other energies, which are discussed in Chapter 2. Under these circumstances outside resources such as the nurse may be indicated to help the family move back toward the desired range of behavior, which is necessary for the health of the total family.

In addition to the family's adaptation to its individual members (subordinate system), it must also adapt to the community (superordinate system). This adaptation is based upon the family's learned ways of maintaining balance, in view of the internal and external demands. If family members have limited education they may be forced into low-paying jobs and the family members adapt to the income in a way consistent with their goals and past learning. As a result, they may have an inadequate diet, unsafe housing, shabby furniture, and a lack of facilities for privacy. Their attempt to adapt to their income may maintain a precarious balance for them with health. Depending upon the time of entry into the family system by a community health nurse, the nurse's plans may involve preventing and/or working with disease processes. For further discussion of the process of health and levels of preventive interventions, see Chapter 9.

Exchanges with subsystems of the community may assist the family in maintaining its homeodynamic balance or in moving away from it. For example, a pregnant woman who has increased dependent psychological needs creates a change in the family system. If family members are unable to meet this need because of work and other pressures, this may upset the family balance, or the woman may meet this need by turning to the extended family, friends, and others in the larger community. Meeting this need, incidentally, is important for health reasons because it is believed that the mother who is unfulfilled in this need will be unable later to meet the needs of the newborn. Thus, if the community fulfills this need, we have an instance where community relationships have helped to maintain a family balance toward health. However, this pattern of meeting the mother's needs through community relationships will affect other family members (see parts affecting the whole in this chapter) by weakening the marriage ties and strengthening those beyond the family, by the mother's taking the children out of the home more often or, by her being away from the children more often. In the instance previously mentioned—that of community relationships affecting the family balance in a negative way—the husband may be under extreme pressure at work and, thus, because of his psychological reaction to the work situation he may be unable to relax at home. His way of dealing with this tension may be to use the defense mechanism of projection (ascribing repressed mental processes to the external world) and take out his frustrations on the family members. If this is a sudden change and the family does not understand the dynamics or lacks the psychological strength to cope with this behavior, it may create problems for the family. Or, the husband may become so engrossed in community relationships that he is rarely at home and upsets the other family members by his absence.

Just as there may be excesses or deprivations of individuals' needs within a family, which affects the whole family as a result of overly rigid or overly loose role structures, there may also be excesses and deprivations affecting family growth, resulting from exchanges with the community. If the family continues on welfare, its members will not adequately develop their own resources as individuals and as a family (entropy). Likewise, if the father spends most of his time at work, he is not likely to develop close relationships at home where children need a father and there should be a sharing of decision making and emotional support with the wife. Although families may adapt to these patterns through the process of feedback (to be presented later), all members may be affected by this established pattern at a later period. The children who lack a role model (unless there is a substitute role model from the community) may have difficulty establishing their sexual identity later in life. The wife may feel overly burdened and undersupported in home responsibilities. The husband at some point may feel left out and not a part of the family. Sheehy in *Passages* discusses this particular feeling which occurs in males in middle life.[25]

Other families may fail to grow adequately because of underutilization of community resources (exchange). For example, some families who lack financial resources to meet their basic needs may fail to use social services even when needed.

Thus excesses and deprivations of exchanges with the community may affect family development. Because there are numerous reasons for families to overuse or underuse community resources when a need exists, community health nurses should always determine the basis for the behavior observed, as a basis for interventions. One family who needs financial assistance may fail to use social services because they are unaware of it and another family may be too proud to use it. Therefore, before nurses can plan to initiate changes to assist family adaptation, they must identify the basis for the behavior observed (see Nursing Process, Chap. 6).

Although we have discussed the homeodynamic range of families and their attempt to maintain a steady state through rules about acceptable behavior with family roles, it seems important to reemphasize that, at any point in time, a family establishes a balance of relationships and behaviors within the family and outside the family to help maintain autonomy. This balance results from internal and external demands upon the family at that particular time and the experiences of the group (education, social-cultural, psychological development, etc.), which has given the family the resources to cope. These resources (knowledge, skills, attitudes, finances) will vary from family to family and, thus, attempts to maintain a balance in light of these pressures will vary. In some families, this balance will move the family toward a higher level of health and in others it will move them adversely down the health continuum. This balance includes, in addition to relationships, such behaviors as eating patterns, personal hygiene patterns, rest and relaxation patterns, use of community resources, and so forth, all of which may move them toward or away from health. These patterns of humans in relation to their environment are discussed in Chapters 1 and 2, which says that multiple factors in individuals and their environment may interact to make humans more susceptible and the environment, including the disease agent, more favorable for a forceful attack resulting in diseases in humans. We also said that we are interested in preventing disease processes before disease agents and humans are brought together, by interrupting processes that are ongoing. Thus, we are interested in assessing these multiple relationships and behaviors of the family and comparing them with established norms of the range of adaptability, as a basis for planning nursing care, which will move families toward health.

ENTROPY AND NEGENTROPY IN FAMILIES

ENTROPIC PROCESSES

In the family entropy is always present because the parts of the system (members) must continually adjust to the input of energy and there is energy lost in the process of transformation and subsequent feedback. However, this loss of energy and tendency toward equilibrium is not detrimental to the family with efficiently functioning parts because there is always enough energy to sustain the family beyond this disorganization to meet the needs of the system (adaptation) and to move it to a higher order and organization (negentropy). This is seen in families that move easily through the life cycle (to be discussed shortly) and in families that resolve crisis easily.

However, families that do not exchange freely among its members and between the family and the community exhibit entropic processes and are often labeled pathologic or dysfunctional. Some classification systems of family functions that could be considered entropic are presented later in this section, and additional family maneuvers that are entropic follow.

Scapegoating. Assigning blame to a person by another (scapegoating) is an entropic maneuver. The object of scapegoating is to release tension and to place it on another, usually a weaker individual, instead of resolving the problem in a healthy manner. Often the scapegoat in a family is a child who is relatively weak and who can be molded to fit the needs of the parents. For example, a father who performs poorly at work may displace his unhappiness (tension) on a child who is criticized for his school performance. At the same time, a wife who is unable to criticize her husband for his poor work performance may instead criticize her child. Multiple tensions resulting from inadequacies of various family members may be displaced upon the one member who assumes the role of the scapegoat. This process helps the family maintain its homeodynamic equilibrium, but in a precarious position.

Scapegoating may also occur in a strict and authoritarian family where each member wishes to rebel, but does not or cannot rebel for various reasons and, instead, places this frustration (tension) on one member who is labeled rebellious. This member is then locked into that role so that the others are not punished for their rebellious thoughts. If the member assuming this role in the family leaves, someone else will be put into the position to maintain the family balance.

A breakdown in this kind of family's defenses may result from the child becoming emotionally disturbed or from community pressure when the child exhibits this behavior in the community, such as, at school. Then outside assistance from the community may force the family as a group to look at their interrelatedness and to move toward a new homeodynamic balance.

The practice of scapegoating in a family is an entropic process because the family as a unit is not working efficiently; that is, there is not enough energy left over from the internal role transactions to allow the family to adequately grow into increasingly higher levels of order and organization. Individually, members who scapegoat are not learning ways of problem solving because they overuse the defenses of projection, denial, and displacement. In addition, by using these techniques they are not looking at their own underlying insecurities, such as poor job performance, and, therefore, they do not learn ways to increase their work performance. This has a never-ending effect on exchanges with the community. Without increasing the work performance (output), there is little increase in money (input) to meet the family's increasing material needs as the family evolves through time. Thus, the family's exchange with the community is at a standstill or it regresses, which hampers the family's movement forward. The child or weak member is also hampered developmentally, and since the family is interrelated with each part affecting all the others, this will affect the development and prevent the family's movement toward increased order and organization.

Doll's House Family. Langsley has identified the Doll's House Family as one in which the wife is a dependent, infantile personality.[26] This family is interlocked within their roles because the wife must continue to maintain the husband's self-esteem and borderline maturity. Increasing independence, or individuality, on her part threatens the husband's security. Thus, each partner is weak and the balance between them is precarious. A major conflict is generated by any significant departure from their expected roles.

Again, like Wynn's schizophrenic family, much energy is expended trying to maintain these roles at the expense of the individuality of the members. This entropic process may lead to psychologic disease for either member and for the family as a system.

Schizophrenic Families. Schizophrenic patients seem to come from homes in which there is inadequate family functioning and relationships. This has led many professionals in psychiatry to talk about the "identified patient" as merely a symptom of a sick family.

Lidz found that schizophrenic patients come from seriously disturbed families in which there was usually at least one schizophrenic or paranoid parent.[27] The other parent contributed to the disordered family by either accepting the unusual behavior or by withdrawing from the family. This left the child with a distorted image of family functions and relationships.

In schizophrenic families, spouses are unhappy, openly hostile to each other, and often compete for the loyalty of the children. This leaves the child confused about family relationships and loyalties. In many cases family roles become further distorted by forcing the child into a parent role to complement the role needs of a dependent parent.

Mothers of schizophrenic children have often been described as domineering, overprotective, and manipulative, whereas, the father has been described as weak, passive, and elusive. Interaction usually takes place between the mother and the child with the father remaining outside the interactional framework.

Maternal Deprivation. Bowlby has reviewed many of the studies on maternal deprivation.[28] In these families there is a lack of a consistent, appropriate, satisfying, and loving relationship with a mother or mother substitute during infancy, which leads to intellectual, emotional, and physical underdevelopment, or death of the child. If children survive, they are marked for life, so to speak. As they mature they are never able to form close emotional relationships with others. Most often in families where maternal deprivation occurs (when not a result of separation), the mother is an immature individual who has not had her own emotional needs met during her lifetime and, thus, is unable to meet the needs of the child. In addition, if the mother is emotionally insecure and self-centered, the husband must complement her role behaviors and, thus, spend a lot of time and energy reassuring the mother. In this family, the child is deprived of love (energy) and does not grow and develop adequately (entropy). The mother uses much energy trying to meet her emotional needs and the husband may use much of his energy trying to meet the immature needs of the wife. In many instances there may not be adequate energy for the family to grow and so the family remains at a steady state or fails to grow at all (entropy).

Low Self-Esteem Marital Partners. Satir discusses partners who marry to meet their self-esteem needs. Each one suffers from low self-esteem and relies on the other partner for complete fulfillment.[29] Because of their defenses and lack of open, honest communication, they do not perceive each other as they really are. After marriage their differences create anxiety and tension, so they complement each other by continuing to be someone other than who they really are. This creates a very precarious balance when faced with internal and external demands for change. When a child is added to the family they attempt to mold the child to meet their unfulfilled needs and may compete for the child's attention, casting the child into an abnormal role. Thus, the partners use energy to maintain their defenses, and the children use energy fitting into roles for which they are unprepared. Again, the family may maintain a steady state or it may move backwards (entropy).

Poverty. Because financial deprivation makes stability and growth somewhat precarious, **poverty** is an entropic process in the family. "Poverty is a relative term that reflects a judgment made on the basis of standards prevailing in the community."[30] As of 1975, an American family of four in an urban area was considered poor by government standards if the annual family income was $5050 or less. In 1974, there were 24.3 million persons in the United States living in homes where the annual income was below the federally defined low-income or poverty level.[31] Poverty in families has been labeled with various names in the literature ranging from multiproblem and hard-core families to disorganized or disadvantaged families. Such families also receive a higher proportion of community health nursing and other community service time (family–community exchange) because they have a higher proportion of chronic diseases, births, infant mortalities, and have poorer health standards and environments in which to live. They also may underutilize some necessary health services, such as, preventive services.

In poverty families there is a higher incidence of abandonment of wives and children, which reinforces the matriachal family and contributes to family disorganization. Children who lack an adequate father figure as a role model may develop weak egos and confusion about sexual identity. Because of limited resources (material goods) they may experience more rivalry and competition for what little is available to them and grow up to be impulsive, unable to defer gratification, and may have strong feelings of inferiority and helplessness.

Because of limited material comforts and time to meet more than the most basic of needs, poverty families experience deprivation and are unable to grow into increasingly complex individuals and families with the skills necessary to meet increased demands. Such families often perpetuate themselves from one generation to another.

NEGENTROPIC PROCESSES

When families are not exhibiting entropic processes or a temporary steady state they are evolving toward increased order and organization. Members periodically grow (as outlined in Chapter 2) and the family system is flexible enough to allow for and to adapt to this growth. At the same time these families have the energy to go through the increasingly complex tasks of the family life cycle.

Functional families as opposed to dysfunctional families are most able to meet the task required as they go through the life cycle. Functional families have limited fixed roles, which allow them to accommodate to internal and external demands for change and growth. These families have companionship but not to the exclusion of individual identities and differences. Members know the source of their pains and can recognize and communicate needs and feelings to each other. Members are allowed to handle their own problems, if able, and all learn to solve problems. Power is equally distributed and the family is open to new ideas about family policy and patterns that will facilitate change as needed. Some rules are fixed, but children are allowed the freedom to develop their own identities. Although children are nutured, independence and interdependence is fostered.

Some characteristics of these families that allow optimal growth (negentropy) of both children and adults include (1) fostering autonomy (2) demonstrating physical affection (3) limiting fixed rules and giving reasons for expected behavior (4) not blaming, criticizing, or discouraging (5) flexibility in different situations (6) not punishing physically or emotionally, and (7) not using power struggle, revenge, or conflict maneuvers.

Glasser and Glasser identify the following criteria of adequate family functioning. These criteria facilitate individual and family growth (negentropy) within the family unit. The criteria include the following:

1. Internal role consistency among family members.
2. Consistency of family roles and norms and actual role performance.
3. Compatibility of family roles and norms with community norms.
4. Meeting the psychological needs of family members.
5. The ability of the family group to respond to change.[32]

Family Life Cycle. The normal course of development for most families has been divided into stages. The transition from stage to stage in the life of the family is particularly stressful and threatening to the family's existence the same as the transition periods for individuals moving from stage to stage may be stressful (see Crises, Chap. 10).

The pattern of development of families is consistent and sets a standard for observing families encountered in community health nursing. For example, we might question whether or not a family is adequately meeting the developmental tasks for the particular stage they are in or whether they need assistance with the transition from one stage to another. The concept of resources presented earlier is useful here.

The family life cycle includes both the individual developmental changes of family members and the cyclic changes of the marital relationship. Various authors describe a variety of stages, ranging from four to twenty-four stages, that make up this cycle. One author uses four stages in the cycle consisting of the married couple, young children, children as adults, and the elderly couple. Another author uses five stages consisting of marriage, expulsion, dispersion, independence, retirement and death.

Duvall's eight stages of family development are most commonly used in nursing and are discussed here.[33] These stages include married couple, childbearing, preschool-age, school-age, teenage, launching center, middle-age parents, and aging family members. From our point of view completing the tasks of these stages in development leads to increased order and organization for most families and, thus, represents negentropy for them. Other families such as the communal family, the homosexual family, or the single-parent family requires modifications in the stages and tasks.

As a family moves from one stage to another, there is the potential for crisis as new adaptations to the new responsibilities are required. At the same time, there are new opportunities for growth. For example, the married couple must establish a mutually satisfying marriage, adjust to pregnancy and the promise of parenthood, and fit into the kinship network. Other critical periods and the adjustments necessary by the family are discussed in Chapter 10 in the section on crisis.

Tasks that traditional families as a group must master at each stage of development and establish and maintain include variations of the following:

1. An independent home
2. A mutually satisfactory system for getting and spending money
3. A mutually acceptable pattern of division of labor and accountability
4. Continuity of mutually satisfying sexual relations
5. A system of intellectual and emotional communication
6. A workable relationship with relatives
7. Ways of interacting with friends, associates, and community organizations
8. Competence in planning, bearing, and rearing children
9. A workable philosophy of life

Nontraditional families must also master several of these tasks. A communal family must often work with all the tasks, while the homosexual couple may work with all the tasks, except childbearing and rearing. In some instances, homosexual couples have been awarded child custody from the previous marriage of one of the partners and, thus, may need to develop competence in childrearing. Single parents with children must also fulfill the above tasks.

At each stage of family development these tasks change. For example, during the married-couple stage the family establishes an independent home. In the childbearing stage, they reorganize housing arrangements to provide for the small child. During the preschool phase, they supply adequate space, facilities, and equipment for the expanding family, and during the schoolage stage they provide for privacy, quiet, and order in the home. During the teenage stage, housing facilities are provided for widely different needs, whereas, during the launching stage they must meet the costs involved in helping children leave the home. During the middle years, the couple maintains a pleasant and comfortable home, and the home is again readjusted to the aging years.

In addition to the life cycle of families, which all families go through over time, Zimmerman says that over time families will go through cyclic changes because of changes in civilization.[34] His premise is that the family and society constantly interact and cause changes in each other. He identifies three main types of families. They are (1) the trustee (2) the domestic, and (3) the atomistic. In the trustee family, the welfare of the family is paramount and individuals do not have rights, but are family property. Members' welfare is always subordinate to the family group. In the domestic family, the individual's rights are recognized but the family unit remains strong. This is an intermediate family type in which the state (government or other legal body) creates the concept of individual rights to be maintained against family authority. In the atomistic family, individual rights are predominant with minimal family authority and frequent divorce. He believes this leads to hedonism, feminist movements, childlessness, delinquency and widespread adultery.

Zimmerman judges the present day American family to be in the atomistic phase. He predicts that when the atomistic-type family continues for a period, changes will come about to again reemphasize the trustee-type family.

CLASSIFICATION SYSTEMS USEFUL FOR ENTROPY–NEGENTROPY ASSESSMENT

Feldman and Schery have tried to identify families on a continuum that from our point of view range from families showing negentropy to entropy.[35] They classify families as adequate—chaotic, neurotic, and psychotic.

The adequate family has a history of good adaptation to ordinary problems of life. This family is identified by a community agency when confronted by an externally induced crisis (death of parent, acute illness). The family soon develops ways of coping with the stress and establishes a new steady state. This family usually experiences negentropy.

The chaotic family has many problems including a lack of clarity about role expectations, little sense of direction and family goals and is thus unpredictable and impulsive. From an entropic–negentropic point of view, this family loses much energy from the system and experiences many periods of entropy. With outside professional assistance, the family members can possibly increase their feelings of adequacy and experience increased negentropy.

The neurotic family is characterized by continuous anxiety that causes unhappiness and uneasiness. They often perform many tasks well but have great difficulty focusing upon one, in particular. This family can experience more negentropy than the chaotic family because a minimal number of functions are affected.

The psychotic family may have a psychotic member, may operate in bizarre ways or show evidence of psychotic symptoms in some respects, but not others. Since the family is interrelated, this family, too, is likely to experience more entropy than negentropy.

Voiland has also developed a classification system for families.[36] She identifies the perfectionistic family, the inadequate family, the egocentric family, and the unsocial family. Because all of these families are dysfunctional and use a lot of energy to maintain their defenses, they are characterized by a high degree of entropy.

The **perfectionistic family** is concerned with being faultless and does not express open friction. Self-analysis and criticism is characteristic of all its members and when an external event or stress affects the family, they view the family responses as a lack of measuring up to perfectionist standards and achievements. This leads to anxiety and uncertainty in the members.

The **inadequate family** has an overreliance on others outside the family for encouragement, directions, and support when faced with problems the average family could resolve itself.

The **egocentric family** is characterized by self-centered and opinionated parents and their narcissistic needs set the tone of the family. The problems of the children are either denied or each parent blames the other spouse.

The **unsocial family** remains aloof or does not exchange socially with the community. Usually more than one member is personally maladjusted and requires the attention of community, social, or legal institutions.

FEEDBACK IN FAMILIES

Self-regulatory processes in the family require that the family maintain a steady state (entropy–negentropy) at times, by the use of role behaviors and rules about these roles, so that it can continue to perform the functions of the family as a whole. However, these processes also require that the family be able to readjust its roles and role behaviors as the family as a whole (or its individual members) moves to a new stage of development (see Chap. 2) or as it is faced with other internal and external changes, such as, a change in its structure through additions or losses (discussed earlier), or through the loss of a job (external). Buckley postulates that families as any social system must be capable of changing their basic structure, organization, and values in order to remain viable.[37] Hill says that these changes may "take the form of changes in inter-component relations (greater autonomy and decreased constraint); qualitative changes in the nature of relationships (such as between a sexually maturing son and his mother), changes of governing values, purposes, and standards; basic changes in internal and external input operations (as in the increased earning power of the adolescent); and the ascendance of components or subsystems with new and different properties in the governance or management of the system (such as may occur in family governance when adolescents graduate into young adulthood while still living at home)."[38]

Thus, the family system must be capable of maintaining a steady state at times and changing to new steady states at other times. The process whereby families maintain a steady state has been discussed earlier and the process whereby it moves to new steady states follows.

Duvall says that families who are best able to withstand stress and maintain a homeodynamic balance are able to (1) approach problems in a unified manner as a family (2) have a nonmaterialistic orientation (3) share tasks frequently between husband and wife (4) perceive the nature of the problem adequately (5) have a democratic orientation with diffusion of leadership regarding problem-solving tasks.[39]

At any point in time the family demonstrates patterned role behaviors, which have been learned and adapted to in order to meet its goals. When the family is faced with internal pressure for change (transition to new stage for members or family as a group) or any external pressures (loss of job, illness), the family experiences tension and conflict that must be reduced. Said another way, the family sees a mismatch between its output (what the role behaviors are) and the internal standards and values in relation to the need for change.

The family will go through various maneuvers and try out various role behaviors, in an attempt to obtain a fit between the output and the internal values, to relieve the tension and conflict.

Coercing is the most universally used maneuver and involves the manipulating of present and future punishments. This may be in the form of overt attack or threat of attack in the future and varies in intensity from mild manipulation to physical torture. If successful, the conflict is resolved through submission, although individuals may neutralize the effect of coercion by defying.

A second maneuver is **coaxing** whereby there is a manipulation of present and future rewards. In this maneuver there may be asking, pleading, promising, begging, and tempting, and if the members succeed, it is to gain present or future rewards. This technique can be neutralized by refusing or withholding.

Evaluating usually follows coaxing and coercion and may be a counterattack. In this maneuver, behaviors are identified and categorized in a value context by praising, blaming, shaming, approving, or disapproving. Value judgements such as fool, mama's boy, sissy, and so forth, may be used.

Mashing, another maneuver, is more indirect than any of the above because correct information is withheld, or incorrect information pertinent to the settlement of the conflict is withheld. This may involve pretending, censoring, evading, lying, and distorting.

Another maneuver is **postponing** with the expectation that others will change their minds in the interval by "sleeping on it." Another technique is **role reversal** whereby individuals put themselves in the role of others.

Any of the above maneuvers are unilateral decisions in which some give in or submit to others. Consequently, there is a unilateral decision or accomodation to another with role changes.

Change can also be initiated in the family by *de facto* decision making where agreement is made in the absence of dissent, rather than active decision making. Some members may not accept but will go along with the decision.

It is usually best when role changes are indicated for all family members to explore together ways to solve the problem. In this maneuver, agreement is reached and all decisions from the group are given equal assent and all feel equally committed without reservation or resentment. A compromise in which there is a change for all parties is usually the outcome. Following the compromise, the family members are able to adjust and to work through the new roles, to internalize them, and to learn how to reward others in the family in their new roles.

Following the above maneuvers or attempts to retain or change role behaviors, the family either maintains its steady state or moves to a new one in which all are affected. For example, if a child becomes more independent as a result of growth, the mother must change her behavior to provide less physical care, but she may need to give more emotional support. In her additional time, she may take over other role behaviors or she may get more involved in the community. She may also need additional support from the husband or other family members.

Obviously the family's decisions to maintain or move to a new steady state moves them toward or away from a healthy balance. If the family decides to maintain a steady state when members need more freedom to grow, the family members will be stifled in their development (negentropy) or they may upset other members if they refuse to remain in a fixed position. Thus, as indicated earlier the families who are most adaptable to change (not overly rigid or loosely structured) provide the most healthy and viable family for all members and the community.

As a result of the nursing assessment, community health nurses may at times need to help families resolve role conflict when change is indicated in the family system. The process of confrontation, resolving role ambiguity and role conflict, is discussed in Chapter 8 for use by teams, which may be useful for families seen by the nurse.

COMMUNITY HEALTH NURSING AND FAMILIES

Community health nurses must view the family as a totality that is made up of individual members (subordinate system) who interact with the community (superordinate system). Nurses must observe the exchanges of individual members (food, oxygen, love, and so forth) with others and the environment and compare with established norms to determine if there are actual or potential health problems. The nurse must also assess each individual member for actual or potential health problems. Many of the guides available are useful during this process, such as, the Denver Developmental Screening Test, Erikson's guidelines for psychosexual development, and so forth. The nurse should also determine the basis for the observed behavior so that the best support can be given the family members to maintain or change the observed behavior. (See Chap. 6 on the nursing process for a discussion of this concept.)

The nurse looks at the family as a unit and determines if it is at an appropriate level for family developmental tasks and if the members are coping adequately with their actual or potential health problems. This assessment forms the basis for assisting the family in maintaining or changing their health-related behaviors, which is discussed further in Chapter 6.

The nurse also looks at the exchanges between the family and the community and the family's adaptation to these changes. From this assessment it is determined whether the adaptation is producing a precarious or a long-term balance regarding health and how interventions can improve the family's balance toward health. Concepts of health, autonomy, and resources presented earlier are useful in looking at family and community relationships. Thus, this view of the family allows nurses to use nursing processes with families to help them maintain or regain health.

Because the community is a superordinate system of the family, and the family is a subordinate system of the community whereby each influences the other, nurses must maintain a two-way focus while working with families. Nurses must look at the family as it influences community health, and at the same time look at the community as it influences family health. Likewise, a two-way focus should be maintained between the individual members of the family and the family as a unit because each influences the health of the other. Thus, a family member with a communicable disease should be isolated from other family members to protect the family's health; also, a sick family should be isolated from the community. On the other hand, the family should also be protected from illnesses in the community that are communicable, and individuals in a family may need to be protected from abusive or mentally ill individuals in the community or family.

REFERENCES

1. Benson R, McDevitt J: Community Health and Nursing Practice, p 229. Englewood Cliffs, Prentice-Hall, 1976
2. Freeman R: Community Health Nursing Practice, p 109. Philadelphia, W B Saunders, 1970
3. Murray R, Zentner J: Nursing Concepts for Health Promotion, p 347. Englewood Cliffs, Prentice-Hall, 1975
4. Sussman MB: Family systems in the 1970's: Analysis, policies and programs. In Hymovich, Barnard M (eds): Family Health Care, pp 18–37. New York, McGraw-Hill, 1973
5. Rae S: The family as a system: A network of relationships. J Psychiatr Nurs and Mental Health Services XII, No. 2: 17, 1974
6. Leininger M: Nursing in the context of social and cultural systems. In Mitchell P (ed): Concepts Basic to Nursing, p 35. New York, McGraw-Hill, 1973
7. Koos E: The Health of Regionville. New York, Columbia University, 1954
8. Hill A, Helvie C: Community Health Nursing Course Outline, The University of California, School of Nursing, 1964 (unpublished)
9. Sussman MB: Nontraditional Family Forms in the 1970's. Minneapolis, National Council on Family Relations, 1972
10. Burden S, et al: The Single Parent Family. Proceedings of the Changing Family Conference. Iowa City, University of Iowa Press, 1976
11. Anderson R, Carter I: Human Behavior in the Social Environment, pp 106–110. Chicago, Aldine, 1974
12. Ibid
13. Sussman MB: Family systems in the 1970's: Analysis, policies and programs. In Hymovich, Barnard M (eds): Family Health Care, p 25. New York, McGraw-Hill, 1973
14. Leitch C, Tinker RV: Primary Care, p 5. Philadelphia, F A Davis, 1978
15. Bredemeier HC: Social systems integration and adaptation. (unpublished) Cited by Shirley A. Smoyak: Toward understanding nursing situations: A transactional paradigm. Nurs Res 18:407, Sept–Oct 1969
16. Koos E, op cit
17. U.S. Department of Labor: Employment and Earnings. Vol. 26, No. 7. July 1979
18. U.S. Bureau of Cẽnsus. Statistical Abstracts, Table 321. Washington, DC, 1968
19. Cooley CH: Human Nature and Social Orders, pp 152–153. New York, Charles Schribner's, 1902
20. Caplan G: Principles of Preventive Psychiatry. New York, Basic Books, 1964
21. Erikson E: Identity and the Life Cycle. Psychological Issue Monograph, 1, 1959
22. Duvall E: Marriage and Family Development. Philadelphia, JB Lippincott, 1977
23. Hirsch S, Leff J: Abnormalities in Parents of Schizophrenics, p 20. London, Oxford University, 1975
24. Glasser P, Glasser L: Families in Crisis, pp 3–12. New York, Harper & Row, 1970
25. Sheehy Gail: Passages: Predictable Crises of Adult Life. New York, EP Dutton, 1976
26. Langley D, Kaplan D: The Treatment of Families in Crisis. New York, Grune & Stratton, 1968
27. Hirsch S, Leff J, op cit, pp 16–18
28. Bowlby J: Maternal Care and Mental Health and Deprivation of Maternal Care. New York, Schocken, 1967
29. Satir V: Conjoint Family Therapy: A Guide to Theory and Technique. New York, Science and Behavior Books, 1967

30. Kosa J: The nature of poverty. In Kosa J, et al (eds): Poverty and Health. A Sociological Analysis, p 2. Cambridge, Harvard University, 1969
31. U.S. Department of Health, Education, and Welfare. The Measurement of Poverty. Washington, DC, Government Printing Office, 1976
32. Glasser P, Glasser L: Families in Crisis, p 291. New York, Harper & Row, 1970
33. Duvall E, op cit
34. Leslie GR: The Family in Social Context. New York, Oxford University, 1973
35. Feldman F, Scherz FH: Family Social Welfare, pp 47–51. New York, Atherton, 1967
36. Voiland A, et al: Family Casework Diagnosis, pp 115–289. New York, Columbia University, 1962
37. Buckley W: Sociology and Modern Systems Theory. Englewood Cliffs, Prentice-Hall, 1967
38. Hill R: Modern Systems Theory and the Family: A Confrontation. Social Science Information, pp 7–26. International Social Science Council, Oct, 1971 Reprinted with permission.
39. Duvall E: Family Dynamics. Philadelphia, JB Lippincott, 1971

4

The Community as a System

The community is a major focus of community health nursing activities. The emphasis is upon reducing mental, physical, and social disease among community populations. At the administrative level, continuing community assessment of health needs, and the availability and adequacy of health services to meet these changing needs provides the basis for establishing health priorities. Community health nursing practice is influenced by these health priorities. Although nurses may work in small areas of the community, as a basis for their practice, they must always be aware of the ways in which family and group health interrelate and influence community health. Community priorities influence nursing practice through policies that administratively determine the groups or categories of families to be sought out in the community (casefinding by the nurse and others) and to determine to whom nursing care is delivered. Benson and McDevitt say that the patient in public health is not just a person, or even a few families, it is the community.[1] Commenting on the community health agency's role they say that the public health agency examines the result of organized community effort for the community health. Its role in this effort varies: it may carry out direct services, or, as is more frequent, it may act indirectly as coordinator, potentiator, or change agent.

Because the community is one focus for nursing process in community health nursing, a concept of community is important. Definitions of community and the theory of the community as a system follows.

DEFINITIONS OF COMMUNITY

Several ways of viewing the community have been offered in the literature. Peal defines a **population** as "a group of living individuals set in a frame that is limited and defined in respect to both time and space."[2] Although Pearl refers to population, this definition is equally applicable to a community. In this definition, space may refer to a political or geographical boundary, and time may refer to a specific point in time or an interval of time. Within these limits of time and space, health problems can be enumerated, health services provided, and health laws enforced. This boundary defines the opportunities for taxation to support health services and the group of people who must be represented in decisions involving both continuation of health

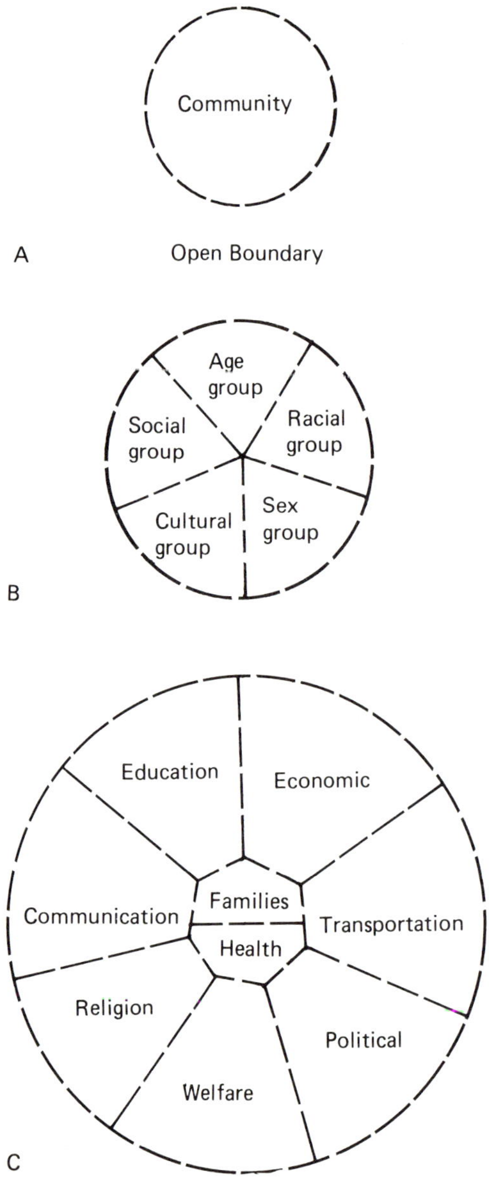

Figure 4–1
Community diagrams. **(A)** Geographical, political area. **(B)** Demographic approach. **(C)** Social systems approach.

laws and services and proposals for new ones. The time and space aspect of the definition, coupled with statistical concepts, allows community-wide evaluations of changes in population structure, morbidity, and mortality rates, and other health-incident and prevalance rates between two points in time related both to populations and their environment. Although this definition provides a framework for viewing health problems within a specific area, the community is an open system and will be influenced by events outside the area.

This definition of the community may be utilized by community nursing to plan and evaluate total community services in smaller units of the community. Nursing services are potentially available to all people within the community. However, the usual pattern is for a staff nurse to focus on high-risk groups in a subdivision perhaps as small as a census tract in a densely populated urban area, or as large as a county in a sparsely populated rural area.

A second closely related method of viewing the community is to consider it as a collection of actors. The emphasis here is upon descriptive categories of people such as preschool children, senior citizens, Mexican–American residents, social-class groups, and so forth. This demographic approach is useful for planning services and for carrying out epidemiologic studies. Categorization of the population by age, race, sex, social class, and other demographic variables shows unequal distributions of diseases and health conditions among the population and shows where services need to be provided to high-risk groups. For example, Taylor, using the demographic approach to the community as opposed to the individual approach of the private practitioner, says, "A woman is either pregnant or not pregnant; a community is about 3 percent pregnant. A patient has or does not have heart disease; the community always has heart disease, though the rate may go up or down."[3] Thus birth rates, morbidity, mortality, and other rates categorized by subpopulations of the community at risk are important for planning and evaluating services. See Figure 4–1 for a diagram of ways of viewing the community.

Categorization of subpopulations may also provide clues to causal factors when the specific attributes of these groups are examined. For example, at one point in history, large numbers of young children in certain areas of the community were admitted to hospitals for lead poisoning. Concentrations in city hospitals where financial eligibility established lead-poisoning victims as coming from lower-class social groups led to investigations of the behavior and environment of this group of children. It was found that lead used in the paint for the interior of these dwellings was being ingested by the children who were at an age when everything went into their mouthes.

Although these definitions of community contribute to our understanding, an emphasis upon the place or demographic characteristics, as a basis for health planning, does not ensure improved community health. First, the preceding ways of conceptualizing the community do not consider the people who are assisted with services. Hanlon points out that there is an increased need for voluntary public participation in health programs if we are to be successful, and that there are many sociocultural forces that affect the utilization of health resources.[4] It follows from his findings that planned health services must be acceptable to the people for whom they are intended, and that health personnel must explore group attitudes, values, and beliefs before providing services. If the health problems of a group pose a major threat to the community, however, understanding is not enough. Health personnel may need to function as change agents to align attitudes, values, and beliefs with community values for the benefit of all. Another alternative in this instance might be to impose new health laws, but this method has not been very effective.

Previously identified ways of conceptualizing the community have also been deficient in their lack of dynamics for viewing evolving community health resources to meet the growing health needs of humans from changing relationships with the environment. These dynamics in addition to ways of viewing changing population structures, health problems, and so forth are important in a concept of the community. Concepts of the community from a systems point of view fills this gap.

From this perspective, the **community** is defined as an arena of interaction, with individuals, groups, and institutions participating in an ongoing performance. Definitions consistent with this view have been presented by Tinkham and Voorhies and Klein.[5,6] Tinkham defines community as "a social system . . . where people band together for their mutual protection and common good," and Klein defines community as "patterned interaction within a domain of individuals seeking to achieve security and physical safety, to derive support at times of stress, and to gain selfhood and significance throughout life."

Both of these definitions imply interaction within a community to meet individual needs and because humans collectively evolve and their environment is continually evolving and changing, and because society is becoming so specialized in knowledge, skills, and functions, any theory of community based upon these definitions must be dynamic and allow for interrelated services such as education, health, welfare, and protection. Systems theory which is presented in Chapter 1 can also be applied to a community and shows this dynamic interaction.

We have viewed community in terms of a place, a collection of people, and as a social system, and each of these views is relevant to community health nursing. Likewise, each of these concepts will fit within a systems-theory framework. Community health patterns and resources are continually evolving, and viewing the community as a closed system with a boundary (geographical or political), at any point in time, allows the nurse to evaluate actual or potential health hazards. This may involve enumeration of factors such as age distribution, morbidity and mortality rates, group health behavior or the number of people exposed to questionable environments. These data may serve as a guide for planning services and may give an indication of the population balance toward or away from health. The demographic approach looks at subgroups of the population, subsystems of the community, and the changing effects of these subsystems on the total community. Because the community is continually evolving it is also important to view the community as an interrelated system (family, health, welfare, economic) in which change in one will affect the others, and change in a subsystem will affect the total system. In addition, because the community is an open system, change may be affected by forces or systems outside the community. Changes in systems either in or out of the community may tip the balance of health in favor of humans, or changes may put humans in a less favorable position. For example, a strike in a community (economic) may create a state of disequilibrium and affect human health (groups of families) if this change is not counterbalanced by other systems (welfare, health), either locally or from outside sources; this is another way of saying that changes in systems (health, education, welfare, and so on) affect the health of families (another part of the system). These dynamics refer to the social systems approach to the community and are discussed in greater depth when we look at the community as a system.

COMMUNITY DEFINED FOR COMMUNITY HEALTH NURSING

Again refering to our definition of a system in Chapter 1, and considering some definitions of community presented earlier in this chapter, we can define a **community** as a whole that is made up of interrelated parts, which functions as a whole as it continues to exchange with the larger system. The whole of the community is defined in relation to geographical or political boundaries and can be a census tract within a community, the whole community, or an institution, such as, a school or industrial organization, depending upon the focus at the time for the particular nurse. The interrelated parts are the communities' subsystems, such as, education, welfare, health, and families. Because groups of families, which make up the community population, are one of the subsystems of the community that is both influenced by and influences the community, we focus on this group in providing nursing services. However, because within the total group there are varying socialcultural backgrounds, age groups, values and beliefs, our demographic approach is important in looking at this subsystem to identify groups for priority of services. Other aspects of the definition such as interrelated parts functioning as a whole and the whole exchanging with the larger system are incorporated into systems theory and will be clearer as we now look at the community as a system.

THE COMMUNITY'S PLACE IN THE HIERARCHY

Because community health nurses look not only at a particular system but also at the subordinate and superordinate systems, these will be identified for the community. The **subordinate system** of the community is defined as the interrelated parts that make up the system, such as, health, education, welfare, recreation, and families. Many of these subsystems are used as resources for families with whom we work and are discussed in relation to families in Chapter 3.

The **superordinate system** of the community is defined as the state and nation that exchanges with the community and affects the health, autonomy, and resources of families or the community population. For example, if there is a communicable disease in an adjoining community, this may spread to the disease-free community if not counteracted by immunizations and other health measures. In addition, nurses may attend state and national meetings and read national nursing and health journals to further their knowledge about communicable diseases. They are also licensed by state organizations and must meet minimal standards of care. These factors from outside the boundary of a community influence the quality of care provided. Other examples will be elaborated upon when we look at these exchanges later in this chapter.

BOUNDARY OF THE COMMUNITY

Although the community is an open system exchanging with the state and nation, it has a boundary and can be distinguished from its environment because of the greater concentration of energy within the system than immediately around it. The boundary of a community, like the family, may be more difficult to grasp than the boundary of individuals. However, there is greater interaction and interdependence within the community than between the community and other communities outside the boundary. The boundary of a community can vary depending upon the nurse's focus, for we indicated in our definition of the community that the nurse may focus on a school, on a census tract, or on the whole community. There will be greater interaction and interdependence in the smaller units than the larger units as each unit becomes more loosely joined. For example, there will be more interaction and interdependence in a small school than in a census tract or neighborhood, and more interaction and interdependence in a neighborhood or census tract than in a total community. However, the concepts of the dynamics of systems remain the same and can be applied to any nursing focus. The focus of this chapter will be on the community as a whole. Nursing in other communities such as a school or an industrial plant will be discussed in Chapter 6.

CITY VERSUS RURAL BOUNDARY

The **standard metropolitan statistical area (SMSA),** designated as a city, is a county or group of contiguous counties containing at least one city of 50,000 people or more. In 1978 the Census Bureau estiamted that there were 281 SMSAs in the United States. From the known census statistics in 1970, there were 228 SMSAs. Sixty-nine percent of the population in the United States lived within a SMSA. Of this 69%, 37.6% lived outside a central city and 31.4% lived within the city. On the other hand, 31% of the U.S. population lived in areas that could be designated as rural.

EXPANDING-CONTRACTING BOUNDARIES

Like the family, the community expands and contracts its boundary at times to meet the changing needs of its population during its life cycle. This is necessary to maintain its self-regulatory processes. For example, over time, a community may move from a young population with many children to an aged population with a lack of facilities to provide preventive and curative services for this population. If the community also lacks the manpower and financial resources to provide such facilities it may expand its boundary to recruit new professionals or it may obtain resources from the state and federal government. A comparable situation also exists when a strike in a community puts many individuals out of work and the various subsystems (welfare, health, education) are unable to counteract the effects of the strike (by meeting the economic, health, and educational needs of this segment of the population). Again, the community could expand its boundary and turn to the state or national government for assistance in maintaining its population.

STRUCTURE OF THE COMMUNITY

Just as the family system begins with two or more people (*e.g.*, a married couple, a communal group, or two homosexuals joining together), the community also begins when a group of families locate in a specific area at a specific time having decided that it is more economical to pool resources and divide labor tasks. As the community grows in population (families) and the group identifies the need for further assistance from outside the family, there will be increased specialization, and a variety of subsystems such as education, welfare, recreation, and health will evolve.

NEIGHBORHOODS

The community population (family subsystem) may be composed of several neighborhoods or census tracts. Each neighborhood may have its own social-class values, beliefs, cultural heritage, and health problems (demographic), but it interacts with other neighborhoods that make up the community. Neighborhoods may vary in size from small to large groups of families that have similar characteristics.

Neighborhoods may be old, well-established areas with a sense of unity and rapport, or they may be relatively new with a transient population and with little sense of unity and rapport. Nurses should be aware of the history of their particular community as a basis for determining if there are leaders and other resources that can be quickly mobilized to assist with health problems or whether the area is new and unsettled.

SUBSYSTEMS OF THE COMMUNITY

Currently, the interrelated parts of the community, which make up the whole community structure, encompass the following subsystems: family, economic, political, religion, education, health, welfare, communication, and transportation. Sanders uses only 5 subsystems of a community: family, economy, government, religion, and education.[7] However, he has several subcategories, for example, transportation, banking, agriculture, industry, commerce, medicine, and organized labor are under economy. Since health, welfare, and transportation are important components of community health nursing, it seems beneficial to look at these as separate subsystems. However, banking, agriculture, industry, commerce, and organized labor can more easily be subsumed under the community subsystem of economy.

The structure of the community also includes the roles or structured patterns of behavior within and between the subsystems, which are relatively stable aspects of the subsystems. Although these roles may be vacated and refilled by different people over time, those filling these roles have been socialized into them through special educational programs and, thus, the roles remain relatively stable. For example, a staff community health nurse has special roles within the staff-nurse subsystem and between this subsystem and the other subsystems of the community. Within the subsystem, the nurse is responsible to a supervisor for knowing and adequately providing nursing care to assigned families. This includes knowing their health needs, developing plans to meet these needs, knowing community resources, setting priorities, having a knowledge of health and illness, and a knowledge of the principles and skills in providing nursing care. In addition, the staff-nurse role involves meeting with the supervisor periodically, following up on suggestions offered, and participating in other staff activities assigned, such as, immunization or well-child conferences.

Between the nurse's subsystem (health) and the subsystem of the family, the role also involves assessing, planning, implementing, and evaluating nursing care. Concurrent with this process, the nurse relates and communicates with families and groups. Underlying this role is the knowledge, skills, and attitudes developed as part of the nurse's education program and experiences since graduation.

Within patterned role behaviors there are also established methods of communicating, decision making, lines of authority and other processes that facilitate community functioning. Some role behaviors include a decision-making component that influences several people, whereas others influence a few. For example, supervisors or directors often have sanction to make decisions influencing many staff nurses, whereas staff nurses usually lack this sanction. Likewise, supervisors and directors usually have more authority than staff nurses. Individuals occupying various roles know the extent of their authority, their decision-making potential, and the channels of communication. They also know the influence of those above and below them in the organizational hierarchy. These aspects of role behavior influence relationships within and between community organizations.

Figure 4–2
Health subsystem of the community.

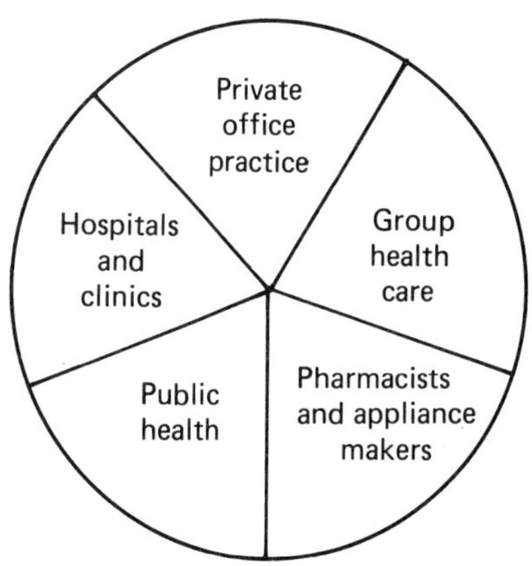

Health Subsystem Structure. Sanders has identified 5 types of health structure or subsystems of the health subsystem of the community.[8] These are pictured in Figure 4–2. They are closely related but distinct enough to be analyzed separately and include the following:

1. Private office practice of health personnel
2. Group health care such as schools and industry
3. The world of hospitals and clinics
4. Public health
5. Pharmacists and others who sell materials and appliances required by humans

Sanders says that the structure of each differs because the group situation varies. For example, the physician would not diagnose in the drug store, nor would a surgeon perform surgery in the Public Health Director's office.

Sanders also says that the health subsystem of the community and all subsystems of the health subsystem have identifiable characteristics that are the following:

- A structure or related series of agencies, organizations, or establishments
- A set of functions—patent and manifest
- People who are responsible for promoting the interest of the system or major part of it
- Ideology or rationale which provides the justification for the continuation of the system
- Necessary equipment and material resources to carry out the expected activity
- Links with other systems within and outside the community

PROCESS IN THE COMMUNITY

FUNCTIONS

The outcome of all processes (internal and external exchanges) in a community are to provide certain things for the population. Warren says the community has the following functions:[9]

- *Production–distribution–consumption.* This includes the service activities of the subsystems such as industry, business, religion, education, government.
- *Socialization.* The process of transmitting knowledge, social values, and behavior patterns to members in settings such as the schools.
- *Social Control.* A check-and-balance system for gaining compliance to group norms regarding behavior. These norms will vary from community to community and are enforced by governmental agencies such as the police and courts.
- *Social Participation.* Provides opportunity for community members to participate in religious and voluntary organizations in the community.
- *Mutual Support.* Support provided to community members by such agencies as social agencies, hospitals, and health departments.

Klein uses a list of community functions that is very similar.[10] His list of basic functions includes the following:

1. Providing and distributing living space and shelter and determining use of space for other purposes;
2. Making available the means for distribution of necessary goods and services;
3. Maintaining safety and order, and facilitating the resolution of conflict;
4. Educating and acculturating newcomers (*e.g.*, children and immigrants);
5. Transmitting information, ideas, and beliefs;
6. Creating and enforcing rules and standards of belief and behavior;
7. Providing opportunities for interactions between individuals and groups.

These functions are based upon established patterns of interaction and revolve around "differentiation of roles, allocation of social status, and the provision of acceptable means for social mobility."[11]

Sanders' list of community functions is also similar, and it includes the recruitment of new members; communication; differentiation and status allocation; allocation of goods and services; social control; socialization; social mobility; internal accommodation and adjustment to forces outside the system.[12]

The functions of a community are carried out by the subsystems of the community interacting internally and externally with systems outside the community. For a community to continue to exist these functions must be met.

EXCHANGE WITH THE ENVIRONMENT

Because of the complexity of the community, it is easier to look at the exchange between subsystems of a community and the environment (surrounding communities, the state, and nation), than it is to look at community-to-community exchanges.

Health Subsystem. A first exchange between the health subsystem and the environment involves health. If there is a communicable disease, such as influenza, in the community, nurses are concerned with preventing its spread within the community by treatment and preventive measures and also preventing its spread to other communities and to the nation. Nurses recognize the potential of this biologic energy for exchange. We also do things to protect the community such as setting up mass-immunization clinics and mass educational programs to help the population protect itself from influenza.

Another exchange between the health subsystem and environment involves information. For example, as graduate or student nurses we belong to professional organizations and subscribe to professional journals. We may publish articles that influence the practice of other nurses outside the community or we may implement ideas in the community from articles we read. We also participate in professional organizations at the local level, which influences state and national organizations. We in turn are influenced by the state and national organizations. For example, as members of organizations we may be elected as delegates to state or national conventions and may take resolutions to business meetings which if passed will influence our practice. On the other hand, other groups from other districts of the state (community), or other parts of the country, may also take resolutions which if passed influence our practice. It is important that students and graduate nurses belong to these professional organizations so that they can have input into decisions that affect their practice. Certain checks-and-balances at the federal and state level are implemented in an attempt to maintain and improve the health of families and individuals at the community level. Among these are state board examinations and licensure practices, the code of ethics, standards of practice, and procedures for dealing with nurses who do not live up to the set standards and codes.

Each discipline in the health subsystem also has ties outside the local community. These disciplines both influence and are influenced by these exchanges.

In addition, the concept of resources (presented in Chap. 3) is useful for looking at the exchanges between the health subsystem and environment. If the community health subsystem discovers an increase in the incidence of lead poisoning among children, for instance, and lacks the financial and manpower resources to implement a program of casefinding, prevention, and treatment, it may turn to the state or federal government for the needed resources. During times of rapid change in a community, such exchanges become imperative if the community is to maintain the health of its population. For example, during a natural or man-made disaster, where food, water, and other necessary basics of life are disturbed, resources such as manpower, finances, immunizations, materials, water, food, and so forth are often needed. As a result of this identified need in times of community crisis, voluntary national resources such as the Red Cross have evolved. The state and national resources for health are so important that they will be discussed later in this section on community exchanges.

Many of the exchanges between the health subsystem of a community and its environment may facilitate or hamper the maintenance or attainment of a higher level of health for the population. For example, if we plan a crash immunization program in a community and have made arrangements with local subsystems (education, communication) and other parts of the health subsystem (physicians), but have not involved those outside the community (state nurses' association, state medical association) in the planning and decision making, this oversight with an important exchange may cause failure of implementation of the program.

Education Subsystem. The education subsystem has exchanges with the environment similar to those presented for health. Again, if the education subsystem of a community lacks resources to provide education, teachers and money may be recruited from other communities (or the state or nation) on a temporary or permanent basis. If we scan nursing journals, we see many advertisements for faculty in various parts of the country, and also graduate programs in nursing often have one bulletin board devoted to available positions around the country. Educational journals will carry similar advertisements for elementary or secondary school teachers.

Likewise, teachers are influenced by journal articles on educational practice and try new approaches and techniques, or they may contribute to journals that influence practice outside of the community. In addition, teachers belong to professional organizations and have conventions and thus influence and are influenced by standards, policies, and resolutions on a national basis.

Other Exchanges. Because most of the exchanges between the community's subsystems (economics, politics, religion, welfare, and communication) and the state and nation are similar in nature to those just presented, they will not be looked at here.

However, it is important to consider the concepts of health, autonomy, and resources when viewing these exchanges.

From the community health nursing point of view we are always looking at other exchanges to see if they facilitate or hamper the maintenance or attainment of a higher level of health for families or groups in our community. For example, the recent emphasis on human sexuality in many education subsystems based on the two-way process of family and community interaction has influenced national norms. This should help students look at, evaluate, and work through feelings in this area of behavior. This learning which is an important aspect of human behavior should facilitate the movement of families to a higher level of health in the future. On the other hand, failure to provide learning in this area may lead to poor adjustment and a lower level of health for segments of the population.

An interesting exchange between the political subsystem and the community is presented here as it accounts for change (moving away from the steady state—a part of self-regulatory processes) in communities. At any point in time, there are established patterns of behavior for populations, but over time these may change (positive feedback). For example, in the past, deviations from the nuclear family were not tolerated well in communities and this pattern was maintained by laws against unmarried adult people living together, and so forth. However, as segments of society change their values and beliefs, the process is available to change laws, which allows for new behaviors. The process may be through initiating referendums on the ballot locally which, if passed, may be picked up by other communities, or it may be through individual lawsuits moving from the lower courts to the Supreme Court. Thus, communities do not remain the same but change over time partly as a result of changes in laws which are passed in one community and then apply to the nation and are then enforcable in other communities. Recently attempts are being made to provide equal rights for women: a change that would affect all communities. These efforts were preceded by efforts to obtain equal rights for blacks and are proceeding concurrently with efforts to obtain equal rights for homosexuals. Recently, a lawsuit for material support against a Hollywood actor, following a separation by an unmarried housemate, may have implications for unmarried couples living together and may make this pattern of behavior more or less acceptable in the eyes of the law. Another example of change initiated through the legal system affecting families and the state involved the taxpayers' revolt in California.

Thus, the political–legal system provides the mechanism for moving communities away from their steady state to a different steady state, which is an important part of self-regulatory processes to be presented later in this chapter. This pressure by groups upon the sociocultural system can be likened to pressure brought by individual members upon the family for change.

From nursings' point of view, it is important to keep abreast of these changes so that we can correctly inform families about the legality of observed behavior and help them consider the alternatives and the consequences of their behavior. However, it is important to remember that the final decision about behavior always rests with the client (see Philosophy, Chap. 5).

Nurses should also identify key people in each community subsystem so that they can utilize their services in planning community care. For example, nurses might identify key people in the communication subsystem (radio, TV, newspaper) and use their services to bring health information to the attention of the community, or they might identify key political, religious, educational, and other community leaders in a neighborhood to help plan and implement a particular health program.

Communities Obtain, Retain, Contain, and Dispose. Like the family, a community obtains energy, information, and matter from the environment and retains, contains, and disposes of some of these to the environment. Obtaining refers to the input to the community. Examples of obtaining involve all the supplies needed by the families who make up the population. Such supplies include food and other goods for sale (refrigerators, cars, air conditioners, clothing); goods for building (lumber, bricks); goods for providing medical and health services (medications, blood-pressure cuffs, x-ray machines); materials for heating homes and buildings (fuel oil, coal, wood); manpower and money to provide services if needed, among other inputs.

The community may contain some of these energies and information, preventing them from crossing the community boundary. For example, one community may forbid untrained midwives from practicing in the community, whereas others may allow them. Or a community may prevent certain foods or services from entering a community because there is no demand. Even the size of food cans may vary from census tract to census tract within a large community because of demand. For example, when I lived on Nob Hill in San Francisco, the neighborhood was made up of mainly singles, couples, or small families. Because the grocery stores catered to the local population, the size of canned fruit and vegetable containers was small. However, in another area of the city, the Mission district, which was made up of predominantly large families, the can size of fruits and vegetables was large. In addition, some of the so-called luxury food items may be found in a middle- or high-income area, but not in a low-income area. Or, there may be many laundromats in a neighborhood where the lower economic groups do not have their own washing facilities. Laundromats may be lacking in a higher income area because there is not a demand for them. Likewise, fast-food restaurants may predominate in certain areas of lower class families or areas with many children and teenagers but be missing in upper-class areas, or areas with few teenagers and children. Consequently, community health nurses can learn a great deal about their community (census tract) by observing what is obtained and contained.

The community may also retain certain energy, information, and matter. Often if there is a demand for certain services and goods as previously discussed, they will be retained in a community, otherwise, they will be disposed of. For example, one community may have several people interested in antique shops. As these shops evolve, there must be a population to support them. If the community is without financial resources or it does not value the past, the shops will go out of business and be replaced by other shops that more closely meet the needs of the particular population. Likewise, if the individuals who opened the antique shops wish to continue in their business they may be forced to move to another community to provide for their financial needs. Otherwise, through the process of feedback they may match their behavior with their values and goals by changing their values and goals about making a living.

The community also provides output in the form of waste products (sewage, industrial waste), goods, and services. One community may be a coal-mining town and thus export coal. Another may be an agricultural community and export fruit and vegetables. And yet another may be a university community and produce individuals who have expertise (learned behaviors) in a variety of areas. Communities most likely have multiple products that may include prepared leaders from universities, goods, and services.

Whatever the processes of obtaining, retaining, containing, or disposing of energy, information, or matter found in a community at any point in time, it is the community's way of maintaining a degree of balance toward health for the population. These patterns are based upon the community's learned behaviors for coping as a community and, in reality, may help or hinder the health status of the population.

STATE AND NATIONAL HEALTH ORGANIZATIONS

Many of the exchanges between the community subsystem of health and the environment are with state or national health organizations. Often these organizations have evolved as a result of emergencies and crises rather than from long-range planning by state and national health groups.

National Health Organizations. The United States Constitution provides the framework for involvement of the federal government in health services. Although the Constitution is broad and general, its statements have been interpreted to include the health of all individuals. For example, Article 1, Section 8, Paragraph 1 of the Constitution gives the federal government power to regulate commerce with foreign nations and among the states and this has been interpreted to include such health matters as international and interstate quarantine, sanitary supervision, and vital statistics. In addition, Congress has enacted legislation involving the federal government in health. For example, Public Law 89-239 provides for the establishment of regional centers to work with clients having one of the three major health problems in the country—heart disease, cancer, or stroke.

In general the health programs of the federal government have three focuses: services to the general population, services to special populations, and involvement in international health. Services provided by the federal government are usually those that cannot be provided by states. Services for the general population include such things as protection against hazards, advancement of health and environmental sciences, augmentation of health facilities and selected health personnel, collection and dissemination of vital and health statistics, and support of disaster relief and civil defense. Services provided to special populations include such things as protection of workers from hazardous occupations or adverse working conditions, services for children, the aged, the retarded, the economically deprived or vocationally handicapped, special services for farm families, hospital and medical care for government employees, and the purchase of medical care for special groups. The federal government also has an interest in international health, which is demonstrated by involvement in the United Nations, the Pan-American Union, the North Atlantic Treaty Organization, and other international organizations. The government also provides money for research and health training to people in foreign countries.

U.S. DEPARTMENT OF HEALTH AND HUMAN SERVICES. The Department of Health and Human Services was created in 1980 from the Department of Health, Education and Welfare to promote general welfare in health and human services. Programs of the department are administered by agencies such as the Public Health Service, the Social Security Administration, the Office of Human Development Services, and others.

The Public Health Service is the one agency of the Department of Health and Human Services given specific responsibility for protecting and improving the health of the U. S., although all agencies have health-related aspects in their programs. The public health service is broken down into bureaus including the National Institute of Health and the National Institute of Mental Health. Functions of the bureaus of the Public Health Service include conducting and supporting research and training in health and public health sciences and administration; providing hospital and medical services to authorized personnel; aiding hospital and health facilities development; preventing the introduction of communicable diseases into the United States; and assisting states in applying new knowledge in preventing and controlling disease, maintaining a healthy environment, and developing community health services.

OTHER FEDERAL AGENCIES. Many other federal agencies have health functions related to their main tasks. For example, the Army, Navy, and Air Force Departments administer medical services for military personnel, the Veterans Administration provides medical care for veterans, and the Justice Department provides medical care for prisioners. Other agencies are concerned with safety, industrial hygiene, employment of children, animal diseases, and control of atomic energy.

STATE HEALTH SERVICES. Although state health services will vary from state to state, each has the general responsibility for protecting the health of its population. These general responsibilities, which are provided for by state constitutions, are supplemented by specific health laws and statutes passed by the state legislature as new issues are faced. Thus, states will vary in their regulations for licensure of health personnel, safety, education and employment of children, legal adoption, marriage, divorce, and so forth. However, most states have provisions for reporting births and deaths, reporting certain communicable diseases, for environmental and food sanitation and for preventive services. These programs supplement the efforts of local health departments.

INTERNAL PROCESSES

Subsystem Change. In the community the various subsystems mentioned earlier form the interrelated parts, which function together as a whole. These parts are interrelated and there are various attempts to maintain the steady state or the *status quo*.

Internally, the community needs periods of time where a steady state is maintained and there is organization of its parts to meet its needs and goals. Each of the subsystems, which are joined together, is composed of organizations and individuals. Individuals function in roles within these organizations and these roles are relatively fixed or patterned at any particular point in time. However, the roles may change over time. With a specific role there are certain demands and also certain freedoms and privileges. This structure of roles within organizations, which makes up the subsystems of the community, helps the community to maintain its steady state.

We are all familiar with these roles, which are usually layered from the lowest position to the highest. Each position is supervised by someone in a higher position who provides checks-and-balances on the role behavior. As with the family, there is a range of acceptable behavior that may vary from organization to organization within a subsystem or from subsystem to subsystem. However, if individuals try to move outside this range of acceptable role behaviors, there are counterforces to try to maintain the steady state. In addition to supervisors who provide a check-and-balance on role behaviors, peers and subordinates may also counteract behaviors, which deviate from an established role. For example, students may pressure a teacher to perform better if they feel they are not receiving the instruction they expected, or patients may pressure nurses for more attention in the hospital if they perceive that as part of the nurse's role. Likewise, peers and supervisors may pressure staff to maintain role behaviors if they deviate from the established range. At times, if individuals do not conform to established norms, they are subject to removal from their positions. At other times, however, with the process of feedback and maneuvers used in bringing about a change away from a steady state, it is always possible that deviation outside the established range will lead to a new steady state. For example, as a nursing student I was not allowed to marry or to live outside of the dormitory. I was also expected to stand up when an instructor entered the classroom, or when a doctor or a supervisor came onto the hospital ward. If it were not for individuals deviating outside these established norms of patterned behaviors and the eventual acceptance of new patterned behaviors, the student role would still be the same today.

A change in one part of a subsystem of the community affects all of the other parts of the subsystem in varying degrees. Because the parts within a subsystem are more interdependent and have more interaction than they do between subsystems, this change may be more noticeable. For example, if nurses in outpatient departments and hospitals begin teaching diabetic patients about diet, taking their insulin, and skin care, this will affect the roles of the nurses from the health departments, who may have been previously doing this teaching as part of their role functions while in the home. Likewise, if nurses take over teaching in the outpatient departments they may have less time to assist the physicians, which will affect their primary role. Also, while they are teaching, they may discuss community resources and, thus, take over a role behavior previously occupied by the hospital social worker.

Because a change in a part of a subsystem affects all the other parts, joint planning and coordination are necessary to ensure that the clients needs are being met, but not duplicated. Such planning involves frequent communication among the various parts of a subsystem (nursing) and between subsystems (nursing, social work, medicine). Most communication by nurses is verbal, however, some commmunications may be written in the form of directives or policy changes.

A change in a major subsystem also affects all of the other subsystems of a community in varying degrees. For example, changes in the law (political–legal) regarding compulsory vaccination prior to school enrollment leads to changes in school policies (education); requires programs for immunization (health); may require financing (economic); may require changes in family practices (family); and may require enforcement (law). These changes may or may not be initiated depending upon the willingness of the community to change (see Feedback later in this chapter). For example, breakdown of the plan may occur because of the family's religious beliefs against immunization; because of a lack of manpower and funding to carry out the program; because of a lack of school personnel to check records, and so forth. Such breakdowns may require new plans on the part of the health team to meet the health threat, which was the prompting factor in initiating the program. It should also be remembered that because the community is an open system, the health team can turn to the state or federal government for manpower and finances for the program.

Disruptive changes in a community are usually

kept to a minimum because of the patterned behaviors regarding decision making, communicating, authority, and other processes incorporated into roles. In addition, there are usually built in check-and-balance systems. For example, directors of the organizations of the various subsystems are usually given the authority to make major decisions that will affect other community subgroups, although staff may have the authority to identify areas where decisions are needed and to communicate this information through appropriate channels to the director. Before directors can initiate change they usually have a responsibility to discuss the proposed change with a board of directors, or other groups. Likewise, if change is to be initiated they usually have a responsibility to communicate with other community subsystem directors.

Any one of the subsystems identified previously can initiate change, which will affect other systems. However, because we are most interested in families, which make up the community population as a subsystem of the community, we are focusing the rest of this section on the population and changes that may affect it or how families may affect the community subsystems.

Population Subsystem Change. Over time, the kinds of family groups making up a community may change through immigration, emigration, and movement of existing families through the life cycle. For example, at one point, the population of a community may be composed of predominately young families and children; at another time, aged and middle-year adults may predominate. Services needed from community subsystems (health, welfare, education, political) by the two different populations will vary. Likewise, a change from predominately middle-class to lower-class populations will necessitate changes in services provided. Thus, we must be aware of trends in the community and use our demographic approach discussed earlier to initiate services, which are appropriate to the population from a health point of view. Although we may not be involved in actually making decisions about services we do have a part in this process. For example, over time we may see a change in the population structure of our community, perhaps a census tract, and may identify gaps or duplications in service as a result. We would then have an obligation to present this information to our supervisor who would feed the information through appropriate channels so that the data is available for decision making.

Health problems may also change because of population changes. If we see a rise in the incidence of communicable diseases, for example, in our community, we might focus on casefinding, teaching families about prevention and might also discuss the problem with our supervisor to see if a mass immunization, screening, or educational program would be appropriate at this particular time.

Changes in other community subsystems may also have an effect on a family's health. As the welfare system changes its requirements for eligibility, some of the families in the nurse's caseload may be left without financial assistance or with only limited assistance. Or a strike in the community which may leave large segments of the population without work, may also affect our families. Likewise, a change in the political officers or communication leaders (in newspaper, radio, or television) who do not favor certain health programs may affect families.

Any of the changes within a community can move families toward or away from a health balance. Often such changes are counterbalanced by other changes, which maintain a health balance. For instance, a strike in a community that leaves families without financial resources may be counterbalanced by increased funding from welfare on a local, state, or federal level, so the basic needs can be met. These families may also be eligible for food stamps. And perhaps funding would be available from the local, state, or federal government to provide free health care for this population, which was previously able to manage on its own.

The community health nurse's role is to bring nursing and community resources together to solve family problems created by changes in community subsystems. If community resources are unavailable because of increased demands, nurses should report these deficits to supervisors so that the data can again be fed into the decision-making process at the upper levels. In the meantime, nurses may need to help families look for alternative ways to meet their needs. For example, if family income is limited due to a strike and social service funds are unavailable, nurses may need to help families look at their budgeting, low-cost housing, or other ways to meet their goals with limited financial resources.

Types of Population Subgroups. A community at any point in time will be made up of various family subgroups and these will change over time. Although we could look at cultural or ethnic groups, we will look specifically at the social classes of families. Often as a neighborhood ages, the middle and upper class families move out and it is taken over by the lower classes. The social class of a particular group has relevance for the community health nurse because the knowledge, attitudes, beliefs, and behaviors of groups vary. Families are often grouped into upper, middle, or lower classes and this determines the life style of the family, which governs environmental exposure, customs, and habits that affect health.

People of the middle and upper classes usually enjoy better health, are more self-sufficient regarding health matters, avail themselves of the best medical and health care, and because of a higher educational level and values in health respond better to appeals to modify behavior in a positive health-related way. For example, they are more likely to receive dental care, reduce or quit smoking, receive immunizations, follow prescribed diets, and so forth. The lower classes usually have the worst health outcomes and are the most difficult to persuade to obtain treatment. This is partly because of their income level, which leads to poor housing, inadequate diets, crowding, and other conditions, which reduces their resistance to disease agents. Their thinking is also often present-oriented rather than future-oriented and they understand concrete ideas rather than concepts and abstract ideas. With a present orientation rather than a future orientation, they are less likely to utilize preventive services.

Warren says that on the average people of different social classes vary in their aesthetic tastes, in the books and magazines they read, the way they vote, the size of their families, the way they spend leisure time, and even in their sexual morality.[13]

Studies of Class Behavior. Various studies have been carried out on class values, attitudes, and behaviors and these are valuable to the community health nurse working with families as subsystems of the community. Watts compared some characteristics of lower- and middle-class people and found that lower-class people are more oriented to the present rather than the future.[14] They also take advantage of what is immediately available rather than plan for a future they can't visualize. On the other hand, the middle class is more future-oriented and defers gratification by planning ahead and saving for a desired goal. It also values cleanliness, work, and self-discipline.

Koos categorized his population studied into social classes and asked each group if the following symptoms were significant and required the attention of a doctor: loss of appetite; persistent backache; continued coughing; persistent joint and muscle pain; blood in the stools; blood in the urine; excessive vaginal bleeding; swelling of ankles; loss of weight; bleeding gums; chronic fatigue; shortness of breath; persistent headaches; fainting spells; pain in the chest; lump in the breast; and lump in the abdomen.[15] He found the higher social class was consistent in recognizing the symptoms as important, the skilled workers were less concerned, and the lowest class was indifferent to the symptoms. He concluded that there were obvious differences between the social classes concerning their attitudes toward symptoms.

Research has confirmed that when symptoms are considered normal, no action for seeking health care follows. In addition to social class, other factors may also influence health behavior. Koos found that people afraid of surgery, where indicated, would ignore the most pressing symptoms to avoid going under the knife.[16] In addition, cost was often a deterrent to seeking care, especially when the cost was an unknown factor and the family income was meager. A third variable involved the need for treatment and the age of the person needing treatment. Some symptoms were given importance if they occurred in a young person but disregarded if they occurred in a middle-aged or elderly member of the family. The cultural content of the family's social group was also a factor in seeking treatment. One lower-class housewife told the interviewer she would be "hooted out of town" if she consulted a doctor about a backache.

The implications of this research for community health nurses are the following:

- Before individuals will take health action they must recognize that they have a problem (lower class is less likely to recognize this; different people have different concepts of and values in health).

- For health action involving a problem, sometimes the fear of treatment must be less than the fear of the consequences of not having treatment.
- In some instances, especially in low-income families, the cost of care should become a known factor.
- Health action is tied closely to the overall belief system of people.

Nurses can help subgroups of the population by working with their concepts of health; by explaining treatment and the consequences of not obtaining treatment; by explaining the cost of care and financial assistance available; by determining the belief system of the family and working within it; and by connecting new ideas of care with old ideas of the particular family.

Closely related research on motivation in health action was done by Rosenstock.[17] He found that before people will take health action they must feel (1) that the problem does or could affect them (2) that the problem will not subside on its own (3) that medical help will make a difference because there is knowledge and treatment for the condition, and (4) that the treatment is less threatening than the consequences of no treatment at all.

Again, community health nurses must make symptoms and conditions explicitly known to families; they must discuss the course and outcome of the condition and the medical or health treatment.

Another research study on beliefs and attitudes toward health and health practices and the use of medical and other personnel in the treatment of disease was carried out by the National Opinion Research Center and sponsored by the Health Information Foundation.[18] The sample comprised 2379 adults and a representative sample of the American public. Variables of age, sex, region of country, size of community, occupation, education, income, and family structure were obtained and because of the sampling technique the results can be generalized.

In relation to the expectations of illness, each respondent was asked to agree or disagree with certain statements regarding health. These include statements such as the following:

- No matter how careful a person is, he has to expect a lot of illness during his lifetime.
- Aches and pains are not important—you just get used to them.
- People understand their own health better than most doctors.
- You shouldn't go to the hospital unless there is no other way to get care.

It was found that people with low education and low income showed the highest agreement that people should expect a lot of illness and that one should get used to aches and pains, and so forth. This was in marked contrast to the upper levels of income and education.

Knowledge about disease also varied with social class. Dunnell and Cartwright found that the proportion of people giving four or five correct answers to questions about whether diabetes, anemia, bronchitis, tuberculosis, and polio were "catching" fell from 82% for people in Social Class I to 53% in Social Class V.[19] Their results confirmed earlier results by King.[18]

In a similar study at Cornell where patients were interviewed about their conception and knowledge of their health problems and their expectations of personnel, it was found that lower-class patients lacked knowledge, seemed to have a need to understand their condition, and yet made no effort to obtain this information.[20] These patients also failed to criticize the doctor for not giving them the information, which suggested that this group perhaps did not expect the doctors to fulfill their educational needs.

Mechanic also says that lower-class groups have less information and knowledge about disease and are more likely to hold irrational ideas about illness.[21] They also rely more on folk medicine and fringe practitioners, and they delay seeking medical treatment more than middle- and upper-class groups. Some of the reasons for delaying treatment from physicians or for seeking help outside the organized health care system (folk medicine) were discussed earlier.

Interaction of Families With the Community. There are various points of interaction between families (community population) and the community. These can be categorized in the following way:

I. Points where the official community and families interact regularly
   A. Taxes (daily)
      1. Supermarket
      2. Transportation
      3. Postman
   B. Services
      1. Public welfare
      2. Police
      3. Fire
      4. Government hospitals
      5. Health department
      6. Government employees
         a. School
         b. City/county/local government
II. Points where the voluntary services community and family interact regularly
   A. Private enterprise
   B. Private investigators, security patrol
   C. Fire department with supplemental volunteers
   D. Private physicians, hospitals, health groups
   E. Organized employees
   F. Private schools, inservice educators
   G. Churches
III. Emergency points of interaction with any or all of previous categories
   A. Regional or area disaster
      1. Natural—Hurricane, tornado, drought
      2. Man-made—Kepone poisioning, radiation
   B. Local disaster affecting families
   C. Familiar crises requiring intervention (Method of intervention)
      1. Low income– Pregnancy (WIC program)
      2. Fixed income over age 65 (Special bus rates; drugstore rates; movies rates; old-age survivors insurance)
      3. Child–wife–elderly abuse (Police department)
      4. Fire in home (Fire department)
      5. Veneral disease or other epidemic (Health department)

Thus, the interaction between families in the population and the community cuts across all subsystems.

ADAPTIVE PROCESSES IN THE COMMUNITY

When change occurs in one part of the community system, the whole system is affected and other parts will try to counteract the change to maintain a steady state (one aspect of feedback process). For example, in the example presented earlier regarding compulsory vaccination prior to school enrollment, the schools may refuse to check student records for proof of vaccination claiming that they do not have the time and personnel. Families may also refuse to get the vaccination saying it is against their religious beliefs. Or, more likely, families will pressure key people in the political system to have the decision reversed. Likewise, the economic subsystem may indicate that money is not available to provide this service. There may be unending attempts to maintain the status quo, that is, to keep things as they are and not to enforce vaccinations prior to school enrollment.

As indicated earlier, the community may always turn to the state and federal governments to initiate change that will benefit the community. In the vaccination example, the health subsystem of the community might request funding and manpower to provide the vaccinations.

The community at any point in time is made up of various groups and organizations, which are for or against things as they are. Thus, although the system as a whole remains intact, there is stress and strain in parts of it. Other parts will adapt to these stressed parts and, although the community system may not be as efficient as it should be, it will continue to maintain itself as a system. For example, some families may be opposed to pre-school enrollment immunization because of religious beliefs but will accomodate to this practice because they want their children to have an education and because it is strictly enforced. When many families attempt to pressure the political system for change, other groups may pressure the system to maintain things as they are. Often, depending upon the amount of pressure or the number of people who are unhappy with the way things are, a change will be proposed on the ballot during an election to be decided upon by the majority. This change if initiated may create stress for another segment of the population who through the process of feedback will need to rectify their internal standards and values with new behaviors. For example, as Blacks gain equal rights in the nation and can live wherever they want, some whites who have negative feelings and values may have to work these feelings through. This is through the process of feedback which reduces the tension in the individual system when confronted by a mismatch of internal values and external behavior.

Many of the changes in a community may move families toward or away from health. Although we are health-oriented, groups in other subsystems may be more motivated by other goals than health. For example, recently in our area of the country people were developing symptoms of kepone poisoning as a result of working with this chemical. In addition, the chemical plant was dumping large quantities of waste into the rivers and contaminating the fish. The plant's motivation was only to make a profit, but this had a marked effect on the health of the population and on the economy. For example, as a result of contaminated fish, rivers were closed to fisherman who earned their livelihood by catching and selling fish. However, the danger to the population at that point warranted the closing of the rivers at the expense of putting the fishermen out of work.

Thus, it is important that community health nurses be aware that not all groups have health as a top priority. This awareness will allow them to look at things realistically and at proposed changes to determine what patterns are beneficial or harmful to families and what are the possible outcomes of the proposed changes. The concept of balance-and-risk, which will be presented in Chapter 6, is useful for this purpose because there is risk involved in both initiating change and in leaving things as they are. However, the nurse should weigh the risk of either, as a basis for decision making.

A community, like the family, can experience excesses and deprivation in its exchanges and thus fail to grow adequately. For example, if a community is functioning to capacity but fails to receive an adequate share of its taxes back from the state and federal governments, it may not be able to continue with adequate health, welfare, transportation, and other services to meet the needs of the population. On the other hand, communities may become too dependent upon these exchanges (money, manpower) and fail to develop their own resources.

ENTROPY AND NEGENTROPY IN THE COMMUNITY

ENTROPY

In the community, entropy is always present because the subsystems must continually adjust to the input of energy and information and because some energy is lost in the process of transformation. For example, organizations often employ new members who must be oriented to their role and learn to relate to co-workers. During this process, the subsystem is not working as effectively as possible. Or, new people may have ideas about changes they wish to institute, which may or may not be initiated depending upon the complemental fit of other employees and the employer. During the process of determining whether or not to make the changes, one or another part of the organization may be disrupted and so not function at its fullest. Likewise, information that is initiated at the top of the organization may create problems for some parts of the system, which again will not function at its maximum. However, this loss of energy and tendency toward equilibrium is not detrimental to the subsystem and community as a whole because there is enough energy to go beyond this disorganization to meet the needs of the system (adaptation) and to move it to a higher order of organization (negentropy).

Various factors in a community may, however, lead to entropy to varying degrees. Some of these may be temporary and some may be more permanent. For example, during a recent blackout in an eastern city, there was widespread looting and burgularies. This increase in crime could not be handled by the available police force (counterbalance) and led to loss, disorder, and disorganization. This entropy was of a temporary nature and equilibrium was restored in a short time. Such temporary periods of entropy may also follow disasters, strikes, or riots, when the community is not prepared to counterbalance these incidences with additional resources from the subsystems (health, welfare, police, and so forth).

More permanent entropy may result from the loss of the economic base in a community. For example, in a community where there are limited job opportunities, the young may move away leaving a void for replacing people who retire and causing a lower birth rate and a higher death rate among the aging population. Or, one factory in an area may move out of the community to a new location leaving an economic void for the community. Since other community subsystems such as health and welfare are usually unable to counterbalance this change indefinitely, families will move away and the community will die, unless it can attract other industry. Some of the gold-mining towns in the western part of the United States had a large influx of people during the gold rush and then died when people moved on.

Certain areas or neighborhoods of a community (the nurse's community) may also show entropy. For example, if middle- and upper-class families move from the center of the community to the suburbs or surrounding communities the corresponding loss of the tax base in the center city portion may lead to a loss of subsystem services such as police and fire protection, health and social services. Such an area would be blighted and would move toward entropy.

Discrimination. Communities that are not using their resources to their fullest or fail to provide means for social mobility for certain members also may experience entropy to a lesser degree. For example, communities that do not provide equal opportunity for women, Blacks, and other minority groups are not utilizing their human resources and growing to their potential. In a 1979 newspaper article, a reporter from New York said that women in the job market are currently no better off then they were at the turn of the century, according to a survey by an antidiscrimination group.[22] The study said that while 60% of Americans are female or members of a racial minority, white males still dominate business, government, education, health institutions, and the media. Of 441 occupations listed in a June 1978 census classification report, the study said, the majority of working women are found in only 20 of these.

Other findings on sexism showed that the median weekly income of full-time working women was 73% of the men's salary in professional/technical jobs, 64% in clerical jobs, and 45% in sales jobs. For college graduates, the median income for white males was $17,891, whereas the female counterpart earned $10,861.

In relation to racism the article said that the Black family income rose to 61% of the White family income in 1970, but fell to 57% in 1977. In addition, Blacks made up less than 4% of the professionals in medicine, law, and engineering. Milio looks at many of these prejudices in communities involving decision-making opportunities, access to health care, and access to education for minority groups.[23]

The Bureau of Census says that in 1974 low-income Blacks constituted 31% of the Black population, which was more than three times the comparable proportion of 9% for the White population.[24] The majority of these families had a female as the head of the household. Of black families below the low-income level, 14.2% had males as heads of households, whereas 52.8% had females as heads of households.

Prejudices that prevent communities and segments of the population from reaching their full potential are also detrimental for all people. Those who are denied access to equal rights take energy from the system (lost energy) as a result of the feelings engendered by the inequality, and those with equal rights may lose energy in their effort to constantly justify why things should remain as they are. In the end, the whole community suffers from this process because it is not realizing the full potential of all its citizens.

Like the family, a community with subsystems that are tightly knit and attempt to maintain the status quo will fail to meet the needs of the population as change occurs leading to entropy. At the other extreme, the community with subsystems that are loosely joined and fail to communicate and accomodate or counterbalance changes in other subsystems, will fail to meet population needs and also experience entropy. Thus, like the family, the community needs subsystems that are flexible in role functions and are willing to change goals and objectives to meet the changing needs of the population. These communities will continue to exist and grow (negentropy).

In a community population, humans are more prone to entropy at some periods in their development than at other periods; that is, they are less able to adapt to energy exchanges because they lack the acquired and learned mechanisms of adaptation. For example, early childhood and old age are two periods of development in which entropy is more likely a result of stress and will affect large numbers or segments of the population. Infants must rely solely on acquired mechanisms of adaptation because they have not learned ways of assisting their body to adapt, and the aged have suffered so many periods of entropy that their regulatory mechanisms function at a lower level. Also, for the aged much energy is used in trying to maintain functioning of the body when parts have changed because of irreversible damage during such periods. Vital statistics give us some indications of periods of development when specific age groups are more susceptible to environmental excesses and deprivations at a time when the body is least able to adapt. These periods change from time to time (refer to discussion of current high-risk groups in Chap. 11).

NEGENTROPY

Growth of the population in a community is usually a sign of a prosperous and healthy community. Along with growth of the population, there is an increase in the size of the subsystems, such as, schools and services to meet the increased needs of the population. And there will be an increase in the tax base (*e.g.*, taxes to support public services and to supplement private services). Although there may be some disorganization between the time of need and its fulfillment for the population, a flexible community adapts to the changes.

Doxiadis describes the evolution of cities through history using five stages differentiated by the distance a person can travel within a certain span of time.[25] His A-level community's size was 2 × 2 kilometers, with less than 50,000 people. No more than 10 minutes is required to walk from the center to the periphery of the city.

B-level communities are 6 × 6 kilometers in size and have more than 50,000 people in the population. Walking time was no more than half an hour and paved roads and horsedrawn carts moved people. These communities were difficult to govern and mobs frequently controlled them.

The C-level community depended upon subways or elevated trains to move people. Later, freeways were built to accomodate automobiles. D-level communities are modern cities with major problems and the megalopolis is made up of E-level communities, which continue to have the problems found in the D-level communities.

Miller says that the "universal city" or "ecumenopolis" is the ultimate city and requires centralized planning.[26] In this system, technology would solve the problems of transportation, waste collection, distribution of supplies, and so forth.

No pattern for community evolution other than cities has been identified, but it seems likely that any community follows a similar pattern. Most communities probably grow in density of population, geographic area covered and availability of services and other specialized functions.

One generalization about the growth of cities has been advanced in the concentric zone theory. Although the city may have various forms, basically as the middle and upper classes move further from the city's interior, they are replaced by the lower classes. Thus, the city is made up of circles or some other pattern around the central business district. Next in line are wholesalers, light manufacturers, then low-class residential areas. These are followed by lower middle-class residential areas, high-class residential areas, heavy manufacturing and outlying business districts. Beyond these are the residential and industrial suburbs.

Some of these patterns are recently being reversed because of energy shortages, inflation, and efforts to rehabilitate centers of cities. Reilly says that "the rising cost of resources has begun to have an impact upon Americans' budgets, ways of life and ways of thinking."[27] He goes on to say that Americans paid little for foreign oil in 1965 and by 1970 the average family paid $35 for imported supplies of oil. However, in 1975, the cost was $350 and in 1980 every family pays $500. Thus, some middle-class Americans have moved back to the center of the city. At the same time, there have been efforts to rehabilitate these areas. For example, Reilly says that in 1975 almost half of 260 cities surveyed by the Urban Land Institute reported housing rehabilitation, property improvement, and other efforts to build up older sections of the center city.[28] Altogether, such activities are ongoing in about 75% of all cities over 500,000. In addition to the energy crunch high-interest rates, sewage connection moratoriums, slowed growth policies in communities, and the high cost of new housing have facilitated a return to the city's center and rehabilitation of existing houses. Specific examples of communities which have changed the appearance of their central area can be found in Ficker and Bourne.[29,30]

Eldredge sees several alternatives for the individual in cities.[31] One alternative is the megalopolis, which is currently with us and which offers a variety of life styles. Another alternative is the metropolitan area (center city; 500,000 and up), which is currently being redeveloped to attract middle-class taxpayers back into the city. Another alternative is the smaller central city which is similar to the metropolitan central city but on a smaller scale or the small central area of a town. He also suggests satellite cities near the large cities, near inner and outer suburbs and near exurbia and quasi-rural areas. It is obvious that alternatives to center city living must be considered in view of population growth. For example, Davis says, "If the urban proportion were to continue to rise at the 1950–1970 rates . . . 100 percent would be living in (urban) places by 2031."[32]

Whether a community grows and becomes increasingly more complex is dependent upon a surplus of opportunities for the population. If jobs and other opportunities are readily available, a major portion of those living in an area will remain, and new people will immigrate to the area.

As people immigrate and the population increases, there are increased demands for goods and services and all of the subsystems also grow. Or, if new services are required, new organizations within the subsystems evolve to fill the needs. As these subsystems continue to change to meet the changing needs of the population, they grow and become more complex.

From a health point of view, it is believed that a growing city or community that has flexible subsystems is most healthy because the tax base exists to provide services needed by the population, and the resources are developing in organizations and families. However, it should be remembered that resources include the optimum use of minorities by the community.

FEEDBACK IN COMMUNITIES

When change is introduced into a subsystem of a community, others must also change if the community is to remain viable. As mentioned earlier, other subsystems will attempt to maintain the status quo or steady state (one part of the self-regulatory processes). If the change is minimal or if there is enough pressure for change, other subsystems may cooperate. Thus, when change is initiated in one subsystem, others may cooperate, accommodate, or resist.

In a community, there will be patterned behaviors associated with roles of individuals within subsystems and between subsystems that are almost automatic and thereby reduce the energy required to carry out these roles. When change is initiated in one subsystem, which affects the other subsystems, these patterned behaviors no longer work adequately and tension rises in the other subsystems. In addition, more energy is lost from the whole system during this period.

In an attempt to reduce the tension in the system, certain maneuvers will be tried within and between subsystems. (Several of these maneuvers were discussed in Chap. 3.) For instance, in the example about compulsory school immunizations presented earlier, the members of the health subsystem could have bargained with the school subsystem to obtain adequate personnel to check records to see that this change was implemented. They might have suggested that if the school members go along with this change (which is necessary for community health) they will go along with the next change proposed by the school. The leaders in the health subsystem also have to work with the economic subsystem to finance the program. This may be done by presenting and defending the budget to the city council. Part of the defending involves politicking for the funding because there are several subsystems in the community simultaneously trying to obtain limited funds. Various maneuvers can be tried with each of the subsystems involved until the change is initiated or rejected.

If the goals of the subsystem are important in the eyes of the members of the subsystem, they will continue to work for the change even if rejected initially on the local level. In this instance, they may turn to the state or federal government for funding or other resources to provide materials for immunizations, for personnel to check school records, and so forth.

Thus, if the goals are important and members of the subsystem are committed to the goals, they will pressure and use various maneuvers with other subsystems equally affected to bring about the change (one part of the self-regulatory processes). Otherwise, they may be content to forget the goal and remain at its steady state (another part of the self-regulatory processes).

This same process is followed in placing a referendum before the voters of a community, and in eliciting votes for the proposed change in meeting a goal of a special-interest group. Often the mass media or communication subsystem is used to bring the information before the particular population and to attempt to influence their vote. Or, one-to-one interviews and discussions between members of the special-interest group and members of the population may be used. Often, the key people in a community in various subsystems are visited by members of the special-interest group, and the maneuvers discussed in Chapter 3 are used to influence them. These key people, in turn, are expected to sway other members under their leadership in the subsystem.

Thus, depending upon the strength of the goal underlying the change and the pressure brought to bear upon the affected subsystems, the steady state may be maintained or it may be changed to a new steady state (self-regulatory processes). Following change, the tension in the system eventually subsides and new patterns of behavior evolve and become partially established. During the process of moving to the new steady state, some energy is lost from the system because of the need to consciously focus upon the new patterns of behavior, but once mastered, they again become automatic and facilitate role behavior without loss of energy.

FOCUS OF COMMUNITY HEALTH NURSING IN COMMUNITIES

Community health nurses must focus upon the community population (total, census tract, school, or industry) and its subordinate and superordinate systems to use the nursing process effectively and in the interest of the community population. At any point in time, nurses work with actual or potential high-risk segments of that population to help maintain or regain balance and purposeful direction in individuals' lives. To help high-risk segments of the population maintain balance, nurses may do casefinding in their particular community for unsupervised prenatal mothers, unsupervised well children, and other high-risk groups, and help them secure any needed medical and health care. They may also set up classes on growth and development, nutrition, accident prevention, or other relevant areas for particular high-risk groups, for those individuals referred from community resources such as hospitals or well-child clinics. In some instances, they may visit the homes of this particular segment of the population. Various categories of high-risk groups are usually identified by different health agencies. For example, prenatal mothers are often considered to be high risk if they are from a lower socioeconomic group, they are under 16 years or over 40 years of age, they have had complications in the past, they are having their first child, or they have a chronic or an acute health problem that would endanger the health of the mother or child.

To help segments of the population regain balance and purposeful direction, nurses may do casefinding for diabetics, children with symptoms of lead poisoning, or whatever other conditions are prevalent in the particular community population. Nurses may work with groups of poorly controlled diabetics to teach them nutrition; administration of insulin; care of equipment; prevention and treatment of wounds; signs and symptoms of insulin shock or diabetic acidosis. They may also work with groups of parents who have children with lead poisoning by teaching the signs and symptoms of lead poisoning; by teaching environmental control; available community resources, and prevention. Nurses may also give bedside care at home to segments of the population with chronic or acute illnesses, if this is within the scope of the particular health agency.

Nurses must, over time, assess changes in the population structure and changes in the mortality and morbidity rates of the particular community, so that nursing services continue to meet the needs of the particular population. Also, to identify increases or decreases in the incidence and prevalence of diseases, nurses may compare current rates with past rates and also compare these rates with other communities, as well as with the state and the nation. If there is any increase, this should be discussed with the supervisor to determine if additional services or a change in priorities in the community is indicated. At times, the changing conditions within the population can be dealt with by short-term intervention; mass programs such as screening and immunization may be effective.

Nurses should also be aware of potential increases in the incidence and prevalence of diseases in the community. For example, during the winter months various flu epidemics usually spread from community to community. If there is advance notice and immunizations are available, a mass program to immunize all or high-risk segments of the population such as the aged, children, and those with chronic conditions may be effective to maintain the balance of the population.

If there is a change in the population structure of the community, nurses should also evaluate nursing services. To determine population structure changes it is usually necessary to compare the current structure with previous data for the area, such as a year ago, five and ten years ago. If there is a change in the social-class structure, age structure, race structure or other demographic factors a change in preventive and treatment services by nurses may be indicated.

Community health nurses should also look at the relationships between subsystems of the community and the population to determine if these relationships are assisting populations in maintaining health or moving them away from it. For example, are the communications subsystems presenting adequate, informative data to the nurse's community on health and health issues? Can nurses work with key people in the communications subsystem to improve the quality of health information? Can nurses be used for public information of special health programs such as mass immunization programs, blood pressure screening programs, or classes on growth and development or nutrition to be given at various locations as needed throughout the community. In addition, nurses may use the services of various subsystems with segments of the population to maintain or regain balance. For example, nurses may refer the unemployed to social services, vocational rehabilitation or unemployment services, or they may refer groups of understimulated lower-class children to Head Start or child development programs to help them maintain balance.

As changes in the subsystems of the community occur, nurses should continually assess the effects of these changes on the health of the population and on the nurse's practice as a basis for planning nursing care for the population. For example, the Crippled Childrens Bureau of the state and local health departments may reduce categories of children who are eligible for services through the program. Families who have children with conditions eliminated from the list of eligible services will still need care for these children. Nurses may help this segment of the population budget money so that they can pay for private or clinic services, may help them locate part-pay services, may help them locate sources for financing, and so forth. Should there be an increase in the incidence of the eliminated conditions at a later time, nurses may channel this information to supervisors and others in an effort to have the service reinstated. As indicated earlier, the nurse must be continually aware of changes in subsystems of the community, as changes have an effect on their functioning with the larger population.

Nurses should also be aware of the exchanges with the superordinate system of the community and its effect on the community. Examples of the spread of disease and its effect on the nurse's functions were discussed earlier. Nurses should also continually evaluate their performance in light of accepted standards and the code of ethics, and should continually upgrade their performance through reading, attending national or state meetings and workshops.

REFERENCES

1. Benson E, McDevitt J: Community Health and Nursing Practice. Englewood Cliffs, Prentice-Hall 1976
2. Pearl R: On biological principles affecting populations: human and other. American Naturalist 71:50–68, 1937
3. Mattison BF: Community health planning and the health professions. Am J Public Health 58:1019, June 1968
4. Hanlon JJ: Public Health Administration and Practice. St Louis C V Mosby, 1974
5. Tinkham C, Voorhies E: Community Health Nursing Evolution and Process, pp 194–195. New York, Appleton-Century-Crofts, 1977
6. Klein D: Community Dynamics and Mental Health. New York, John Wiley & Sons, 1968
7. Sanders I: The Community: An Introduction to a Social System, p 133. New York, Ronald Press, 1975
8. Sanders IT: Public Health in the Community. In Freeman H, et al (eds): Handbook of Medical Sociology, pp 411–412. Englewood Cliffs, Prentice-Hall, 1972
9. Warren RL: The Community in America, p 9. New York, Rand McNally, 1973
10. Klein D. Community Dynamics and Mental Health, New York, John Wiley & Sons, 1968
11. Ibid
12. Sanders I: The Community: An Introduction to a Social System, p 345. New York, Ronald Press, 1975
13. Warren RL: Studying Your Community, p 351. New York, Free Press, 1975
14. Watts W: Social class, ethnic background and patient care. Nurs Forum 6, No. 2:155–162, Spring 1967
15. Koos E: The Health of Regionville. New York, Columbia University, 1954
16. Ibid
17. Rosenstock ZM: What research in motivation suggests for public health. Am J Public Health March 1960
18. King S: Perceptions of Illness and Medical Practice, pp 122–123. New York, Russell Sage, 1962
19. Dunnell K, Cartwright A: Medicine Takers, Prescribers and Horders. London, Routhledge & Kegan Paul, 1972
20. Reader GG, et al: What patients expect from their doctors. Modern Hospitals July 1957
21. Mechanic D: Illness and Cure. In Koso J, et al (eds): Poverty and Health, p 207. Cambridge, Harvard University, 1969
22. The Virginia-Pilot and The Ledger Star, Norfolk, Jan 21, 1979
23. Milio N: The Care of Health in Communities: Access for Outcasts. New York, Macmillan, 1975
24. U.S. Department of Commerce. The Social and Economic Status of the Black Population in the United States 1974, p 43. Washington, DC, Bureau of Census, July 1975
25. Miller J: Living systems: The organization. Behavioral Science Vol. 17, No. 1:116–119, Jan 1972
26. Ibid
27. Reilly W: Conservation, Community and Personal Responsibility. Vital Speeches of the Day, p 202. Jan 15, 1976
28. Ibid
29. Ficker VB, Graves HS: Social Science and Urban Crisis. New York, Macmillan, 1978
30. Bourne LS, Simmons JW: Systems of Cities. New York, Oxford University, 1978
31. Wentworth EH:Alternative Possible Urban Futures. Cities in Change, pp 488–499. Boston, Allyn & Bacon, 1977
32. Kingsley D: World Urbanization 1950–1970, Vol II. Analysis of Trends, Relationships, and Development. Berkeley, Institute of International Studies, Population Monograph Series, No. 9, p 52, 1972

5

The Evolution, Characteristics, Goals, Philosophy, and Ethical Basis of Community Health Nursing

HISTORICAL FOUNDATIONS

Throughout history community health nursing has been influenced by the dynamic health needs of community populations and by the nature of organized community efforts to meet these needs. Concurrent with and influencing these relationships has been the evolving knowledge of the natural history of diseases and the practices necessary to control and treat them in conjunction with the prevailing ideologies of the particular period.

Over the centuries, the types of diseases affecting mankind and the severity of their effects on populations have changed. The effects of early epidemics on populations were reduced or eliminated as their causes became known, and this knowledge in turn led to more effective control and treatment. Throughout this process the attention paid to health and disease was influenced by the ideologic concepts that dominated society at the time. These influencing ideologies varied from theologic, economic and political, to social.

Community health nursing evolved as the need for care in the home was identified. Early rules were recorded for such care by the Hebrews in the book of Lev. 12:15.[1] These rules were based upon cleanliness and community responsibility to health, such as, with leprosy and the believed uncleanliness of women following childbirth. Underlying the care given by religious orders at that time was the religious ideology of service to God.

Later, Christians followed the example of Christ and formalized charity by creating groups that cared for the sick as a service to God. This formalized structure was directed by the church, and widows and nuns prayed for and stayed with the sick to meet their needs. About 60 A.D. Paul, the apostle, described Phoebe as a "deaconess" who was assigned to care for the sick in their homes. Phoebe is considered to be the first visiting nurse.[2]

For over a thousand years following the time of Phoebe, the care of the sick in their homes was motivated by the religious ideal. Care continued to be carried out under the direction of the church and included prayer, remaining with the sick, and in some instances isolating them from those that were not ill. This was based upon the prevailing belief that some of the common epidemic diseases, such as, leprosy, typhus, dysentery, diarrhea, or scurvy were caused by divine or demonic wrath and a variety of environmental causes, and were for some unknown reason contagious.

During this period hospitals had their beginning. As the Crusaders traveled specific routes, monasteries opened along the way to aid the sick and weary. Nursing care was provided as part of this service.

Around 399 A.D. Fabiola, the daughter of a great Roman family, established a hospital in Rome for the care of the sick, and sought out patients in the streets. It seems possible that this might have marked the beginning of casefinding in community health nursing.

During the 16th and 17th Centuries, care for the sick and poor moved away from the monasteries in some countries. In England, Henry VIII did away with medical care in monasteries and assigned the responsibility for it to local governments. This was based upon an economic and humanistic ideology. For example, with an increase in trade and the rise of a new social class, the bourgeoisie, the notion of wealth no longer consisted solely of land but of commodities of trade. Concomitant with increased economic activity was the rise of the nation-state and it was realized that the more money a state accumulates, the more powerful it becomes. To ensure this steady economic growth, the state had to protect and care for its citizens. At the same time the humanistic concepts of the brotherhood of humans and of the freedom and equality of humans had been gaining acceptance.

As a result of this ideology various measures were presented to the English Parliament to deal with poverty. In 1601, these measures were consolidated into the Elizabeth Poor Law which did not treat health matters specifically, but stated the responsibility of the state for the lame, impotent, old, blind, poor, and those unable to work. This statement was interpreted loosely and was expanded to include medical and nursing care.

Other countries, such as France, continued to give care in the hospital and home under the direction of the church. These efforts were usually sporatic and short-lived. For example, in 1610, St. Francis de Sales organized a nursing service for the care of the sick in eastern France. This care was to be given by orders of nuns drawn from women of the upper class. After 5 years this care was discontinued because of the cloistering of the nuns.

In the 18th and 19th Centuries, several societal forces stimulated further interest in community health nursing. There was a growing sense of humanity and a deepening consciousness of the social problems (poverty, inadequate housing, child labor, lack of educational opportunities) affecting individuals and families caught in the movement of a society from rural to urban living because of industrialization. At the same time there was a growth of knowledge in the medical sciences on ways to promote health, prevent and cure diseases. These needs led to the recognized need for educated nurses.

The practice of visiting the sick and poor and offering nursing care on an organized nonreligious basis was introduced in England and America at the beginning of the 19th Century. People performing these duties were largely untrained, but William Rathbone of Liverpool, England, recognized the need for training and, supported by Florence Nightingale, began the district nursing service in Liverpool, in 1859. Under this plan, a nurse and a "lady" visitor were assigned to each district and a total of eighteen districts covered the city. This plan became successful and was later adopted by other cities in England.

At the same time, there was a movement to utilize nurses to teach hygiene in homes. This was probably the beginning of the health-teaching and counseling role of the community health nurse. This effort followed attempts to distribute health information by pamphlets, which was aimed at elevating the poor, the infirm, and the feeble, physically, socially, morally, and religiously. In 1862, the Manchester and Salford Sanitary Reform Association decided to employ people to make day-to-day visits among the poor, to teach and to help. The duties included the following:

TEACHING HYGIENE AND CHILD WELFARE

> They must carry with them carbolic powder; explain its use and leave it where it is accepted; direct the attention of those visited to the evils of bad smells, want of fresh air, impurities of all kinds; give hints to mothers on feeding and clothing their children.

> SOCIAL SUPPORT
>
> Where they find sickness, assist in promoting comfort of the invalid by personal help.
>
> TEACHING OF MENTAL AND MORAL HEALTH
>
> They must urge the importance of cleanliness, thrift and temperance on all possible occasions.[3]

Later this voluntary venture was incorporated into the Manchester Public Health Department and this practice soon spread throughout England. Because of the lack of uniformity in training, functions, or titles of this group, the London County Council set up regulations governing qualifications and certification in 1909. Training Centers were established and examinations were developed and administered.

In the United States, nursing care of the sick in their homes by a graduate nurse (Frances Root) began in New York City in 1877. These services were organized by private citizens who saw the need and consequently founded the beginning of the Visiting Nurses' Association. These services soon spread to other cities.

In 1882, Robert Koch reported studies that demonstrated that tuberculosis was a transmissible disease caused by a specific organism. This new concept of disease brought a new approach to the control of tuberculosis—that of public health measures. It was quickly recognized that the community health nurse could make a contribution to disease treatment and control.

In 1898, Los Angeles became the first city to officially employ a nurse to care for the sick at home. With the new concept of disease causation—the germ theory—nursing gained a broader range of duties. They became responsible for casefinding and caseholding, for teaching patients and their families, and for providing pre- and posthospital nursing care under the auspices of the official health agency. As nurses recognized other problems in these homes and as knowledge about preventive measures evolved, nurses moved into other specialized programs such as school nursing, maternity nursing, and child health programs. These programs expanded under the auspices of the specific health department.

In 1902, Lillian Wald organized the first school nursing program by public health nurses in New York City. Lina Rogers, the first school nurse, evolved a plan to solve some of the health problems of the school-age child. As a consequence of her work, twelve public health nurses were employed in the New York City Health Department to carry out her plan. This pattern spread to other states although some transferred the responsibility of the health department to the State Department of Education. Currently, we still have these two plans of responsibility for school nursing services and in some instances they are shared by the health and education departments.

Other specialty areas of community health nursing evolved at this time. Occupational-health nursing programs, which were initiated in 1895, preceded slightly the school nursing specialty and both were followed by the venereal disease nursing specialty in 1909. Maternal and child health programs evolved as a nursing specialty in 1912 and 1913 when health departments started maternity services and child-health conferences under the leadership of the Children's Bureau.

Another important development took place in 1909 when Lillian Wald persuaded the Metropolitan Life Insurance Company to begin home nursing services for its policyholders. This was initiated through a working arrangement with the Henry Street Settlement, which had become a model and training center for community nursing. This program was highly successful and with some modifications was adopted by other insurance companies in the following years. These programs in which insurance companies paid full costs for nursing services placed community-health nursing agencies on a firm financial base. Later, services were provided to non-policyholders on a fee-for-services basis among those able to pay. This practice contributed to the growth of privately supported visiting nurse agencies and at the same time changed the notion that community nursing services were only for the poor.

In 1910, the first academic program for preparing community nurses was begun at Teachers College of Columbia University. Prior to this movement, the academic world saw nursing training as a kind of apprenticeship such as the type that was established at the Henry street settlement. Although other colleges and universities followed this pattern, it was soon recognized that community health should be an integral part of the preparation of all nurses rather than a specialty. In 1923, the Yale School of Nursing was founded as a collegiate school and was the first to include community health as part of the preparation of all nurses. Slowly other schools adopted this pattern, but it was not until after World War II that community health nursing became an integral part of all basic collegiate curriculums and a requirement for a school's accreditation by the National League for Nursing.

This trend toward community health nursing being an integral part of all nursing curriculums was carried over into community-health nursing practice. Here, also, there was a shift from specialization to generalization. Under this pattern, staff nurses became responsible for all kinds of services in their district, and the agency provided them with consultant services. This generalized concept of nursing was fostered by the National Organization for Public Health Nursing, which was organized in 1912.

After World War II, there were increased demands for nursing services at a time when the supply was limited. Wider use of the team concept and the use of auxiliary personnel under supervision was tried in agencies to meet this increased demand. Teams are still being used and the concepts of team delivery-of-care are presented in Chapter 8.

With the growing number of health agencies employing nurses, there was also an effort to prevent duplication of services by official and voluntary agencies in communities. One method was to combine agencies whenever possible, for example, the health department and visiting nurse association. This had the effect of further generalizing the nurse's work to include a wide range of ages, conditions and settings, and also to use the total spectrum of prevention in their work; that is, instead of focusing on bedside care or teaching health maintenance and promotion, nurses were involved in teaching and counseling for the prevention of disease and the promotion of health as well as bedside care of the sick at home and rehabilitation, where indicated. These activities are elaborated upon in the next section and in Chapters 6 and 7.

CHARACTERISTICS OF COMMUNITY HEALTH NURSING

Often a valuable way of familiarizing yourself with the characteristics of a new practice area is to relate it to a known one. We have found this useful when introducing nurses to the characteristics of community health nursing, that is, to relate community health nursing to nursing in institutional settings such as hospitals and nursing homes.

We believe differences exist in the two settings (community and institution) that alter the nurse's role and make additional concepts, theories, and models imperative for effective practice. First, the patient groups that receive nursing services in the two settings may be different from one another. In the hospital, the nurse sees a selected sample of the communities population: people who have recognized an illness and have been motivated to seek, expect, and accept medical and nursing services. The nurse in the community, on the other hand, works with a population that has various ideas and values of health and illness. In addition, they are motivated by forces (economic, social, and so on) other than health, which may take precedence at that point in time. This may not be the case of hospitalized patients who are motivated to recover and who are legitimately exempt from other responsibilities. Whatever the concepts and values of health and the motivating forces of the individual and family at home, their behavior will reflect these values. Although the ultimate goal of nursing services may be the same in both settings, the nursing concepts and approaches in attaining it will be different.

Second, the length and intensity of nursing services rendered and the physical and mental condition of the patient varies in the two settings. In the hospital, the patient is usually acutely ill and requires intensive nursing care, often of a highly technical nature, over a short period of time. Here the emphasis may be on assisting patients to regain their adaptive skills (biopsychosocial) through therapeutic interventions. In the community, some members of the family may be acutely ill; some chronically ill; other members may appear well at any point in time, so that continued nursing services are needed over a longer period of time. Nurses in this setting are concerned with the more subtle and nontechnical factors and forces that may influence health and illness over time and the nurse must be highly sensitive to these subtleties. In this setting, the nurse may be primarily concerned with assisting individuals and families to maintain and increase their adaptive skills (physical, psychological, social). Each setting requires a different framework for assessing and using resources for health care. For example, in the hospital, nurses more often use their own resources in giving direct patient care and in helping patients regain their adaptive skills; whereas in the community, nurses may strengthen family resources through teaching and problem solving with the intent of helping them maintain or increase their adaptive skills, or nurses may complement the family and community resources to provide health care to the family.

Another important difference is the area of responsibility of each of the institutions. The hospital is primarily responsible for actions within the institution, and its goal is health—the treatment and recovery of patients. On the other hand, the public health agency has responsibility for all health concerns within a geographic area and its goal is health at all levels of prevention from primary to rehabilitation (see also Chap. 9).[4]

Nurses working in the community must use a framework that allows them to elevate community health by working with families and groups. To do so they need an understanding of the influence of the family on the community, and the influence of the community on the family in relation to health, resources, and autonomy. The systems theory related to individuals, families, and communities provides this framework (see Chaps. 1 through 4). Nurses must also use a systematic process in assessing family and group health problems and patterns (see Chap. 6) and must consider the multiple, interrelated factors that influence health and behavior, if they are to effectively focus upon primary, secondary and tertiary preventions concurrently (see Chap. 9). They must also consider the consequence of their actions before proceeding with services and plans, if they are to maintain and improve health in the population.

The differences between hospitals and community health can be further elaborated on by the following comparison of the role of the general-duty staff nurse in the hospital—a role that is familiar to all nurses—and that of the first-level community health nurse in the community. This contrast was published by myself and other coworkers in Nursing Outlook in 1968 and is reproduced as follows:[5]

UNIT OF SERVICE

Hospital staff nurse—Unit of service has a single focus: the individual hospitalized patient or patients in a ward unit.

Community health nurse—Unit of service has a double focus: the small group; the family (micro approach). Individual is always considered in relation to other family members and to the community. Second, the nurse is concerned with groups of people or subgroups in the community (macro approach). This may involve specific age groups (child health conference), specific health problem (venereal disease), specific condition (expectant parents), or specific places (school or industry).

HEALTH FOCUS

Hospital staff nurse—Focus is on treatment and care of the sick patient and on restoring the individual's balance toward health. Nurse responsible for nursing care of patient. She may delegate responsibility to ancillary workers. Contact with patients is over a short period of time.

Community health nurse—Focus is multiple: on promoting health, maintaining a degree of balance toward health, early detection of disease, and care measures (restorative, habilitation, and rehabilitation).

Focus is on assessment of the impact of socioeconomic and cultural factors affecting health measures that must constantly be dealt with and often take priority in order for family to assume health measures.

Nurse's goal is to assist patient, family, or caretaker to assume nursing care responsibility. Nurse may give partial nursing care or delegate responsibility to ancillary worker. This may include temporary treatment before, during, or after hospitalization, partial assistance as an occasional bath to an aged person with a chronic disease, or partial service, such as administering medication or changing dressings.

Contact with the individual or family continues for a long time.

RANGE AND VARIABILITY OF WORK

Hospital staff nurse—works with disease classification in hospital units, as in medical-surgical, or with age groups, as in pediatrics. Problems are identified and the nurse works with identified diseases as priorities.

Nurse works with acutely ill patients.

Variability is restricted to one ward or service.

Community health nurse—Works with the entire spectrum of health and illness conditions, from optimal health to minor or severe disease conditions, from acute to chronic illnesses.

Works in all kinds of settings—home, school, clinic, industry.

Variability in one day may include all age groups.

Services cut across all areas of living, not just physical or mental health. This may include such areas as recreation, nutrition, or budgeting.

BOUNDARIES OF SERVICE

Hospital staff nurse—Deals with one hospital or one institution. Institution's goal is health—treatment and recovery of its patients.

Community health nurse—Deals with all institutions, those whose primary goal is health, and those with other goals. Works in schools, where primary goal is education, or in industry, where the primary goal is production. The nurse deals with both community and world agencies.

The legal responsibility of the official health agency may cut across jurisdictional lines. (If an individual with a communicable disease moves from one county to another, there is a legal responsibility to notify the receiving county.)

COORDINATION

Hospital staff nurse—Coordination must be achieved between all personnel responsible for patient care within the institution, such as doctor, social worker, physiotherapist, x-ray personnel, lab technician, and clergy.

Coordination with community nursing agencies to achieve continuity of nursing care for the patient on discharge.

Community health nurse—Coordination must be achieved among a variety of medical and nonmedical personnel within the health agency and with those outside, such as sanitarian, plant foreman, teacher, social worker, and rehabilitation worker from the hospital.

Focus is on continuity of health care, including nursing care. Coordination of other agencies and efforts in achieving this goal must also be obtained.

The nurse is in touch with community lay groups as well as official agencies, such as parent groups, Salvation Army, Senior Citizens, welfare and probation departments.

This contrast can be further spelled out by comparing some of the unique characteristics that affect nursing services and activities in the hospital and community. They include the following:

LEGAL AND MEDICAL AUTHORITY

Hospital staff nurse—Legal authority underlying the nurse's work in the hospital is derived from the policies of the institution and state laws regulating nursing practice.

Medical authority is available for medical direction. The patient is always under medical care. The diagnosis and treatment orders provide the framework for many aspects of nursing care activities.

Community health nurse—Legal authority underlying the nurse's work in the official health agency is vested in the health officer and is founded on health regulations and laws. It encompasses all health concerns within a political jurisdiction.

Medical authority frequently is more distant and indirect. It may be vested in the health officer, medical program director, private medical practitioner, or general agency policies. In certain settings, such as the school, medical direction may be contained only in general policies.

Frequently there is no medical diagnosis, nor is the patient or family under medical care. The nurse may make the health assessment, decisions about the need for securing medical care, and referral to medical resources, or initiate the families' contact with them.

NURSING AUTONOMY

Hospital staff nurse—The physician is the medical authority. The nurse relates the patient's condition to him and he makes decisions about further medical treatment. Workload is regulated by hospital admissions.

Nurse is assigned responsibility for several patients or for certain tasks for a large number of patients such as giving medications or certain treatments.

Has autonomy for planning and implementing nursing care measures for patients in hospital unit.

Community health nurse—Medical autonomy may be delegated to nurses. They thus represent medical authority in the home, school, or plant.

They may make decisions for medical treatment in the immediate setting. The nurse shares medical management with the private physician and others.

The health needs of the population in the community regulates the nurse's work. Nurses are responsible for management of caseloads in the district or the population groups served.

Have autonomy for planning and implementing nursing care measures for patients and families. They have extensive authority for making decisions and for developing or initiating various health and group activities in the community, and share this planning with various community groups.

FAMILY AND PATIENT AUTONOMY

Hospital staff nurse—Individual autonomy of patient is restricted. The patient must fit into the hospital routine. His family is restricted by visiting hours and hospital policies.

The patient has consented to hospital services on admission, and he expects nursing services as part of his care.

The patient is not functioning in his usual activities or with the same control over his environment.

Community health nurse—Family has complete autonomy and control, except for communicable diseases.

The patient or family may not have asked for or consented to nursing services. They may not be aware of nursing services in the community. Family may resent services, as in tuberculosis where the health department has a legal responsibility.

Family or individual is functioning to some degree with control over his environment. Nurse may give partial assistance; the family the rest, or the nurse may make known available resources and leave the contacting to the family.

PREDICTABILITY OF EVENTS

Hospital staff nurse—The course of events is primarily focused on treatment of the individual patient in one place and time.

Factors in the patient's home environment are not observed by the nurse.

Community health nurse—There is an interplay of multiple factors in daily living that affect family and community health in the home environment, such as social, physical, emotional climate, and cultural background. These multiple factors are in constant movement and may change direction of health at any time, such as, father losing job or mother getting sick. These multiple factors may be directly observed and the nurse must be alert to their being associated with one another.

SPHERE OF INTIMACY

Hospital staff nurse—The patient is stripped of his clothing and privacy.

The hospital setting is an artificial environment for the patient and limits the nurse's observation of family relationships or other indicators of health.

Community health nurse—The home is the most private sphere of life in which intimate relationships may be directly observed.

There is no restriction on the usual behavior of the family members in the home.

Other indicators of health may be directly observed such as housing, sanitation, and neighborhood.

SCOPE OF PROFESSIONAL RELATIONSHIPS

Hospital staff nurse—The nurse's relationships are in the main limited to hospital personnel. She reaches into the community when implementing plans for continuity of nursing care for her patient.

Community health nurse—Nurse has professional relationships with people in various disciplines other than medical. She is responsible for assisting patients and families to coordinate health care, which necessitates contact with personnel from health, welfare, and other significant community agencies.

ACCESSIBILITY OF NURSE TO STIMULATE NURSING ACTIVITIES

Hospital staff nurse—The focus is on the health of the individual patient or a group of patients within the boundary of the hospital.

The nurse may interest and stimulate activities of the outside community for additional services to patients. For example, she may initiate a friendly visiting service to patients.

Community health nurse—In the home the family unit offers a pivotal point for the following:

Integration of health services of the community to individuals and families.

Integration and stimulation of new activities and community resources needed for the health of the family or population group.

CASEFINDING AND CASEHOLDING

Hospital staff nurse—Casefinding is determined by hospital admission policies and cases are held until they have regained a degree of adaptive skills. This is usually of a short-term nature and is determined by the hospital physician.

Community health nurse—Cases may be channeled to the nurse from a variety of agencies dealing with high-risk community groups or nurses may identify high-risk cases in their community. They carry these families until there is no longer a need for assistance with maintaining and increasing adaptive skills. This decision is usually made in conjunction with the supervising nurse and agency policies, although in some instances (communicable diseases) the physician may make the final decision.*

GOALS OF COMMUNITY HEALTH NURSING

Four major goals of community health nursing follow. These include (1) helping individuals, families, groups, and the community (systems) reach the highest level of health compatible with human potential and desire (2) providing comprehensive care to these systems (3) preserving the autonomy of the system, and (4) improving nursing and public health practice.

GOAL ONE—HIGH LEVEL WELLNESS

The first goal of community health nursing is to help individuals, families, groups, and communities reach the highest level of health compatible with human potential and desire and within the socioeconomic environment. Although people and situations vary over time within communities and the family household, nurses strive to reach this goal by working with exchanges in the family and community system and its environment, as they exist at any particular time. Nurses at any time may be working at the tertiary end of a continuum of preventive services giving physical care and psychological support to individuals, groups, and families who lack the physical and emotional ability to meet their own needs. Or, they may relieve a busy mother periodically on whom the total care of the family falls. This helps the mother maintain her adaptive ability (physical, psychosocial) without being overloaded. In both instances, the energies of the nurse are used to assist others to regain or maintain their energy level (health) and balance. At another time or concurrently with the above activities, nurses may teach signs and symptoms of illness, preventive care, aspects of diet, personal hygiene, the need for rest, and community re-

*Copyright 1968, American Journal of Nursing Company. Reproduced with permission from Nursing Outlook, Vol. 16, no. 8, Aug 1968

sources available to assist the family or group when they lack the resources to cope with threats. This will increase the family's mental ability to cope with future stress situations and will move them to a higher level of order and organization (negentropy).

At other times, nurses may identify environmental energies that pose a threat to community groups. For example, they may identify sickness caused by a water supply or by food and would consult the sanitarian who would check on biologic excesses in these mediums. If confirmed, the sanitarian and nurse would take steps to prevent further illness.

Or, nurses may find attitudes in community groups that are nonconducive to a higher level of health and would work as a change agent to bring these attitudes into alignment with healthful attitudes, based upon scientific knowledge. For example, nurses may find groups who are opposed to fluoridation of water or immunizations. Based upon their knowledge, they know that both are helpful for a higher level of health by preventing dental cavities and a variety of diseases. Through the nursing process to be discussed in Chapter 6, nurses can work to change these attitudes.

Interrelatedness of Family and Community. It should be clear from the foregoing that the family and community are closely interrelated. The level of health of the family can affect the total community, and vice versa. For example, a communicable disease such as tuberculosis or venereal disease in an individual or family poses a major threat to others in the community, and if unchecked may run rampant through the community lowering the level of the community's health. This is clearly shown in one of the many examples of struggle and partnership among man and disease agents in *Mirage of Health* by Dubos, who says,

> The destructive power of tuberculosis when it first strikes a population is well illustrated by the epidemic among the Plains Indians of Western Canada. In the 1890's the annual death rate from tuberculosis in the Qu'Appelle Valley Reservation of Saskatchewan reached the fantastic figure of close to ten percent of the total population. More than half the Indian families were eliminated in the first three generations of the epidemic. Moreover, some twenty percent of the deaths in the surviving families were caused by tuberculosis.[6]

On the other hand, the community may also affect its families. For example, if a community lacks the necessary resources for giving preventive care services such as immunizations, food and water inspection, or garbage disposal, the population may suffer additional diseases, which another community with such services would avoid, and would thus be at a lower level of health because of the community.

Ordinarily when groups in the community lack resources to meet their own health needs, whether preventive or curative, they turn to the community for such services. Therefore, their resources are closely tied to those of the community. Since families are also evolving in a dynamic environment, the need for assistance from community sources varies depending upon the health situation of the family. For example, when a family member gets sick, others must take on additional duties. If the illness is of short duration and of minor consequence, families may have the resources to deal with the illness. On the other hand, if it is a long-term major illness, the family may need assistance from the community for medical care and perhaps part-time nursing care. This should be available to help the patient regain his adaptive abilities and balance and the family members maintain theirs.

Another area where family and community are closely interrelated and which may influence the level of health is individual and group autonomy. This, too, is constantly shifting as new diseases, knowledge, and so forth evolve. Isolation of cases, immunization, food inspection, pasturization of milk, and garbage disposal are examples of community autonomy. When new threats are posed to a community population, humans may lose some of their autonomy for the preservation of the group. Without community autonomy the level of health would not reach its potential.

Families and community are closely interrelated, then, in terms of health, autonomy, and resources. Because humans and their environment are continually evolving as is health knowledge, then health, autonomy, and resources should also be seen as dynamic concepts.

Major Focus on Family and Groups to Meet Goal. Recognizing the interrelatedness of the family and community, community health nurses focus primarily on families and groups (micro and macro approach) to elevate total community health. By working with families, nurses identify actual or potential health hazards and assist families to regain or maintain health. Likewise, they are able in this setting to measure family resources against those in the community. If they find gaps in community services, nurses take this back to the supervisor who channels the information to the administrator who, in turn, assists in initiating new community resources. The nurses then take this knowledge back to the families. Or, if nurses find individuals (*e.g.*, cases of communicable disease) who are putting their own autonomy before that of the community by refusing to remain isolated, they must work with them as well as with the supervisor who may use legal action to preserve community autonomy and, thus, increase the level of wellness in the community.

In one model in Chapter 9 we discuss two types of action that are used in primary prevention: interpersonal and social action. The community health nurse is involved primarily with interpersonal action and only indirectly with social action. As part of nurses' epidemiologic functions, they may identify situations that call for further investigation, which may ultimately lead to social action, however.

Major Focus in Families and Groups Is on Primary Prevention. The health care given by the community health nurse involves a wide spectrum of activities aimed at high level wellness. It involves working with individuals, families, and groups at their level on the health continuum within their socioeconomic and environmental limits, and may involve focusing on any of three levels of prevention (primary, secondary, or tertiary) to assist families in maximizing their potential or improving their level of wellness. At any time, they may help a recuperating stroke patient strengthen muscles to regain independence, or nurses may help families learn about preventive measures and problem-solving methods. Although nurses deal with families on all levels of the preventive-curative continuum, their major focus is on primary preventive activities.

The concept of levels of prevention and the knowledge needed to intervene at various stages in the health or illness process is presented in Chapter 9. The goal of **primary prevention** is to put humans in a favorable balance of health, by making disease agents less potent, making the environment less favorable for the interaction between humans and the disease agent, or making humans more resistant to disease agents. Because individuals, families, and communities are interrelated, the overall community goal is to help the community maintain or attain a higher level of health by reducing the incidence and prevalence of diseases.

With **secondary prevention,** the goal from a community point of view is to identify and treat the disease process early to reduce the length and severity of the illness for significant numbers of the population and to prevent the spread to others if the disease is communicable. During the **tertiary stage of prevention,** the goal is to increase the proportion of the sick population who are able to return to a level of health, which is as useful as possible, through treatment and rehabilitation.

GOAL TWO—COMPREHENSIVE CARE

A second goal of community health nursing is to provide the best possible health care to the greatest number of people in the community, consistent with agency priorities and policies. Comprehensive nursing care is often referred to in the literature and is one way of providing the best possible care. It may be defined as the provision of personal care, medically prescribed treatments, teaching, emotional support, environmental manipulation, and other activities such as are needed to promote comfort and optimal health of the family and protection of the community.

Comprehensive care is a broader concept than comprehensive nursing care and may incorporate team relationships with other health members for the benefit of families and community groups. It can be defined as "care that is provided to the patient according to his needs in an appropriate, continuous and dynamic pattern."[7] By "appropriate'' is meant care that is geared to the health needs of the particular client and/or family in whatever setting they happen to be at the moment. It is not a ready-made plan to be applied to all clients, but rather an individualized plan based upon an assessment of the physical, social, economic, and psychological needs and resources of the particular client and his family.

An important aspect of comprehensive care that is relevant to a discussion of ''appropriate'' continuous care is the concept of continuity of care. This concept is familiar to nurses from an individual client's point of view such as moving patients from acute-care to long-term facilities or to home as their condition warrants, but how often do we consider family members in this transition? Starting with the hospital setting, how often do we use the client's family in our nursing care plans? Is this not appropriate and would it not at times best meet the patient's needs? Perhaps the client's wife has given some nursing care in the home and helped to meet the client's psychological needs prior to hospitalization. Is this care disrupted at the time of hospitalization when the patient most needs the continued support of those close to him? And wouldn't the help of the client's wife in this case provide the needed continuity of care and perhaps increase her resources for coping with and caring for illness in the home, if supplemental teaching is provided (negentropy)? Or again, how often do we admit cardiac clients to hospitals or long-term care facilities who have taken medications at home for years and upon admission have their medications taken from them? If our objective is to provide for continuity of care and appropriate continuous care, then we should help to keep clients as independent as possible by letting them continue to administer their own medications if our assessment proves that they are alert enough to assume this responsibility. I have suggested using family resources and using the client's resources to provide continuity of care when a client is admitted to a hospital. Although these plans must be based upon a total assessment of client and family—if our goal is appropriate continuous care, which increases client and family resources and keeps families as independent as possible, our role may be assessment of client and family needs and resources and only supplementing these resources as needed.

As the client moves from the hospital to home again we need to assess client and family needs and resources. What care does the client need? Are family members able to physically provide this care? Are they psychologically prepared to have the patient at home? Do family members have the intellectual capacity to provide care and have they been taught the essential knowledge and skills? Has the client been prepared for discharge? If family resources are not adequate to meet these needs at home, community resources may be needed. This may require placing the client in a nursing home or providing supplemental nursing services to the patient and family at home. Again, appropriate care must be individualized and based upon an assessment of client and family needs and resources.

The usual pattern of supplemental nursing services at home is to provide part-time community health nursing services. It seems possible in some situations that movement of a particular hospital nurse, with whom the client had established a close relationship, to the home on a part-time basis might more appropriately and continuously meet the patient's needs. A few years ago a colleague and a friend at the University of California in San Francisco wrote an article on complemental nursing care that suggested a pattern of care in which the nurse followed clients prior to, during, and after hospitalization and was also available to them by phone when not with them. This pattern seems to provide the most appropriate care and continuous care when a good relationship has been established. However, with the exception of private duty nursing, other nursing groups are not organized for this type of continuity. Is it possible that something would be lost by this pattern of care? For example, community health nurses have traditionally focused on many aspects of care besides bedside care. They may focus on immunizations, food patterns, values and attitudes toward health, patterns of health care, and so forth. However, at the point of the client's movement from hospital to the home, do these benefits outweigh the value of the therapeutic relationship established between clients and their hospital nurse. Most of the above questions cannot be adequately evaluated without adequate studies, but we should not become rigid and follow usual patterns until we can prove, with further studies, that they are the most appropriate for families.

A **continuous pattern,** which is the second part

of the definition of comprehensive care, refers to a continuity of services to clients or families regardless of the facility in which they are located. Since this is related to appropriate care previously discussed, it will not be elaborated upon further.

A third part of the definition, a **dynamic pattern of care** means that care plans must continually be readjusted in the light of changes that occur in clients and their families. This involves an ongoing process of assessment, planning, implementing, and evaluating, which is discussed in Chapter 6. However, recognizing that health is an ongoing, ever-changing adjustment of humans to their changing environment, we can see the need for continually assessing, planning, and implementing. For example, as clients become comfortable in the hospital environment and adjust to their illnesses, they may require less emotional support. Or, as they adjust to (establish an equilibrium with) or ward off disease organisms, they may be able to assume more responsibility for their own physical care. Likewise, as they become more knowledgeable about the care of a colostomy, dressings, and so forth, they become more independent in this area. Each change in the client's energy level requires new nursing care plans.

Comprehensive care, then, can be viewed as a galaxy of services that can be called upon as needed by the client or family. According to the report of the Division of Chronic Diseases this can be diagramed as in Figure 5–1.[8] The innermost circle is the client and his family. The next circle represents an assessment of the client and family on four dimensions: physical, psychological, social, and economic. This evaluation determines the setting in which the client should be placed. A second evaluation determines the modalities used in the care of the client, such as, the patterns of service, and the degree and extent of care. Included in the first circle (the client and family) is an area for re-evaluation in light of any changes taking place.

Once evaluation or re-evaluation have been carried out the appropriate facility must be notified. Further, because of changes in client and family conditions, communication and free flow between agencies must be brought into the picture so that clients can easily move from one facility to another.

The setting in which care is to be given makes up the second circle surrounding the client. This includes home, inpatient, and outpatient care. Inpatient care includes all institutions such as general or specialized hospitals, long-term care facilities, half-way houses, and so forth. Outpatient services include outpatient departments, ambulatory programs of rehabilitation centers or patient visits to physicians, while home care may include nursing services, homemakers, meals on wheels, or other appropriate programs.

The last circle surrounding the client includes the individualized services, which may be brought together in varying patterns depending upon client needs and agency staffing patterns. Services needed for comprehensive care may include medical, nursing, social, dental, nutritional, occupational and other related services. These services may be provided in simple programs of nursing care given to the client at home or programs may be complex as in rehabilitation centers, where all disciplines may be involved.

Supportive items to a community-based comprehensive-care program are outside the client-family diagram. These necessary aspects of support include personnel, facilities, funds, administration, and coordination.

Certain principles necessary to provide continuity of care have been identified. First, administrative leadership is a fundamental ingredient in the operation of a continuity-of-care referral system. Since it is necessary to have free flow among agencies to ensure the smooth transition of clients from one facility to another, administrative leadership can facilitate this. In some areas, the Community Health Council has assumed this role and has drawn representation from professional groups, health and welfare councils, civic and service clubs, and frequently influential persons. The council strives to bring about understanding and action on community problems by keeping the agencies informed of one another's programs, to deficiencies and blocks in community services, and to the need to extend or reduce health services. In some areas, the public health director has assumed this responsibility for coordinating community services, identifying gaps and overlapping of services, and so forth.

In whatever administrative structure is provided for coordinating services, nursing should be represented. The role of staff nurses may be to inform the administrative structure of any obstructions to continuity to care, gaps in services, and so forth

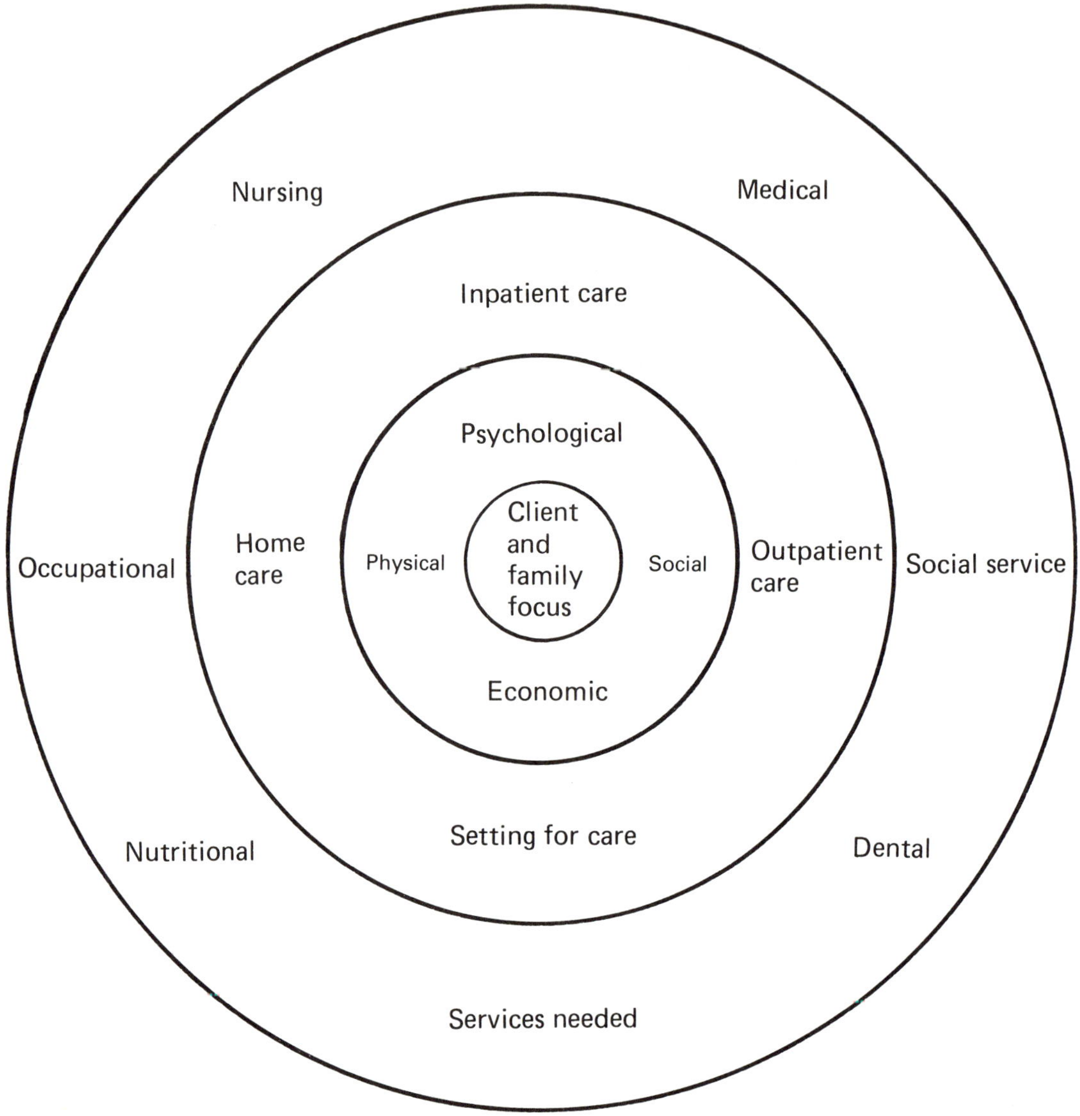

Figure 5–1

Comprehensive care for clients and their families. (Adapted from Lilienfeld A, Gifford A (eds): Chronic Diseases and Public Health, pp 184–186. Baltimore, Johns Hopkins, 1966)

identified during their work with families and groups.

A second principle says that one person must be in a central coordinating position with basic responsibility for intra- and interagency referrals. Although everyone in an agency should be free to initiate referrals as indicated, there should be one overall coordinator to supervise continual care, stimulate interest in continuity, serve as a liaison with other agencies to keep the system going, and so forth. This person is often a nurse because nursing is usually a part of all health-care activities.

In addition, one person should be in a central coordinating position with respect to the multitude of services that may be provided to a client or family in any setting and in any location on the health continuum. For example, a client at home may need, in addition to nursing care, other care such as medical, nutritional, homemaker, welfare, physical therapy, and so forth. Because nurses represent the one discipline on the health team that continues to care for the client and family over a long period of time, they are in the best position to observe changes in the client and family from multiple biologic, social, psychological, and economic forces, and as a result should coordinate the services.

A third principle says that if a system is to be effective in providing continual comprehensive care as clients move from one setting to another, effective administrative procedures and tools are essential. These set the stage for transmitting information in any direction. We should be able to answer questions such as the following: How are referrals to be initiated? How does information get from one agency to another? How are new staff oriented?

Wolff says that certain questions are recommended before making a referral.[9] She says that we must ask (1) "Is there mere in it?" For example, are we referring the patient at home to his physician for a minor complaint, which the physician does not want to be bothered with? (2) "Is it practical?" For example, some mothers may need to take all her children with her when she goes to the hospital clinic. This may involve getting them cleaned and dressed. If she must take a bus, she must manage getting them on and off; this also requires extra busfares. If this is her first trip she needs to get directions, watch for the hospital, and watch her children at the same time. At the hospital she may have a long wait with the children and then finally must make the trip home. (3) "Does the referral fit the person's individuality?" For example, have the parents of a retarded child who are referred to a parent discussion group of these problems come to grips with the problem? (4) "Is the patient's right to say 'no' respected?" This is a basic right as part of the patient's autonomy and should be respected without repercussions by the nurse.

Although much of the discussion has revolved around long-term chronically ill patients who require movement from one setting to another and who constitute a minor part of the community-health nurse's caseload, these concepts are equally applicable to any group at any level on the health continuum. Comprehensive care in the home demands that the nurse continue to assess all plans with families, and to implement these plans. At times, this may mean bringing in other disciplines with knowledge and skills beyond the nurses, to assist with family situations. At such times referral and open communication are important. The dynamics of this as it applies to comprehensive care is conceptualized in Chapter 4 where the system of health and its subsystems are discussed.

Over the last 20 years there has been an interest in adding additional skills to the nurse's repertoire and in extending the nurse's role, which has been discussed in the journals. Some of these role changes involve skills previously performed by the physician. Nurses with additional educational preparation and an internship (usually with a physician) have functioned effectively to provide well child care and emergency care to children, to identify acute and chronic conditions in children and make referrals, to manage health care in stabilized medical clients, and to provide prenatal, postpartum, and labor and delivery services to women without pathologic complications. Brown and also Browning and Lewis have written informative books on the expanded nurse's role.[10,11] Expanded roles for nurses may facilitate comprehensive care as a health worker by increasing the range of skills. This may prove to be a more effective approach to health-care delivery than the previous attempt of coordinating a variety of services and disciplines.

Expanded-role skills should benefit clients seen by community health nurses in the home, clinic, school, or occupational health setting. In addition, some nurses are providing expanded-role services in private practice, group practice, and in corporations.[12,13,14] The expanded-role functions will be discussed further in Chapter 8.

Community health nurses must also plan their work to ensure the greatest good to the greatest number of people consistent with agency policies. This means that nurses must set priorities for visits to families within their caseload and must plan visits at times when they can be most productive. For example, an age-group priority may be mothers and children because of the opportunity to influence this group at a time when they are developing and learning health habits. Or, nurses may want to visit families experiencing crises because of the belief that families are more receptive to change at this time. (This is discussed further in Chapter 10.) Nurses also need to set priorities within a specific category within the caseload. For example, they may have many prenatal mothers and will need to decide which ones need visiting more often or which ones can be taught in groups. Many agencies have set guidelines for these priorities of service based upon groups at highest risk, such as, young mothers, mothers having first children, mothers with previous complications, and so forth. Some of these high-priority groups are discussed in Chapter 11. Nurses use their knowledge of health to determine priorities of service after they have made an assessment of the family.

GOAL THREE—AUTONOMY

A third goal of community health nursing is to preserve the autonomy of the individual, family, or groups within the limits of community autonomy. Each contact the nurse makes with families or groups should provide an opportunity to help them maintain or attain a higher level of health, which will help them remain autonomous. Autonomy may be preserved by assisting them in learning problem solving, by teaching the signs and symptoms of illnesses and the ways to avoid illness, or by teaching the dietary needs of the body at various stages of growth and development. Each contact should help the family move toward self-sufficiency and a higher level of health. Since the concept of autonomy is discussed later in this chapter under Philosophy and is related to nursing process in the next chapter, it will not be further elaborated upon here.

GOAL FOUR—IMPROVED NURSING AND PUBLIC HEALTH PRACTICE

A final goal of community health nursing is to improve nursing and public health care provided for individuals, families, and the community. Through the process of self-evaluation, peer and supervisor evaluations of performance, individual nurses should have a good knowledge of how they perform as compared to other nurses with similar backgrounds and experience. In addition, a plan for improving performance based upon the identified weaknesses (self, peer, or supervisor) should improve the quality of care provided (see Chap. 12). Beyond these efforts to improve nursing practice, theory development and research should be an ongoing aspect of nursing in-service or education settings to make nursing care timely and of the highest quality as nurses interact with a dynamic society.

PHILOSOPHY OF COMMUNITY HEALTH NURSING

Wiedenbach says, "Philosophy, an attitude toward life and reality that evolves from each nurses beliefs and code of conduct, motivates the nurse to act, guides her thinking about what she is to do and influences her decisions. It stems from both her culture and subculture and is an integral part of her."[15]

Dunn says, "all persons need a personal philosophy—that is, a way of life . . . Social organizations need a philosophy too. The family, the community, the work organization, the church, the nation—all of these must have a philosophy. . . . If a philosphy is to be meaningful, it must be consciously lived. . . . It must be something which you try out, experience, and acquire self confidence in doing."[16]

The nurse's philosophy, then, is an integral part of the framework for community health nursing. It influences how the nurse will function with families, groups, and co-workers in a community and is based upon beliefs about the individual, family, and community, beliefs about health, and about nursing. A philosophy is also essential in setting goals for an individual or group.

Nurse's philosophies are influenced by the system of which they have been a part, that is, their family, church, community, education, and so forth. Because the beliefs, attitudes, and values that underlie a philosophy evolve in a variety of systems, conflict among competing values is possible. These in turn may conflict with the values underlying community health and community health nursing. Recognition of such conflicts may be accomplished by making explicit the philosophy of community health and the values underlying it. Evaluation and resolutions of conflicts by the nursing student should be encouraged during educational and clinical experiences. This should later provide some consistency in how the nurse functions which in turn should have a positive effect on the health of families and the community in which the nurse works.

The philosophy of community health nursing derives from acceptance of certain concepts and facts as a foundation for working with people. Among these are (1) the essential dignity and worth of the individual, (2) the possession by individuals of potentialities and resources for managing their own lives, (3) the importance of freedom to express one's individuality, (4) the great capacity for growth within all social beings, (5) the right of the individual to basic necessities (food, shelter, medical care) without which fulfillment of life is often blocked, (6) the need for individuals to struggle and strive to improve their life and environment, and (7) the right of the individual to help in times of need and crisis. These concepts and the values underlying them will be discussed more fully below.

PHILOSOPHY CONCERNING INDIVIDUALS AND GROUPS

Human Life Is Valued and Health Is Essential. The philosophy of community health must be consistent with the overall national philosophy. In America, the national philosophy of a democracy emphasizes the needs and rights of the majority. This framework allows services to evolve as needs are identified and plans for meeting these needs are supported by the majority. Systems and services that continue to meet the needs of the majority are perpetuated in some form as part of the social system. A view of the purposes of these existing systems gives us an understanding of the underlying cultural values.

Underlying the health services in our culture are the values we place on human life and health. When humans began living in groups, they recognized that what affected the individual or family, directly or indirectly, affected the total community. In early times their attention was primarily focused upon communicable diseases, which often spread from individual to individual, and community to community. Because these threatened survival they organized to combat them, and as one health problem was brought under control, new ones came to their attention, and they developed new plans to meet the challenges. Societies continual support of the health system indicates the value it places on health and life.

In community health nursing, we recognize this cultural value and believe that everyone has a right to good health and a long, productive life. This includes the right to basic necessities including health care in times of need and crisis. This belief is reflected in our systematic approach (nursing process) to the client (individual, family, community); in our activities, which aim to put the client system in a favorable balance of health; in our efforts to provide comprehensive quality services to all social, cultural, and racial groups; and in our efforts to continually improve health services offered (preventive and curative) by coordinating those that exist, or initiating new ones in a manner acceptable to the population being served.

Humans Are Basically Good and Are Capable of Thinking and Controlling Their Environment. In our culture, individuals are recognized as human beings who have the intellectual capacity to meet their basic needs. In the past, individuals as part of a simple agricultural society met most of the basic needs of the family. However, as society evolved into an industrial complex, individuals became increasingly dependent upon the community. This was necessitated by the increased specialization of society created by rapid changes in science and technology. However, despite individuals' increased dependence upon the community, the cultural value in them as basically good human beings who have the intelligence to grow and to control their environment has endured and affected the giving of services.

Recognizing that health facilities and services are available to all, we need to consider how much knowledge individuals need to have in order to function in a complex environment. Because of this complexity and human interdependence we believe that everyone has some kind of health-learning need, and that people sometimes need help in recognizing that they need help. That is, all humans have physical, intellectual, emotional, social, spiritual, and aesthetic needs from conception to death. Human beings vary in their ability to cope successfully with adaptation in these areas on the basis of both genetic endowment and environmental influences. Consequently, part of our role becomes that of a health educator—giving individuals, families, and groups the tools that enable them to control their environment and make wise decisions in relation to health. But in most instances decisions are left up to individuals because of our belief in their ability to think, to grow and to act appropriately.

This belief influences how we use the nursing process with clients (individuals and groups). We help clients solve problems, point out alternative solutions, and provide information that lets the client make sound decisions about health and health care. Thus as a result of our contact with clients, they become more knowledgeable about health, illness, and community resources, and develop more skills in problem solving and caring for the sick and are more independent (negentropy). Hopefully, we have given them the tools to grow based upon our belief that they have this capacity.

This is in opposition to a behavioristic perspective which views individuals solely in objective fashion and manipulates human responses through methods such as conditioning, flooding, and systematic desensitization. Human behaviors would be manipulated by the nurse and the belief is that by changing the behaviors of the individual, the person begins to function differently and view himself differently. The behavioristic model is one approach to treating pathologic behavior and has been particularly successful in treating phobias. But as with any treatment, health workers must not use these methods against a person's will (see the Trust Model, Chap. 7).

Health Is Essential for a Society To Be Productive and to Perpetuate Its Culture. In our society which allows social mobility, individuals are always striving for a higher standard of living. We give support to those movements that provide more leisure time, more education, more money to purchase necessary and leisure items, and so forth. These things that are valued can only be realized if society as a whole is productive and if the culture is perpetuated, and for this, health is essential.

Anderson substantiates this concept when he says,

> The promotion of health has a beneficial effect upon the economy of a nation, which in turn will affect the nation's cultural and social advancement . . . clear up disease and people can feed themselves. At the termination of WWII four out of every five people living in Greece had malaria. Led by the U.S. an intensive program was instituted to eradicate the disease in Greece. With D.D.T. to eliminate the anopheles mosquito and chemicals to treat the cases a near miracle was achieved both in terms of health and the nation's food supply. Agricultural production was increased by 40% so that more milk, poultry, olives and other foods were available to the people.[17]

Community health recognizes that many of the values held by the population can only be realized if society is productive and its culture is perpetuated and focuses on key groups of the population to ensure these goals. In the past we have been instrumental in reducing maternal and infant mortality, infant defects and illnesses, and loss of work by the adult population from illness or disability. We continue to provide services to these key groups in society (see Chap. 11) and add other high-risk groups as indicated.

Variations in Cultural Values. Although we have said that human life is valued and health is essential in our culture, we realize that this pertains to most but not to all of the population. We have a mixture of minority groups within our country from other cultures, societies, and religions who perpetuate their background. This leads to a wide divergence in attitudes and degrees to which health is valued or to concepts of health. Health behavior reflects values and beliefs.

Hanlon acknowledges variations in cultural values of health and says that there are three general categories of identifiable groups in the community consisting of ethnic groups, economic and social groups, and different family groups.[18] Thus, the community must think in terms of what is best for all individuals in the community even though this may mean sacrificing the rights and priviledges of some individuals for the benefit of the total community.

In community health nursing we recognize that there may be conflicting values and concepts of health within segments of the population and try to reconcile these values with the values of the majority; that is, we assess the values of these groups as a baseline for providing services. Although this may be difficult for those of us who value health and have a knowledge of health, it is a necessary prerequisite for effecting change in the health behavior of this segment who are affecting the total community's health. For example, we have learned that if we discuss the basic four with a recent immigrant family from Mexico, we are not likely to change their eating patterns. However, if we evaluate the family's nutrition, and build upon this, based upon their background (likes and dislikes), their physiologic needs, economics, storage space, and other factors, and can point out the need for revised eating habits, change is more likely to occur. This is consistent with the principle of teaching, which encourages starting from where the client is.

Democracy—Autonomy. Within the framework of democracy, humans are viewed as being of dignity and worth and are thus given the freedom and right to achieve their goals in a free and voluntary manner. This implies that they have the right to make decisions regarding health and their mode of life in whatever manner is satisfying to them or seems to maintain a degree of balance for them (individual autonomy). This freedom in turn imposes upon them the obligation to assume responsibility for their decisions.

Because humans choose to live in groups and are aware of the effects of the individual on the group, and of the degree to which health is valued, it is necessary to set limits on individual autonomy for self-preservation of the group. Consequently, laws are set up at the state or national level by way of the majority and carried out at the local level for group benefit (community autonomy). Community and individual autonomy continually shift as dynamic humans and their environment evolve.

In community health, we recognize the dignity and worth of individuals and try to motivate them to positive action in matters that can affect other community members. However, we also recognize that our primary responsibility is to the community as a whole and therefore view individuals, families, and groups in relation to the community. Thus, legal action can be used as a last resort, where indicated, if other methods have proved unsuccessful.

PHILOSOPHY CONCERNING HEALTH

Thus far, we have looked at the cultural values underlying the philosophy of community health and the diversity of these values in minority groups. This diversity of cultural values in the population leads to a discussion of the need for community autonomy within a democratic society as a basis for group health protection. Since our goal of community health nursing is health for the community (individuals, families, community), it is important to look at our philosophy of health.

We believe health and illness are dynamic processes resulting from the interaction (input, output) of clients (individuals, families, and communities) with the environment. Because clients are continuously changing and growing (negentropy) and the environment is continuously changing, the relationships between them are constant shifting states of equilibrium and disequilibrium, which requires that the client adapt to maintain balance and purposeful direction. Failure to adapt may move clients (individuals, families, and communities) down the wellness continuum. Over time clients will move up and down the wellness continuum ranging from high level wellness to death depending upon their ability to adapt (see Chap. 9, Concept of Health for elaboration). At any point in time, the people of a community will fall at various levels on the wellness continuum and professionals in the health subsystem will work with different groups, at various points on the continuum, to help them regain, maintain, or attain a higher level of wellness. For example, some professionals will work with the well population in the community to prevent illness and to improve their level of wellness. Others will work with those who have failed to adapt. Some professionals, such as the community health nurse, may integrate all focuses in providing nursing care.

Over time as the age, sex, race, and social class distribution of the population and the environment (biologic, psychosocial, chemical) changes because of natural or man-made factors, the health and health needs of the population also changes. Assessment of these provides the basis for evaluating health services and planning new ones. In some instances there may be a need to better coordinate services. At other times, there may be a need for new services or there may be a need to help the community see a need for existing services. Because health and illnesses are processes, it is possible to intervene at various levels in these processes to prevent or treat early diseases (see Chap. 9).

PHILOSOPHY CONCERNING COMMUNITY HEALTH NURSING

The primary purpose of community health nursing is to help determine the health needs of systems (individual, family, community) and to offer comprehensive quality nursing services that will help them attain, maintain, or regain a high level of wellness. Community health nursing strives to meet this purpose by using a systematic approach—the nursing process and concurrent processes—to assist clients to meet their basic health needs.

We accept health as a dynamic process and believe that through intervening in this process and using knowledge of the natural history of diseases and also nursing and concurrent processes, we can provide comprehensive care that will move populations up the wellness continuum.

We also believe that as systems and their environment evolve and interact, new disease patterns also evolve, which bring about changes in health knowledge and health care. Community health nursing must be sensitive to and a part of the evolution of new knowledge that facilitates comprehensive, quality nursing care. Other aspects of philosophy for nursing can be found in the Code for Nurses and is discussed later in this chapter.[19]

SUMMARY OF PHILOSOPHY

In summary, the following concepts are basic to a philosophy of community health nursing:

- Everyone regardless of race, creed, sex, or sexual preference has a right to good health and a long productive life.
- Everyone has some kind of health learning need.
- Some people and communities need help to recognize that they need assistance to regain, maintain, or attain a high level of wellness.
- Humans integrate constructs and new knowledge that serve their purposes. Thus, knowledge must have meaning.
- Health and health care enable a society to be productive and perpetuate its culture, which affects the standard of living of its people.
- Health is only one of the competing values of humans and thus holds a different place in their priority system at different times.
- Different cultural groups, religious groups, and groups with different social backgrounds have different concepts and values of health.
- Individual and community autonomy vary over time and place.
- Humans are flexible and change with changing external and internal demands.
- Humans have a strong impulse for growth.
- Health is a dynamic adjustment of humans to their environment.
- Systems (individuals, families, communities) move up and down the wellness continuum.
- The major purpose of community health nursing is to help systems attain, maintain, or regain high level wellness.
- Community health nursing accomplishes this goal by using systematic processes.
- Over time new health knowledge and technology evolve to meet changing health needs.
- Community health nursing remains an effective force in society by utilizing and participating in the development of health knowledge and technology.

ISSUES AND DILEMMAS ENCOUNTERED IN COMMUNITY HEALTH NURSING

Brian Robinson

ETHICAL

After adequate assessment and planning, community health nurses intervene in systems (individuals, families, and communities) to help them attain, maintain, or regain wellness. At times, value conflicts are involved and must be resolved in a way that best supports the client or system. Decisions made by the nurse must evolve from a solid ethical base and the nurse must be accountable for nursing interventions and actions. The Code for Nurses (see Appendix F) provides direction for ethical decisions and actions. Some of the issues and dilemmas encountered in community health nursing follow.

> **Case Study.** As a community health nurse you make your weekly visit to the home of Mrs. Harrison, age 33, pregnant with her seventh child. While talking with her, she tells you that having this child would be too much of a burden economically and emotionally for their family. She goes on to ask for information on how and where to get an abortion. She also states that she and her husband have talked about an abortion, but have not come to a final decision as of yet.
>
> Suppose that your feelings are strongly anti-abortion. You wonder what you should do. Should you tell Mrs. Harrison your feelings and views on abortion and attempt to convince her that the right thing to do is to have the child? Do you supply her with the information she requested and let her decide what she should do, or, do you refer her to another nurse or agency and forget about Mrs. Harrison's problem?
>
> As a community health nurse you are now faced with an ethical dilemma. Ethical dilemmas are those situations that present problems or conflicts and give rise to questions such as, what ought I to do? What is the right thing to do? What harm or benefit will result from this action or decision?[19]

Ethical dilemmas are not new to nursing practice. However, with today's fast-paced and advancing technology, the dilemmas faced by nurses are more complex and far reaching in their implications and outcomes than was the case a few years ago. For example, changes in the legal system, such as, legalized abortion; penalties for child abuse; informed consent; the accepted rights of all citizens and changes in medical and health practice regarding death and dying; organ transplants, and so forth require complicated decision making in ethical areas. These and other changes have also increased the responsibilities of nurses and other health professionals to clients.

Responsibilities to Clients. In our technologically advanced society members of the health care team sometimes lose sight of the human factors involved in health care and rely more on the producers of technology. Christman states, "Humanness can easily take second place to this kind of machine potential. In striving to reach the ultimate in technique, the critical interaction of person to person can be masked by the intrusion of a mechanical apparatus."[20]

Nurses as well as other health care professionals must keep in mind that decisions made in day-to-day practice involve more than just turning knobs on a machine or taking one direction of care over another. It also involves considering the clients' views of themselves, their value systems, and their rights and needs to be active participants in the decision-making process. It also involves recognition of clients' needs for support and guidance and the meeting of these needs where indicated.

When dealing with ethical dilemmas and decision making, the first factor a nurse must keep in mind is her primary responsibility to the client. This point is illustrated in changes that have occurred in the nurses' code of the American Nurses' Association. In 1950, when the code was first adopted, it stressed the nurses "obligation to carry out the physicians orders" and safeguard the reputation of other health care professionals.[21] However, the 1976 revision of the code states nursings' responsibility is to protect the "client and the public when health care and safety are affected by the incompetent, unethical, or illegal practice of any person."[22] Childress says that these changes in the code are "important changes in the self-consciousness and maturity of the nursing profession.[23] Thus, nurses who once saw themselves in a subservient role of carrying our doctors orders without question are now placed in the position of questioning such orders, if indicated, on behalf of their client. The focus, then, has shifted from a physician to a client-oriented focus and has a professional basis for decision making rather than blind obedience.

Because of the competing responsibilities to the client, to the profession, and to other health care professionals, nurses often find themselves pulled between what they feel is best for the client, what is best for professional performance, and how to also remain loyal to other professionals in the health care setting. Thus, although nurses have a major responsibility to clients, the ethical dilemma in client situations involves a weighing of professional values and loyalties as well.

All efforts of the health care team are directed at the specific goal of returning the client to the highest possible level of wellness that is realistically obtainable. However, problems may arise in the way that the goal is reached. This point is illustrated in the case of a client, newly diagnosed, who has terminal cancer. The physician's opinion is that in the "best interest" of the client he should not be told his diagnosis. This opinion is based on the doctor's assessment of the client from observations and discussions during examinations and tests. However, the nurse's assessment and plan may vary from the physicians. For example, after caring for the client for several days and having to sidestep questions (*e.g.*, "I have cancer, don't I?" or "Am I going to die?") the nurse believes it is in the "best interest" of the client to inform him of his diagnosis. The question involved, then, is which approach will best help the health care system assist this client to reach a level of wellness; that is, what will reduce the client's anxiety and help him live out his remaining days in comfort

Ethical Issue—Telling the Truth. The first ethical issue that arises from this example is that of telling the truth. If the information is withheld on the assumption that the client will be harmed by being told the truth, then the health professional is satisfying one moral obligation to the client. This obligation is one of protection from harm. On the other hand, the individual's right to knowledge that will ultimately affect the client's self-determination is violated.[24]

Interprofessional Conflict. A second issue raised in this example is not between the client and the professional, but between the professionals themselves. This problem arises when there is a difference of values in those caring for the client. Because of this difference the nurse has a moral obligation to the client, to communicate to the physician her values concerning the client's right to know his diagnosis. This collaboration between professionals does in the ideal situation allow for the best decisions to be made about the client's care.

Professional Responsibility and Patient Rights. In ethical decision making, professionals must keep in mind that it is the client's problem and the client's right to decide the correct way to deal with the problem. The terminally ill client may refuse surgery for lung cancer, although the nurse and physician believe this refusal will shorten his life. However, the final choice, after alternatives have been presented, rests with the client.[25]

The nurse's responsibility is to aid the client in obtaining the needed information for making an informed decision. This information may include not only the client's diagnosis but also information directed at "probability, value, and risk for each projected consequence" to choices in decision making.[26] It is this information that allows the client to make a decision that is in his or her best interest and that of the family. This responsibility on the part of health professionals is stated in the American Hospital Association's "Patient's Bill of Rights," from a client's point of view. It says that the client has the right to obtain complete and correct information regarding diagnosis, treatment, and prognosis in terms he can understand from the physician.[27] The Patient's Bill of Rights can be found in Appendix G.

Although the Patient's Bill of Rights states that information is to be obtained from the physician, this cannot always be the case. For example, the community health client may be seen weekly by a visiting nurse and by a private physician only once a month, or less, for a short visit. Because of the time spent with each professional, the nurse may be the client's prime source of information about his condition. For this reason the nurse is morally obligated to provide information that is as complete and accurate as possible so that the client may make an informed decision about his condition.

When providing information to the client, the nurse has an additional obligation to avoid value judgements about the subject or the information being discussed. Value judgements can be either a conscious or unconscious act on the part of the nurse and may affect the client's decision about what he should do. An example of the nurse's recognition of value judgements in her work was presented in an earlier case study. Steele and coworkers state, "value judgements seem to evolve from what health professionals suppose a human ought to be and from their concepts of well-being."[28] It is an important yet sometimes overlooked fact that nurses need to be aware of their own value systems and their effects on their work with clients. It is this system that effects the type of information and manner in which it is provided.[29]

Self-awareness prevents the nurse from providing biased information to the client.[30] The concept of self-awareness and techniques for assisting the nurse to facilitate self-awareness are discussed as part of the nurse–client relationship in Chapter 7. In addition to self-awareness, the nurse must also be aware of the client's value system to facilitate their relationships and the client's decision-making processes.

Although ethics is a relatively new area of concern in community health nursing and nursing in general, there are a limited number of articles and texts devoted to this important subject. Interested readers are referred to Davis and Fromer.[31,32]

REFERENCES

1. The Living Bible Paraphrased, pp 96–197. Wheaton, Tyndale House, 1973
2. Polan J: Nursing In Society, p 46. Philadelphia, WB Saunders, 1978
3. Hale R, et al: The Principles and Practice of Health Visiting, p 8. London, Pergamon, 1968
4. Leavell H, Clark G: Preventive Medicine for the Doctor in His Community. New York, McGraw-Hill, 1965
5. Helvie C, et al: The setting and nursing practice. Nurs Outlook Vol. 16, No. 8:28–29, Aug 1968
6. Dubos R: Mirage of Health. New York, Doubleday, 1959
7. Division of Chronic Diseases, Public Health Service: The concept of comprehensive care. In Lilienfeld A, Gifford A (eds): Chronic Diseases and Public Health. Baltimore, Johns Hopkins University, 1966
8. Ibid
9. Wolff I: Referral: A Process and a Skill. Nurs Outlook Vol. 10, No. 4.:253–256, April 1962
10. Brown EL: Nursing Reconsidered: A Study of Change, Part 2. The Professional Role in Community Health. Philadelphia, JB Lippincott, 1971
11. Browning M, Lewis E: The Expanded Role of the Nurse. New York, The American Journal of Nursing, 1973
12. Kinlein ML: Independent nurse practitioner. Nurs Outlook 20:22–24, Jan 1972
13. Greenidge, et al: Community nursing practitioners—A partnership. Nurs Outlook 21:228–231, April 1973
14. Rafferty R, Carner J: Nursing Consultants, Inc.—A corporation. Nurs Outlook 21:232–235, April 1973
15. Wiedenbach E: Clinical Nursing: A Helping Art, p 13. New York, Springer, 1964
16. Dunn H: High Level Wellness, p 4. Arlington, RW Beatty, 1961
17. Anderson CL, et al: Community Health. St Louis, CV Mosby, 1978
18. Hanlon J: Public Health Administration and Practice, pp 58–60. 6th ed. St Louis, CV Mosby, 1974
19. Davis AJ, Aroskar MA: Ethical Dilemmas and Nursing Practice, p 6. New York, Appleton-Century-Crofts, 1978
20. Christman LP: Moral dilemmas for practitioners in a changing society. J Nurs Admin 3:15, 1973 Reproduced by permission.
21. Childress JF: Ethical issues in health care: The moral responsibility of nurses. An unpublished address for the Zula Mae Baber Bice Memorial Lecture, University of Virginia, 1979
22. American Nurses' Association: Code for Nurses with Interpretive Statements, p 3. Kansas City, American Nurses' Association, 1976
23. Childress JF, op cit
24. Davis AJ, Aroskar MA: op cit, p 2
25. Ryden MB: An approach to ethical decision-making. Nurs Outlook, p 705. Nov 1978
26. Ibid
27. American Hospital Association: Patient's Bill of Rights. Chicago, 1970
28. Steele SM, Harmon VM: Values Clarification in Nursing, p 12. New York, Appleton-Century-Crofts, 1979
29. Ryden M, op cit, p 706
30. Ibid
31. Davis AJ, Aroskar MA, op cit
32. Fromer M: Community Health Care and the Nursing Process, pp 111–146. St Louis, CV Mosby, 1979

PART II
PROCESSES IN COMMUNITY HEALTH NURSING

6
The Nursing Process

Although different disciplines in the health subsystem of a community have their own professional jargon and, thus, label aspects of their professional practice differently, the process of assessing, planning, providing and evaluating care to systems (individuals, families, communities) remains the same from discipline to discipline. Physicians talk about patient evaluations which include a history, a physical, and laboratory examinations as a basis for providing care, whereas, nurses and social workers often talk about their assessment of individuals and families as a basis for their care. Health planners talk about the community survey and diagnosis underlying care and other disciplines use other terminology for this aspect of the process.

In addition, different disciplines label the total process using various names. Nurses currently call this process the nursing process; physicians call it patient evaluation and management; health planners call it health planning; researchers call it the research method; and other disciplines call it problem solving.

Although the process remains the same from discipline to discipline, the focus and, in some instances, the goals may vary. Some health workers use the process to focus on the individual, others use it to focus on a family or a community. Some use it as a process for preventing diseases in individuals (systems) and others use it to treat individuals (systems). Others, such as community health nurses, maintain a double focus of prevention and treatment when using the process. In most instances, the goal for using the process is to provide more systematic health care for systems (individuals, families, communities), although researchers may use the process to be more systematic in setting up and carrying out their research. In addition to using this process in our professional practice, we often consciously or unconsciously use the same approach in solving problems in our own lives, whether these revolve around a deficit household budget or the need for health care by a family member.

Although in community health nursing practice we use the **concurrent processes** of relating and communicating along with the nursing process, we shall focus here on the nursing process and consider relating and communicating in Chapter 7. In Chapter 8, we shall look at team development and maintenance processes.

THE NURSING PROCESS DEFINED

Yura and Walsh define the **nursing process** as "an orderly, systematic manner of determining the client's problems, making plans to solve them, initiating the plan or assigning others to implement it, and evaluating the extent to which the plan was effective in resolving the problems identified."[1] Thus, the nursing process provides a systematic approach to any system (individual, family, community). Because this definition is consistent with the approach used in this book it is accepted here.

IMPORTANCE OF THE NURSING PROCESS

The nursing process is considered so important in community health nursing that it is incorporated into our standards for community health nursing practice. The eight standards are the following:

1. A systematic and continuous collection of data about the health status of the system. This data should be accessible, communicated, and recorded.
2. The health-status data provides the basis for nursing diagnosis.
3. Nursing diagnoses form the basis for goals and nursing care.
4. Plans for nursing care include priorities and nursing measures to achieve the goals derived from nursing diagnoses.
5. Nursing actions provide for a system's participation in health promotion, maintenance, and restoration.
6. Nursing actions assist systems to maximize their health potential.
7. The system's progress toward mutually determined goals is determined by the system and the nurse.
8. Nursing actions involve ongoing reassessment, reordering of priorities, new goal setting, and revision of the nursing plan.[2]

STEPS IN THE PROCESS

Various steps in the nursing process have been identified by different authors and in this chapter we will consider four of the steps. These include assessing, planning, implementing, and evaluating.

ASSESSMENT

To determine where an actual or potential imbalance exists in a system (individual, family, community), community health nurses must go through the first step of the nursing process, which is the assessment. Although different authors order the steps of assessment differently, there is usually some attention to the collection of data, interpretation of data for tentative identification of needs, and validation of the identified needs.

Individual Data Collection. Often there is some format for the collection of data so that collection can be done in a systematic way, consistent with the focus of the particular agency. For example, the nurse in community health who has a major focus on primary prevention in families and groups collects a different set of data than the nurse in the hospital who is caring for a patient with a myocardial infarction. Some of these differences, which provide direction for data collection, are identified in Chapter 5.

When collecting data on individuals who are ill there is usually some attention given to the chief complaint, present illnesses, past history, and a review of systems falling into categories such as general health; integument; head, ears, eyes, nose, throat; teeth and gums; respiratory; cardiovascular; gastrointestinal; genitourinary; gynecologic; musculoskeletal; and endrocrine. These data may be obtained by history, laboratory, and physical examination and are covered superficially or in-depth depending upon the education and experience of the nurses involved and their particular role in the health subsystem. In addition, there may be some attention given to the family health history and the personal and social history, such as, occupational history, health habits, marital and sexual history. If the patient is at home, data may also be collected on family resources, which may be used to provide care for the patient.

Some disciplines may collect part of the patient history or one such as medicine may collect initial data with other disciplines following up on certain aspects that are more directly related to their discipline. For example, a patient admitted to a medical ward of a hospital would probably have a complete examination done by the physician with later attention to certain aspects of the history by nurses, social workers, and others. On the other hand, if a patient is admitted to a hospital with problems of a psychiatric nature, there may be less attention given to the review of general body systems and greater emphasis on the neuropsychiatric aspect and the social history, which may be carried out initially by a nurse, social worker or physician. Likewise, if the presenting problem is mainly social, the patient would likely present himself at an institution other than the hospital and be evaluated by a social worker who obtains a social and family history.

In the community, the community health nurse often collects data on individuals sick and well in the home, in the school or in industry and may then refer selected individuals to physicians or others for a more detailed examination. Often this data base follows agency guidelines or standing orders. In other settings where physicians are present such as at tuberculosis, venereal disease, or well child clinics, nurses and doctors may collect data jointly.

Family Data Collection. During the process of collecting data from families, there is usually some attention given to the composition and dynamics of the family, sociocultural and economic factors of the family, environmental factors and their health and medical history. The composition and dynamics of the family include factors such as names, birthdates, relationships to the head of the household, and the occupations of members. In addition, it includes data on the roles of members, decision-making processes, relationships among members, eating patterns, leisure-time activities and sleeping arrangements. Sociocultural and economic factors include data on the education level of members, their ethnic background, religious affiliation, family income, value system, and relationships outside the family. Environmental factors include data on housing, the neighborhood, and accessibility to transportation. Under health and medical history of the family, nurses usually collect data on any illnesses, past or present, dental health, medications taken, immunization statuses, sources of and financing of health care, resources in the family used for health care, and an assessment of body systems and the growth and development of each member.

A family assessment guideline using a systems approach is presented in Appendix A. From these data, health problems are summarized as perceived by the nurse and by the family and they then determine which of these should receive top priority for nursing visits.

Community Data Collection. In the community there is usually some attention to a description of the community, population characteristics, environmental factors, the health subsystem, and other subsystems of the community. A description of the community would include data on the location, climate, terrain, boundaries, density, history, and community changes, past, present, and future. Population characteristics include the number of people in the community as compared to 5 and 10 years ago, population density, and demographic characteristics, such as, the age distribution, sex and race distribution, ethnic groups, religious distribution and socioeconomic characteristics of the group. Most of the demographic data is compared with other communities such as the state and nation and also compared with past data on the community as a basis for planning. Environmental factors include an assessment of housing and sanitation including water, sewage, trash, garbage, and so forth. Data under the health subsystem includes vital statistics for the community (live births, neonatal deaths, infant deaths, maternal deaths, and general deaths), incidence and prevalence of the most common diseases, and the major causes of deaths with numbers and rates. These data are compared with data for 5 and 10 years previously in the community, and with state and national rates. The assessment of the health subsystem also includes data on health resources, manpower, and community health nursing services. Data on resources includes the number of hospitals; kinds of services provided; ownership and accreditation; numbers of nursing homes with ownership; bed capacity and services provided; ambulatory services with numbers and kinds of service; and comparable data for voluntary health resources, occupational and school services, health departments, and so forth. In addition, there should be an inventory of the various health personnel active in the community. Other subsystems of the community include data on the communication, transportation, political, economic, recreational, and other subsystems. (See Assessment Guide in Appendix B.) From each of these categories a variety of data are collected to obtain a picture of the total community and its health and health problems.

One study has been done that looks at the quality of life in communities. This study done by Liu ranks the major communities in the United States in relation to economic, political, environmental, health and education components.[3] Health factors evaluated for each community included infant mortality rates, death rates, education and medical care available and accessible. Environmental factors included the air pollution index, noise levels, the water pollution index, climatological data and recreational areas and facilities. Factors for each component such as health and education were averaged for each community. In addition, an overall rank for quality of life was averaged for each community. Thus, communities in the United States could be related to one another in relation to their level of wellness on a specific component and their overall quality of life. According to this study, the quality of life for a large metropolitan area was highest in Portland, Oregon and lowest in Jersey City, New Jersey. For a medium size area the quality of life was highest in Eugene, Oregon and lowest in Mobile, Alabama, and for a small area it was highest in LaCrosse, Wisconsin and lowest in Pine Bluff, Arkansas. This approach allows us to compare the quality of life or specific components of this index between one community and another.

Other Sources of Data. In addition to data collected from the physical examination, history and laboratory findings, data may also be collected through observation, by contacting other personnel and agencies who have previously seen the patient or family, and from previous records.

Analysis of Data. After the data is collected on the system (individual, family or community), the nurse interprets and interrelates the data to identify needs. At this point, nurses usually look at a complex of factors from the data and relate these to their knowledge of systems (exchanges, entropy, negentropy, etc.) as a basis for determining which complex patterns are normal and which present actual or potential problems that may establish needs. Following this process, they may make a tentative diagnosis or follow up on hunches that they will then validate. For example, a patient may have symptoms of jaundice, a mild upper respiratory infection, a low-grade fever, epigastic discomfort, anorexia, nausea, heartburn and flatulence, and give a history of having eaten shellfish regularly. On examination, a nurse practitioner might also palpate an enlarged liver and spleen and make a tentative diagnosis of hepatitis. Following this diagnosis in the home, the nurse might refer the patient to the hospital for laboratory tests and validation of the diagnosis and patient needs. If the patient were hospitalized a complex of needs would evolve to be met by a variety of health professions. Such needs as special diet, bedrest, emotional support, and so forth might be met by the hospital nurse. In addition, from a community health viewpoint, there would be additional needs such as the location of the source of polluted water or food, tracing of contacts, treatment and isolation of new cases, and preventive care for contacts. Thus, coordination and referral are often important aspects of planning.

Or, the nurse in the home may observe family members who have a 20% or more excess of body weight as compared with standards for their age. The nurse might also test for skinfold thicknesses of more than one inch and dyspnea on exertion. The members might also complain of chronic fatigue. From these data the nurse might make a tentative diagnosis of obesity from high caloric intake. However, it would then be important to validate this tentative diagnosis by getting information on daily food intake, activity level, observing eating habits, and so forth.

Although it is important for the hospitalized patient, it is even more important with families, groups, and the community to look at resources as well as health needs as part of the assessment. Often resources can make a difference in what we initially identify as a tentative need; that is, on first observation a health need may seem to be present but later we find that the family or community is coping well with the problem and there is no unmet need. For example, we might identify the need for physical care, emotional support, directions on taking medications and other related needs for a patient at home following a mycocardial infarction. However, as we view family resources to validate these needs we might find the family members are adept at providing physical care, giving medications as ordered, and meeting the emotional needs of the patient and thus there are no unmet needs in this area. However, other needs revolving around this family might emerge from the data, such as periodic relief of the family caregiver, diet teaching for the family as a whole, teaching about body mechanics and the transfer of the patient from the bed to chair. Freeman has presented an assessment guide that considers family resources while assessing family health needs.[4]

Because the individual, family, and community are all open systems, we also relate health and the resources of each unit in the hierarchy to other units as part of our assessment. At the individuals' level we are concerned about the influence of their health on other family members' health and resources to determine if other needs exist. For example, if there is a communicable disease, there may be a need for preventive measures such as immunizations, health teaching regarding handwashing and other safety measures, adequate rest, adequate diet, and so forth, for family caretakers and close community contacts. In addition, a review of family resources indicates whether or not there is a need for part-time assistance with the giving of care, and whether there are other resources (physical, emotional, economic, mental) to provide the care. If not, do we need to assist family resources by teaching about giving care, allowing the members to ventilate insecure feelings, or turn to the community for financial and other assistance. Thus, nurses supplement family resources by using their own or the communities' resources based upon the assessment of family needs.

Likewise, at the community level, we may look at health and resources both within and outside as part of our assessment. We can ask what health problems beyond our community may pose a threat to us and what are the needs related to these. Or, we might observe what other communities have done to cope with health problems similar to the ones we are experiencing; we would ask similar questions regarding resources. If we validate the need for services in our population but lack the resources in the community (manpower, money) we might determine if these can be obtained from the state or nation.

Another aspect of assessment should include a longitudinal view of the system for patterns. For example, a blood pressure of 100/60 or a temperature of 99° may seem symptomatic of illness until we find that it is a normal pattern for the individual. Or, we might observe the family eating lunch and identify an inadequate diet and the need for diet teaching. However, as we continue to visit we might discover that on that particular day the diet was atypical from a variety of factors and there is no need for teaching (verification). At the community level, we may be concerned over a high incidence of a particular disease. However, after looking at the disease longitudinally we may find that the community characteristically has a higher incidence of the disease at that particular time of year and upon further investigation that it is actually lower at that time of year than it was a year or 2 years ago.

Once the unmet needs of the system are identified we move into the planning stage of the nursing process.

PLANNING

Because it is never possible to meet all identified needs immediately with the resources available, an important aspect of planning is to set priorities among the unmet needs. Other steps include establishing goals, developing and selecting alternate methods to meet these goals and planning the actions to be taken.

Priority Setting. A few models for setting priorities have been proposed in the literature. One model that has been used in this way is Maslow's Hierarchy of Needs.[5] In this model, basic human needs are considered to be those needs that all people must satisfy to enhance their self-image. These needs also motivate behavior. Needs can be seen as on a hierarchy and as one set of needs are met the individual (system) moves up to the next level of needs. The first level of needs are physiologic, including food, oxygen, physical activity, rest, elimination, water and sexual satisfaction. All except the last are present at birth.

The second level of needs comprises safety and security needs such as the need for sameness, familiarity and trustworthiness in people, places, events, and things. The third level includes the need for love and belonging such as affection, warmth, kindness, and consideration in human relations. The fourth level includes the need for self-esteem such as respect, status, prestige, and a good reputation. When the fifth level is reached there is the need for self-actualization.

Thus, using this model for establishing priorities of needs, physiologic needs would supersede safety needs, safety needs would supersede the need for love, and so forth. In broader categories physical needs such as a life-threatening situation (actual or potential) would supersede social and mental health needs.

Hanlon presents a different model for establishing priorities.[6] He uses the following criteria for setting priorities:

1. A problem that affects a large number of people ordinarily should take precedence over one that affects relatively few.[7]
2. However, a disease that is severe in terms of mortality and morbidity should take precedence over those that are not. Thus, in combination (numbers affected and severity) the common cold may affect larger numbers of the population than tuberculosis affects, but tuberculosis is more severe and would thus become the priority.
3. Sufficient scientific knowledge and techniques for preventing or treating the disease process should be available if it is to be a priority.
4. The cost and manpower factors should be considered in arriving at priorities because the purpose of administration is to get the required job done with the least possible expenditure of time, energy, and money that is consistent with agreed upon quality of work. If personnel or money are unavailable to carry out a program—it should not be included in the priority—the priority then might be to locate these resources.
5. The readiness of the population for the proposed program should also be a factor in determining priorities. If one plans to immunize 90% of the children in the community under age 5 for polio and this procedure is not acceptable to the community, the program will fail. Here, the priority may be to work with acceptance of the community for the program.

Hanlon presents a formula based upon these and other factors, which can be used to establish priorities. Although Hanlon's model is directed toward setting priorities in the community it can also be used with an individual or family. Within the community, family, or individual there are a variety of needs which can be prioritized using Hanlon's model.

Another model for setting priorities with individuals and families is presented at the end of this chapter. This model considers the readiness of the system for change, the resources (nurse, family, community) available, the autonomy (nurse, family, community), the threat to the community (potential number to be affected and severity) and the risk of changing the behavior observed versus the risk of leaving it as it is, as a basis for setting priorities.

Establishing Goals. In addition to setting priorities for all unmet needs, planning involves establishing goals for planned programs. For individuals and families, most goals can be stated in terms of achieving, preventing, or maintaining. For example, if accident hazards are noted in a home where small children are present you may want to protect the child from an accident. Your goal is to prevent physical injury. At the same time, you would want to increase the parents' knowledge about accidents and accident prevention. Thus, another goal might be to achieve awareness of the need for accident prevention. At the community level, most goals for primary prevention can be stated in terms of reducing the incidence and prevalence of disease or injury and the mortality and morbidity rates in a population group at a particular time and place for most diseases, injuries, and defects. For example, nurses might want to reduce the incidence of polio in a specific community. For secondary prevention or early casefindings a community goal is written in terms of reducing the number of days of illness for a significant proportion of the population suffering from the illness. For environmental hazards, goals in general terms can be stated in terms of avoiding, reducing, or eliminating the hazards to health. With accidents as a problem we might be interested then in preventing accidents in a home, but would also be interested in reducing the incidence of accidents in the population in a community. For environmental goals, we might be interested in reducing the incidence of heat exposure in industrial populations that work in hot areas by isolating or partitioning off processes that give off heat, by venting, and by protective reflective clothing for those that work in high temperatures. In a home we might have an environmental goal of eliminating the rat population and would probably call in a sanitarian from the health department to advise the family.

Alternatives. The next step in planning is to consider alternate ways of meetint the goals. For example, if there is a sick member in the family who needs care, we might meet this goal by providing the care, by using a family member to give the care, by using a home health aide who is supervised by the nurse, or the patient might be placed in an outside community resource such as a hospital. On a community basis, if we are interested in reducing the incidence and prevalence of polio we might meet the goal by planning a massive one-time free immunization clinic throughout the community, by publicizing and increasing the manpower resources in our existing clinics, or publicizing the importance of immunizations and channeling people to their private physicians.

Most of our alternatives follow from the identification of the specific problems seen in the data. For example, if we wanted to reduce the incidence and prevalence of polio in a community we would need to evaluate the data to determine whether there were adequate facilities for immunization; whether they were conveniently located and able to be used; whether parents know about the services; how they view the services; and if they are able to pay for the services. Should we find that there are adequate facilities, which are not being used because the population is not aware of the need for and the resources available, we would see a need to provide the community with this information. Our alternatives then might be to have nurses make announcements on the radio or television, to do an intensive educational program in the schools, to use key people in each neighborhood of the community to arrange meetings with other people in the neighborhood, to use nurses to go door to door in their neighborhoods to discuss resources and the need for immunization, or to use volunteers to telephone people listed in the phone book.

Judgment is important in selecting the alternative method to be used and for most alternatives there are both negative and positive consequences. For example, using a family member to provide care for a sick member may be more economical because of a lack of nursing time, but it may have a negative effect on the care-provider's physical and emotional health. The provision of care by community health nurses may be more acceptable to families but it does take them away from other priorities. Or, the home health aide may not be acceptable initially to the family, but this plan is most economical of the nurses time.[8]

Likewise, in reaching a goal of community education about immunizations, spot announcements by the nurse may be economical of the nurse's time and may be more accepted because of the nurse's knowledge and authority on the subject than would an announcement by a lay person. However, they may not reach the most important groups who may not have these sources (radios, televisions) of communication. Or, using schools as the source for disseminating information may save the nurse's time over other methods, but does not reach adults who often take the action for their children (take them for immunizations). Using key people in volunteer areas may save the nurse's time and may be influential in gaining compliance, but this may not be the best alternative because key people may not have enough knowledge of health to adequately explain the need. Thus, each alternative must be evaluated for its positive and negative aspects and the selected alternative must be the one that clearly has more positives than negatives.

Actions to Meet Goals. Once an alternative is arrived at, actions to meet the goals must be programmed. Components needed for each action include (1) a target group (2) an activity (3) a time period to reach, and (4) a standard.

The **target group** refers to the individual, family, or community group to be reached by our interventions. The **activity** refers to the planned activities to meet our goal, and the **time period** refers to the point in time in which we expect to have completed our activities to meet the goal. The **standard,** which is more useful in groups than with individuals or families, refers to the proportion of people we expect to reach within the time period.

For example, if our community goal is to reduce the incidence and prevalence of polio in a specific community, our main action to meet the goal might be to immunize (activity) 90% (standard) of all children under age 5 (target group) within 1 year or by January 1, 1982 (time period). Other activities to reach the goal would probably also be necessary. For example, an educational goal might be to reach 60% (standard) of the population of a specific town (target group) with a spot announcement regarding polio (activity) by July 1, 1981 (time period).

To meet the goal of providing care for a sick parent by a daughter at home, our main action might be to teach body mechanics, personal hygiene to bed patients or whatever procedures are needed (activity) to the daughter (target group) within three home visits or by June 1, 1981 (time period). Here, we would leave out the standard. In addition, other actions would also need to be programmed and changed periodically depending upon our changing assessment of the situation.

Evaluation Tools During Planning. During the planning phase it is also helpful to consider methods that can be used to evaluate interventions. On a community basis, this is best done by defining the units by which the activities are to be measured, such as, the number of active cases located, the number of hazards identified, the number of violations corrected, the number of cervical cancers removed, or whatever is appropriate to the goals and actions planned. In the example used previously, the unit for action was 90% of all children under 5 years of age in a particular community. If the magnitude of the population under 5 years is known, we can calculate 90% of this figure and compare with the number of children under age 5 who were actually immunized to get an indication of the success of the program action. This planned action could then be related to the vital statistics for the community on polio incidence and prevalence on a time continuum, to determine if our goal of reducing the incidence of polio had been met by our immunization program. This concept is less useful when working with individuals and families.

Recording Plans. Often it is useful to graph the various factors involved in planning on a time axis. One method proposed in the literature is the Program Evaluation and Review Technique or PERT.[9] PERT involves writing a final objective for each program and breaking this objective down into a series of subobjectives. Then, a network of activities and a time estimate to reach each subobjective is graphed. "One of these (paths) will require more time to transverse than any of the others . . . the critical path."[10] With a PERT chart the planner can evaluate the results at each stage to determine if the anticipated progress is being made or where bottlenecks occur if there are any.

For example, our final objective may be to immunize 90% of all children under 5 years of age in a community. If resources such as facilities, equipment, and personnel for this activity are currently unavailable, the nursing administrator might have subobjectives involving the purchase of land, a contract for a building, the completion of the building, equipment installed, beginning operations and a 1 year period to complete the immunization program. This entire project might take two years from start to finish. Concurrently, a second path might include the hiring and training of personnel. Assuming it takes 3 months to hire personnel and 4 months to train them, a total of seven months will be needed for this path. Since the first path requires 1 year and the second requires 7 months, there is slack in the second path. Thus, the first path is the critical one. These paths could be graphed as follows in Figure 6–1.

Although the PERT Chart is most useful in complex planning, it can also be used as a quick reference in planning with families. For example, if we have a family member providing care for another sick member, we may need to teach other elements of care at each stage in the patient's

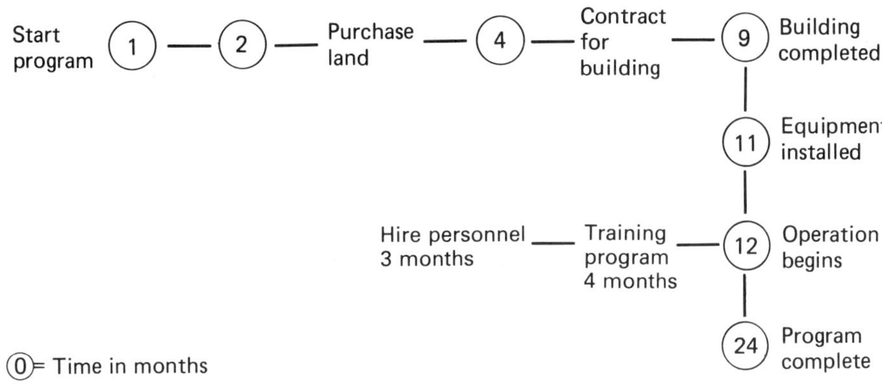

Figure 6–1
Evaluation planning using PERT method.

progress to meet a goal of independence for the patient. The teaching in this instance may focus initially on the individual providing care and later on the patient. Subobjectives might start with teaching personal hygiene, bedmaking, oral hygiene, range of motion and positioning. Other subobjectives might include body mechanics and transfer from bed to wheelchair, as the patient progresses. Later subobjectives could include teaching the patient about mobility in a wheelchair, and later mobility using the walker or crutches, and finally unaided mobility. Concurrently, we might have a subobjective for teaching diet changes over the course of an illness, which would be less critical, but an important component in reaching our goal of independence for the individual (system).

IMPLEMENTATION

The third component of the nursing process is **implementation** and this stage involves the actual carrying out of the planned activities to meet our program goals. Freeman says that interventions may be of three types, "supplemental, facilitative or developmental."[11] "Supplemental intervention means doing things that the family, group or community cannot do for itself."[12] Examples include giving personal care to the sick or newborn at home, giving immunizations in the clinic, or making decisions for families when they lack the resources to cope during a crisis. Facilitative interventions involve "removing barriers to care, whether these barriers are economic, such as a lack of carfare to get to the source of medical care; social, such as a cultural-linked resistance to necessary change; or behavioral, such as a lack of information or motivation on the part of those who are expected to take the necessary action."[13] "Developmental intervention is based on improving the capacity of the recipient to act on his own behalf. Teaching families and groups to make responsible health decisions, supporting them in developing a sense of identity and worth, and guiding them in dealing with predictable crises and points of stress are examples of developmental intervention."[14]

EVALUATION

The last stage in the nursing process is evaluation. As an introduction, it may be helpful to review briefly the preceding stages, which led up to evaluation. From our assessment of the system and its environment we identified problems that reflected a significant departure from established norms. From this assessment, plans were made to meet certain needs resulting from the problem by establishing goals and activities in order of priorities. These plans were then implemented using all available appropriate resources (the individual or family, nursing resources, community resources, and so forth). It was implied that the planned activity would alleviate the identified problem.

Because nurses are one resource used in implementing activities to alleviate the problem, we are interested first in a continuous ongoing evaluation of our own performances. Nurses should continually evaluate their performance to see if they are functioning at a level that is acceptable in practice and consistent with other nurses who have comparable education and experience. A guide for such evaluations can be found in Appendix C. In addition, supervisors also evaluate our performances periodically to see that we are maintaining standards of care and to assist us with any weaknesses. Thus, evaluation of the nurse is an important aspect of this step in evaluating patient care.

A second and equally important aspect of evaluation, relating to the planning process, is known as periodic evaluation. Periodic evaluation consists of four basic aspects identified as follows.

One aspect of periodic evaluation involves the **appropriateness** of the proposed or implemented program. Is this program or goal appropriate in view of all the unmet needs or are other priorities of greater concern? For example, is the program to reduce the number of cases of paralytic polio by vaccinating 90% of all children appropriate for the community or should the planner focus on other unmet needs?

A second aspect of periodic evaluation involves the **adequacy** of the program in meeting the identified needs or problem. For instance, if nurses decide that polio is truly a priority for the community, they must then evaluate whether or not the planned intervention of immunizing 90% of the children under the age of 5 is or ever has been adequate enough to reduce the prevalence of polio, or are there other activities needed to meet the goal? Here, nurses may find that they need to broaden their activities to include immunizations for a wider age range, an educational program to publicize the available services for immunization, and a program to work with parental attitudes about immunization.

A third aspect of the periodic evaluation involves the **effectiveness** of the proposed or ongoing activities to meet the goal. Effectiveness refers to the extent to which the pre-established objectives are met as a result of the planned activities, that is, the changes to be measured should be based largely upon the actual interventions, which follow the planned activities. For example, nurses may ask whether or not the reduction in the cases of polio in the community was a result of the planned activities and interventions (immunization, education, and attitude changes) or did the prevalence of polio decrease by itself when in reality only a small proportion of the target group received immunizations? If such a reduction was noted, it could possibly be related to a change in both the responsible organism and the population itself, and totally unrelated to the interventions. Thus, the program would not have been very effective. Or the nurse may assess an anxious mother with a newborn at home and decide to teach newborn care. However, the mother may first need to express her anxiety and fears about handling the child before she can learn newborn care. Thus, the teaching intervention would be neither appropriate nor effective at this point.

A fourth aspect of evaluation involves efficiency. **Efficiency** refers to the cost in money, time, and manpower of attaining the objectives. Nurses should be interested in meeting the objectives in the most efficient manner possible. Thus, they must determine whether the objectives were met in the most efficient way or whether they should consider alternative ways to meet the goal. For example, if nurses planned to immunize all children under 5 years of age for polio but found that the majority of families could afford immunizations and would have gone to private physicians if the program had been publicized, this approach would have been more efficient. Also, physicians could have been notified of the large numbers of immunizations needed. Or, if a nurse decided to visit a family three times weekly to give care to a bedridden member, she might find that teaching another member to provide the care would be more efficient.

THE NURSING PROCESS AND SYSTEMS THEORY

At the beginning of this chapter the nursing process was described. We will now relate this process to systems theory, which is the focus of this book. From a systems point of view, the purpose of the nursing process is to assist the individual, family or community (system) to regain, attain, or maintain high level wellness where high level wellness means maintaining the self-regulatory processes of the system, that is, maintaining its steady state and movement toward higher levels of organization and order (negentropy) at particular times. Maintenance of self-regulatory processes is consistent with the system's goals and the system may need assistance when goals are not being met. Before we can intervene to help systems meet their goals, we must assess the state of the system at any particular time.

ASSESSMENT OF THE SYSTEM

Assessment is concerned with collecting and analyzing pertinent data about the system, its environment, subsystems and supersystems to identify potential or actual health problems, which have or may interfere with self-regulatory processes. Initially, we might assess the system itself to determine how well its parts are working together and if it is maintaining its self-regulatory processes. With an individual, this may mean comparing the level of growth and development (physical, mental, emotional, ideational) with established norms to determine if growth is within a normal range and the system is growing more complex and organized (negentropy). With individuals we also do a physical and mental health assessment to determine how well the body parts are working together. This can usually be assessed by observing the exterior and actions (behaviors) of the individual, as discussed by Byrne and Thompson.[15] Also, there must be an assessment of body systems, interviewing, and testing using indicators such as temperature, blood pressure, pulse and respiration for signs of deviation from a normal range. If the system is failing to maintain or attain self-regulatory processes (steady states and negentropy), entropy may be present and must be identified as a basis for interventions. In addition to actual entropy in a system, we are also concerned with assessing potential entropy in a system. For example, if an individual smokes 2 packs of cigarettes a day, there is the potential for entropy in the oxygen-carbon dioxide exchange in the lungs and this information can be obtained by interview and observation.

At the family and community level, we also assess the growth and development of the system and look at how well the parts are working together to maintain the whole. Family stages of development and the tasks involved in each state are useful for comparing the observed family's development with established norms. In families and communities, the dynamics of role behaviors, relationships, decision making, communication, and other patterned behaviors are useful for comparing observed patterned behaviors with established norms, in determining how well the system is working and any implications for its health. In addition, if families eating, sleeping, recreation, or other patterns, based upon community exchanges, are not consistent with established norms, there is the potential for entropic processes in its members and the family as a whole. Assessment guides for family and community including these components of internal dynamics are included in Appendices A and B. If families and communities are not maintaining self-regulatory processes, again we must determine if entropy is present and the reason for the breakdown.

Next, nurses must also look at the exchange with the environment and supersystem of the system to determine if there are actual or potential health threats in terms of self-regulatory processes (see Assessment Guides, Appendices A and B). For the family, the type of housing, source and amount of heating, water supply, rodents, and so forth may threaten health and self-regulatory processes of the family members. In addition, their exchanges with the subsystems (economic, religious, transportation, health, social, and families) of the community may facilitate or hamper self-regulatory processes. For instance, if there is a high incidence of influenza among the family subsystems of the community, this may spread to the family we are working with and hamper their self-regulatory process by creating disease and a tenuous steady state. As discussed in Chapter 3, this affects not only the self-regulatory processes of the individual (psychological, mental, social, and physical) but also the family by forcing them to reshuffle their autonomy, resources, and roles. If there are inadequate social-service funds or jobs in a community to meet an unemployed family's basic needs, or inadequate free health services, the members and family as a whole may also experience entropic processes. Thus, a thorough assessment of the system, its subsystems, supersystems and environment is important as a basis for intervention.

Overall assessment of a system by nurses should identify actual or potential entropic processes in the system. Actual diseases and inadequate growth and development of individuals or a family can both be considered entropic processes. On the other hand, inadequate exchanges of a short-term nature while the system continues to function less efficiently could be considered potential entropic processes. If viewed in terms of individuals, the inadequate exchange and potential for entropic processes would comprise a long list such as smoking, inadequate diet, inadequate rest, excessive worry, tightly knit or loosely bound families, which do not allow individuals to grow in their own way, and family roles and relationships as they affect individual members and other factors discussed in Chapters 2 through 4 and found in the Family Assessment Guide in Appendix A. Similar exchanges and their potential for entropy can also be evaluated for communities and would form the basis for interventions.

PLANNING FOR THE SYSTEM

After the individual or family (system) has been assessed, planning by the nurse and the individual or family takes place. The same models for priority setting as discussed in the first part of this chapter are used. If the nurse uses Maslow's Hierarchy of Needs, the physiologic needs are met first. Within these physiologic needs two more categories can be identified for setting priorities. Actual entropic processes would take precedence over potential entropic processes. Thus, in an individual (system) with both lung disease and inadequate diet patterns, the lung disease (actual physiologic entropic process) would take precedence over inadequate dietary patterns (potential physiologic entropic processes).

Additional Concepts in Planning. In the planning stage of the nursing process, we set health need priorities, write goals and actions for meeting needs, and consider and select alternative ways to meet goals. In addition, there are additional concepts that can be considered during this stage, and one concept is that of change.

CHANGE. If the sytsem if showing entropy (actual or potential) nurses are interested in counteracting this process and thus introduce change into the system.

Change can be planned or unplanned. Change is continually taking place in all systems and can be categorized as physiologic, psychological, social, and so forth for individuals and families, while change is economic, demographic, political, and so forth for families and communities. Often there are automatic counterbalances in systems that help to maintain a range of adaptability to these outside changes in the system. However, as systems move outside this range and experience crisis, entropic proceses and disease may result. These changes affecting systems are usually unplanned and often unconscious. For example, we are usually unaware of bodily processes that maintain a constant temperature or blood sugar level and are also unaware of the forces that tend to cause movement away from a steady state.

In nursing plans we are concerned with planned changes that help the system maintain, regain, or attain self-regulatory processes. Planned change can be defined as "a conscious, deliberate, and collaborative effort to improve the operation of a human system, whether it be a self system, social system, or a cultural system, through the utilization of knowledge."[16] Thus, from a nursing point of view the major points of the definition are (1) conscious, deliberate, and collaborative (2) the purpose is to improve operation of the system (individual, family, or community) or to help it regain or maintain self-regulatory processes, and (3) involves utilization of scientific knowledge.

All of these factors should be inherent in the setting of goals, choosing actions to meet goals, and considering and selecting alternative ways of reaching the goal. The planning process should be deliberate and always in conjunction with the particular system. At times, we may also need to collaborate with physicians, social workers, sanitarians, and others on the health team as part of our planning. We must also use scientific knowledge as a basis for our planned interventions to ensure the desired outcome of the planned change, that is, that we improve the operation of the individual or family system by assisting it with its self-regulatory processes. Many concepts of change can be found in the literature and a few of the more appropriate ones are reviewed here.

Bennis and Chin propose 3 strategies for change.[17] The first, **Empirical-Rational Strategy,** is based upon the assumption that humans are rational and follow their rational self-interest once it is revealed to them. This strategy involves dissemination of knowledge by experts who show how the change benefits the system; thereafter, the system changes. For example, if an expert shows that polio immunization prevents polio, the masses will obtain immunization because they are rational beings.

Often, the new nurse in community health nursing uses this approach and becomes frustrated when change does not occur in the individual or family system. However, this strategy is not effective in initiating change unless the system is ready for change.

A second strategy, the **Normative-Reeducation Strategy,** is based upon the assumption that "patterns of action are supported by sociocultural norms and by commitment on the part of the individual to these norms."[18] Change is directed toward increasing the problem-solving and growth potential of the system, which will change when it is able to alter its normative orientation to old patterns and develop commitments to new ones. Normative patterns involve attitudes, values, skills, and significant relationships as well as knowledge. Thus, a change is introduced as the nurse works jointly with individual or family systems to compare how systems see themselves or the problem and how the nurse sees the problem and deals with the attitudes, values, norms, and relationships of the particular system. Next, the nurse intervenes collaboratively with the person or persons to define and solve the problem, paying particular attention to identifying and discussing with them those unconscious elements that impede problem solving. The methods and concepts of the behavioral sciences (value systems, conflict, conflict resolution) are useful in dealing with the problem. This strategy is the better approach to change as it leads to a restructuring of the system and a commitment to the plan of action.

The third strategy, the **Power-Based Strategy,** emphasizes the political and economic sanctions of power; that is, political institutions are used to achieve change and other coercive strategies, such as, manipulating through the use of guilt and shame, may be used to bring about change desired by those in power positions. For example, laws that require immunization prior to school enrollment are based upon the Power-Based Strategy.

A very useful model for planning and initiating change in systems has been presented by Lewin in his Force Field theory.[19] He says, "the existing state of affairs of any behavior is a result of two equal and opposing set of forces that counterbalance each other." For example, if you assess an overweight person in your caseload, the person remains at that weight as a result of the two opposing forces. Although they may desire to go from 180 pounds to 120 pounds, there are **restraining forces** that are preventing the drop in weight. These include overeating because of loneliness and frustration, a lack of knowledge about dieting, a close friend (important to the client) who dislikes dieting, and readily available prepared food at home. At the same time, there are **driving forces** that tend to move the individual in the direction of losing weight. These include wanting the good opinion of friends, feeling better and looking better with a weight loss, and a better self-image. Because these forces, the driving and restraining forces, are equal, the individual remains at the upper weight. Thus, as part of our assessment we should identify the driving and restraining forces of behavior as a basis for planning change. Change is best initiated if we can work with the restraining forces and support the individual during change. For example, in the preceding example, we would want to teach about excessive food intake, plan with the person ways to use time to avoid loneliness, and work with the friend who dislikes dieting and any others who provide extra food to initiate change. It has been found that working with the driving forces is not a useful approach because it tends to bring about increased resistance.

In another family we might find a mother who says that she wants to take the children for their immunizations but has not taken action. Again, we would want to identify the driving and restraining forces. We might discover driving forces such as a desire to be recognized as a good mother, knowing the child's health would be improved by preventing certain diseases, and wanting to please the nurse. At the same time, the restraining forces might include a lack of time, lack of transportation and a babysitter for the other small children, and a lack of knowledge about the location of the free immunizations. These forces are presented in Figure 6–2 for review.

Again, we would need to plan change in relation to the restraining forces of the person (system). We

Restraining Forces	Driving Forces
Lack of knowledge about immunization resources	please the nurse
no babysitter	health reasons
no transportation	"good mother"
lack of time	

Figure 6–2
Driving and restraining forces in attending immunization clinics. Desired: Immunizations for children; existing: unimmunized children.

would need to discuss places where immunizations can be obtained. We would also help the mother arrange for a babysitter and transportation and help her budget her time so that she can arrange for going to the immunization clinic. Thus, we have removed the restraining forces or made them part of the driving forces and tipped the balance in the direction of change.

The Force Field theory is equally useful with any system. For a discussion on its use with groups such as industrial workers, see Bennis.[20]

Kelman says that there are three methods of bringing about change.[21] They are as follows:

1. Compliance—a change in behavior is a result of hoping to gain rewards or avoiding punishment.
   This change may come about when the change agent holds certain rewards or punishments as viewed by the system. This is not a very good approach to change as the system will revert back to the old behavior once the change agent is gone because there is no commitment to the change or restructuring of the system.
2. Identification—a system changes as a result of identification with the change agent and wants to be like the agent or the agent's group.
3. Internalization—a system changes because the idea of change is consistent with the system's values. This is the most long lasting approach to change and often means working within the system's value system.

Paul has an interesting book on interventions in various cultures that were successful when the change agent worked within the value systems of the culture.[22]

Many of the maneuvers discussed under feedback for families and subgroups of the community in Chapters 3 and 4 are used by systems to bring about change. The nurse should be familiar with these maneuvers and techniques and may use some of them to promote growth in the system.

COMPLIANCE. Clients in the community are seen by nurses periodically in the home, school, clinic, or other settings. At other times clients are responsible for their own preventive care and treatment. Because clients' health is interrelated with the health of other systems and the nurse's goal is to elevate the health of the community, the compliance of systems under community health nursing services is important.

From studies on compliance and noncompliance it is possible to identify some factors that encourage compliance of the client system. One factor involves the kind of relationship developed between the nurse and the client. If nurses are distrustful of clients and have a pattern of one-way communications and goal setting, the client is less likely to comply with the planned care than if a trusting relationship exists and the nurse and client openly share concerns and goals for care. A model for developing such a relationship is presented in Chapter 7.

Another factor that influences compliance is a clear understanding by the client of the relationship of the nursing care plan to the prevention or treatment of illness. In addition, the client should have a clear understanding of and involvement in formulating his or her nursing care plan. The client should know the goals of nursing care and the actions the nurse and the client must each take to meet these goals. Contracts between the nurse and client, which are discussed in Chapter 7, may help in this process. Teaching and asking for feedback are other aspects of the process that may facilitate compliance. With these methods the client has the opportunity to hear and see the instructions in writing and to demonstrate understanding through feedback.

Another method for improving compliance is beginning with simple actions and moving toward more complex ones. This way, a client carries out a simple action such as correct tooth brushing before proceeding to a series of simple actions or a complex action, such as, meal planning and preparation. When a simple action is carried out, the nurse reinforces this positive behavior and works with the client on the next step.

Compliance can also be improved if clients are allowed to make changes in their life style slowly. Initial changes should be simple and all changes should be kept to a minimal level that will allow the client to maintain or regain health. Thus, changes, when necessary, should be adapted as much as possible to the client's life style. For example, dietary changes should be planned within the economic, cultural, religious, and psychological framework of the family, if possible. Difficult changes for clients involve personal habits such as smoking, alcohol intake, diet, and physical activity.

Compliance in a family member can also be improved if the family is supportive of the change. Since the family is made up of interlocking members, the family members may need to be involved in the nursing care plan of a member.

Certain groups of clients are considered to be less reliable regarding compliance. These include people who consider themselves less susceptible to potential illnesses, people who have little concern with their health and little confidence in health care, people who are busy with other priorities, people without a home support system, older people, and people from the lower socioeconomic groups. Nurses may question clients about compliance and get some degree of assurance about compliance. Davis found that upon direct questioning over 40% of the patients admitted that they had never planned to comply.[23] These clients should be questioned about their lack of concern in complying, their understanding of the change, and whether or not there are unclear areas they wish to discuss.

COORDINATION. Coordination is another important concept to consider in planning nursing care. Coordination was defined by myself and others as the "efforts made to relate health and welfare systems so that people receive comprehensive continuous services as needed."[24]

Coordination has been necessitated by the specialization and interdependence of the community. The community is made up of an evolving complex of interdependent subsystems, each with their own goals, agencies, personnel, and services. The health subsystem is one part of this complex, which also has a variety of goals, agencies, services, and disciplines. Because health agencies are interrelated and any change in a part of the health system affects the other parts (see Chap. 4), coordination and communication among the parts is important.

Coordination and communication by the nurse with other disciplines and agencies in a community involves two approaches. The first is **horizontal communication and coordination** with others who are involved in the care of the clients. Nurses must coordinate their activities with others who are involved with the family or group, such as, the private physician, school nurse, occupational-health physician, sanitarian, and social worker. At times, the nurse may seek consultation with others such as a nutritionist, social worker, or physician when they need additional insights or information. At other times, they may refer clients to other community resources and disciplines if the health needs are beyond the nurse's scope of competence and area of practice. All of these activities involve coordination and communications. Because of the long-term nature of community health nursing services, nurses are often in the best position to provide coordination. In this role nurses must continue to coordinate the care, keep other involved workers informed, and change nursing care plans in the light of reassessments. For example, the nurse may have a client at home who has had a myocardial infarction. The nurse may perform certain procedures periodically and supervise a home health aide who gives bedside care and cleans and prepares meals. In addition, a physical therapist may come to the home to teach exercises to the client and the client may have to take an ambulance to the hospital for periodic check-ups by the physician. Thus, the activities of the nurse, aide, physical therapist, physician, ambulance driver, and others must be coordinated on behalf of the client. The need for an ambulance, the time of medical appointments, changes in medical orders, and so forth must be communicated to the appropriate people. In addition, as the client begins to do things independently there may be less need for the physical therapist,

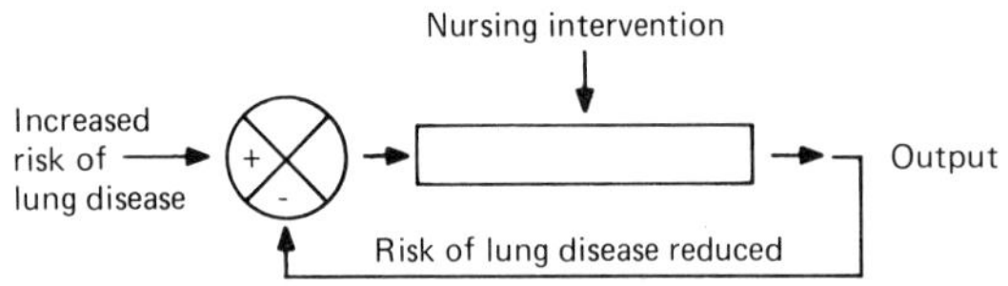

Figure 6–3
Prevention of entropic processes of lung. (Adapted from Crosby M: Nurs Clin North Am 6 No. 3, Sept 1971)

the aide and other personnel and these changes must also be communicated and coordinated.

The second approach involves **vertical communication and coordination** between clients and the health care system. If nurses identify gaps in services to clients, they can report these to administrators. Administrators should then coordinate activities with other agencies and subsystems to plan and provide new services. The information about these services is then communicated to the nurses who take this information to families and groups needing the services.

SYSTEMS INTERVENTIONS

Interventions with systems are attempts on the part of nurses to counteract actual or potential entropic processes in the system to maintain or restore self-regulatory processes. Interventions by nurses can be considered as input into the system to facilitate these processes. An entropic process is positive feedback (see Chap. 1) that tends to move the system away from a steady state. Thus, nursing interventions with individual or family systems aimed at restoring a steady state are then negative feedback. These processes can be diagramed as in Figures 6–3 and 6–4.

In Figure 6–3, the client smokes three packs of cigarettes each day and thus has an increased risk of lung disease (potential entropic process). Nursing interventions are directed toward reducing or eliminating the smoking habit to prevent lung diseases such as cancer and emphysema. If the client is successful, the risk is reduced.

Figure 6–4
Treatment of entropic processes of lung. (Adapted from Crosby M: Nurs Clin North Am 6, No. 3, Sept 1971)

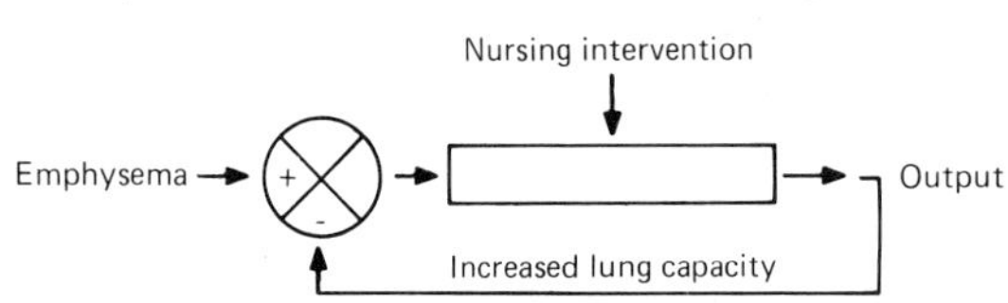

In Figure 6–4, the client has emphysema. If the nursing interventions include postural drainage and deep-breathing exercises, which increases the client's lung capacity, these interventions will tend to move the client away from deleterious entropic processes toward a new steady state.

Working with the learned behaviors of clients is an important aspect of community health nursing. Thus, teaching as a nursing intervention is discussed in the following section.

Teaching as a Nursing Intervention. Following an assessment of the client's learned behaviors regarding exchanges with the environment, nurses may teach them ways they can adapt better to these exchanges and help them either maintain or regain a high level of wellness. Teaching may, thus, be a way of preventing or treating disease processes.

Teaching may be done with individuals or groups and should be based upon a teaching plan. This plan should begin with a statement of the goals and objectives based upon the nursing needs established jointly by the nurse and client. If the client is interested in preparing formula for the newborn the nurse's objective as teacher may be to demonstrate and discuss formula-making and changes in diet as the infant grows and develops. As part of the teaching plan the nurse may have the mother give a return demonstration and ask questions on any points that are not clear.

Feedback from clients following teaching is an important aspect of teaching in view of systems theory as presented in earlier chapters. Because the system has input and output and can contain and retain input, the input and retention can only be evaluated by the output or feedback from the system. Thus, asking a mother to give a return demonstration of a newborn bath or formula preparation or asking a family member to keep a dietary log following a discussion on nutrition allows the nurse to evaluate the input that was retained and used as output. The nurse can then clarify unclear points and increase the knowledge and skills of the client.

Principles of learning should be considered when planning to teach in any setting with any client system. Some important principles of learning are that (1) readiness is a key factor in learning (2) effective learning is based upon a consideration of individual differences (3) learning must be meaningful to the learner (4) the climate must be appropriate for learning to take place, and (5) the learner must have feedback about progress toward goals.

READINESS. Readiness of the learner must be present if learning is to take place. Thus, material to be taught must be relevant, must meet the needs and interests of the client, and must be presented in a way that can be mastered. Nurses should determine the client's interests, needs, and concerns as a basis for teaching. Joint planning between nurses and clients following a comprehensive assessment should also ensure readiness for learning because the nurse will be working on problems that are a joint concern.

At times, the conditions found in a client system gives clues about the readiness for learning. Thus, a prenatal mother may be interested in the anatomy and physiology of pregnancy, the signs of labor, and the process of delivery. Or, a new mother may be interested in learning about care of the newborn, preparation of the formula, and ways of reducing stress on the family.

At other times nurses may identify health problems in the client system that are not of concern to the client. These problems may become long-term plans, which nurses retain until the timing is right to initiate plans jointly with the family to meet them. For example, if a family is uninterested in having an emotionally disturbed teenager referred for counseling, this may become a long-term goal. As the family begins to accept the need for help because the teenager fails in school and has poor peer relationships, the need for counseling may again be discussed using school and peer problems to reinforce this need. Other factors, which may influence readiness, involve improper timing of teaching, such as, teaching when other priorities are demanding the time of the client or teaching when neighbors or friends are visiting the client.

INDIVIDUAL DIFFERENCES. Individual differences must be considered if learning is to be effective. As indicated in earlier chapters individuals and groups learn to deal with environmental exchanges in different social, cultural, economic, religious, and experiential settings. Thus, these factors must be considered in planning teaching activities. If an individual has strong faith in the Christian Science religion, learning may be ineffective if the nurse teaches about immunizations and resources for obtaining these. Likewise, a family with two children who are mongoloid will have different fears and concerns about pregnancy than one that has normal children. Thus, the nurse must be familiar with the client's background if learning is to be effective.

RELEVANCE. Learning must also be meaningful to the learner. Individual differences must be considered, for unless learners see the relevance of the data to their problems, they will be unable to use the data in solving problems. Thus, limitations of experience, background, insight, emotional age, and mental ability may block their perception of the relevance of the data to their problem. Data must be individually tailored to the needs of the client to be meaningful.

At times, nurses may need to relate the data to the problem in very concrete ways. It is also helpful to obtain feedback from clients to ensure understanding because without understanding there is no meaning.

CLIMATE. The climate should also be appropriate for learning. The ideal climate has been described in various ways as supportive, accepting, spontaneous, permissive, and reality centered. The setting should be such that the learner is emotionally and psychologically free to relate the data to the problem. Techniques discussed in the nurse–client relationship in Chapter 7 should be used to create the appropriate climate.

FEEDBACK. The learner must also have feedback about progress toward goals. Feedback is a two-way process that lets the teacher know that learning has taken place and reduces the client's stress level and gives feelings of satisfaction from knowing that he has solved one of his problems. Nurses may ask for verbal feedback or for the return demonstration of such skills as formula preparation, bath of the newborn or sick, or the giving of insulin to a diabetic family member. Misunderstandings should be clarified and the learner should be given verbal feedback regarding his progress and future plans for reevaluation.

NURSING PROCESS IN THE SCHOOLS

Nursing in schools is provided using various administrative patterns. In some schools, nursing is provided by nurses from the local health department as part of a generalized pattern of community health nursing services. In other schools, nurses are employed by the school and give more specialized nursing care. These patterns of nursing care are usually community-wide so that one community may use nurses in schools that are employed by the health department, whereas other communities may use nurses employed by the Board of Education.

When school nurses are employed by the health department, there are advantages such as continuity of care between the school and home, of saving time for nursing in general, and of allowing nurses to use the full scope of their knowledge and skills with all age groups in all settings. Advantages for school-employed nurses include more specialized and in-depth knowledge as the nurse is focusing on one age group and has a better opportunity to integrate health and education since the nurse is in the school full-time and is a part of the school's staff. Both patterns have worked well in different communities.

ACCESSIBLE POPULATION IN SCHOOLS

Hanlon says that there are almost 40 million children between the ages of 5 and 15 years of age and Freeman says there are 55 million persons enrolled in schools.[25,26] This encompasses three out of every five persons between the ages of 5 and 34. "Approximately 35.5 million children were enrolled in elementary schools, 13.4 million children were in high schools, and 6.1 million persons were in colleges or professional schools."[27]

Thus, nursing can reach a large part of this population through the schools at a time when their health patterns and habits are being formed. This will influence the community in a positive way.

FUNCTION OF SCHOOL NURSING

The functions of the school nurse as outlined by the American Nurses' Association fall under the categories of the nursing process.[28] These functions are summarized in the following statement:

> In general, the functions of the school nurse are associated with the establishment and enforcement of the schools' policies and programs for the protection and promotion of health of the pupils; the maintenance of a school environment which is conducive to healthful living; the building of those components of the curriculum which have significance for health; the management of the health service including screening programs and emergency care services; the handling of special problems; and relating the health programs to those of the community.[29]

Thus, the function of nurses in schools include using the nursing process with the school-age population to maintain or improve the health by nursing actions including health teaching, creating an environment conducive to good health, and relating the health of the school population to families and the community. Standards for community health nursing identified earlier can be used in the schools.

The school health program has been defined as "the school procedures that contribute to the understanding, maintenance, and improvement of the health of pupils and school personnel, including health services, health education and healthful school living."[30]

MAJOR PROBLEMS OF THE SCHOOL POPULATION

The death rate for the school-age population is very low. It is less than 1 per 1000 students per year and the leading cause of death is accidents. Of these about one-half are automobile accidents. The second major source of accidental deaths is drowning, and this is followed by burns and firearms. Following accidents are deaths from malignant neoplasms, congenital malformations, influenza and pneumonia, and cardiovascular and renal diseases, respectively.

Despite the low death rate in this age group, there is a high incidence of illness. Hanlon says that there are about 256 acute conditions for every 100 children aged 5 to 14 each year, and about 187 acute conditions for every 100 people aged 15 to 24 each year.[31] Some of these illnesses may result from the psychological adjustment required by leaving the family and attending school and from the increased exposure to disease agents in the school environment at a time when students may be experiencing more stress.

SCHOOLS AS SYSTEMS

Like the individual, family, or community, the school is also a system made up of interrelated parts (students, teachers, administrators) who function together to maintain the whole system. A change in a part, such as a teachers' strike, will affect the whole system. There is also input, output, retaining, and containing within the school system. Input into the school system involves such things as students' attitudes, knowledge, and skills, money from the community to support teachers, money for supplies and equipment, teachers' knowledge, attitudes, and skills, and so forth. Output from the school system includes the knowledge, skills, and attitudes learned by students that can be used in the community. These attributes can be retained or contained by students depending upon their backgrounds and goals.

The school also has goals of which the major one is to educate the school population or to prepare students for coping with their environment. The goals will determine how the school fulfills its self-regulatory processes, that is, when it maintains a steady state and when it moves to new steady states through the process of feedback. All of the concepts of systems related to a community are applicable to the school as a system.

ASSESSMENT IN SCHOOLS

THE SCHOOL POPULATION

Screening for defects or deviations from the normal are done periodically in the school population. Prior to school enrollment, children should have a physical examination to serve as a baseline for further examinations. In addition, they should have up-to-date immunizations.

Thereafter, physical examinations are required three or four times during the school year in certain grades. Ideally, these examinations are done by the family physician and a report of the examination is presented to the school nurse. However, if the examinations are not done by a family physician, they may be scheduled during visits by the school physician. Parents are usually invited to participate in the examination for elementary school children and health teaching may take place at these sessions.

Periodic screening examinations for vision and hearing, skin testing for tuberculosis, or other special testing may also be carried out by the school nurse or other prepared personnel, such as, volunteers, dental hygiene staff, and so forth. Special testing of selected students may also be done by the nurse on self-referred students or on referral from teachers or parents, and on all athletes prior to participation in sports.

In addition to these periodic screening programs, which are initiated at certain times, there is usually an ongoing evaluation of the health status of students and school personnel. Because teachers spend the most time with students, they are usually taught to recognize signs and symptoms of illnesses and refer children who seem to need health attention. Health teaching of teachers and students should, thus, be part of the nurse's role.

School nurses must also be available to assess, plan, and implement care plans when children are injured or when other emergency situations arise. At these times, nurses may carry out established procedures and policies that will resolve the problem or they may need to contact parents and family physicians for direction.

SCHOOL ENVIRONMENT

The school environment is interpreted in its broadest sense and includes the physical, mental, and psychosocial environments within which the school child comes in contact. Aspects of these environments including safety are now discussed.

Safety. Safety is a primary consideration in establishing a healthful environment. Although many people will be involved in planning in schools and supervising children during various activities, the following are some aspects of safety that should be considered from a health point of view. Schools should be built with off-street parking and off-street areas for releasing children from buses or family cars. This reduces the possibility of traffic accidents. In addition, play areas near streets should be fenced off to further prevent injury to children by automobiles. Schools should also be located away from industrial noise and wastes to reduce the hazards associated with these. School plans should include ramps and entrances at the ground level and elevators so that handicapped children can enter and have easy access to upper floors. Special rooms or equipment may also need to be planned for handicapped individuals with hearing or visual problems. These considerations are in keeping with the current trend of keeping handicapped children in regular classes rather than segregating them.

Safety is also an important consideration in school activities. In physical education classes, students should be protected from contaminated water in swimming pools, or from falls and injuries in sports and gymnastics. On the playground, behavior should be supervised to prevent injury, and in metal and woodworking shops students should be protected from the hazards of power machinery. In addition, solvents in print shops or dust and metal particles in masonry shops may be hazardous. School nurses may assess and talk with appropriate school personnel about the hazards and the need to wear protective devices such as safety glasses where appropriate.

Communicable Diseases. Students should also be protected from undue exposure to communicable diseases in the school environment. This may be accomplished by maintaining the immunization level of the school population and by recognizing and exlcuding potential cases of communicable disease from the environment.

Physical Environment. Reading under unfavorable lighting conditions may cause nervous tension and fatigue. The American Medical Association (AMA) recommends 10-foot candles for reading in classrooms, lecture halls, shops, laboratories and libraries. In addition, they recommend 50-foot candles for fine work or partially sighted children.[32] The light should be evenly distributed throughout the room and the ceiling should be painted white with sidewalls painted pastel colors for greatest ease in concentration.

Heating and ventilation should be provided with an ideal room temperature of 68° to 70° and 50% humidity. Since radiation from bodies in the room raises the temperature several degrees, the setting of the room temperature should be adjusted accordingly. Air change of 15 cubic feet per person per minute is usually adequate to provide fresh odor-free air.

Many schools have cafeterias or provisions for student lunches. Although these facilities are under the surveillance of the sanitarian from the health department, the nurse may assess the nutritional value of the meals served, or the overuse of the facilities (crowding) at a particular time and its influence on health.

Psychosocial Environment. The psychosocial environment may also have an influence on the school age child. A curriculum that is too crowded or too difficult or too easy may produce stress. Scheduling should be planned to allow breaks after a short interval of time in the classroom. This is both healthful and conducive to learning.

PLANNING AND IMPLEMENTING IN SCHOOLS

A great deal of the nurse's work in the school involves planning. Initially, nurses collect data on the health and immunization status of children entering school. Plans for obtaining this data involve sending out health forms and parent-information forms on each child. When this data is completed and returned, records are opened on each student and the data is recorded and used as a baseline for further data. If any forms are not returned, nurses must invite these particular parents to school and schedule physical examinations for their children with the school physician.

Thereafter, nurses must plan for periodic physical examinations and screening tests. If volunteers or other health personnel are involved they must be oriented and trained for the task.

Planning and implementing also involved follow-up on defects identified by family or school physicians during physical examinations or as a result of other screening procedures. Follow-up usually involves contacting parents by phone or letter regarding the defect and the need for follow-up care. Forms are usually sent to parents so that a report can be returned to the school nurse. For example, if there is a questionable cardiac problem, the nurse needs to know the amount of activity the student can participate in so that physical education and other appropriate personnel can be notified. Following notification of parents about defects, records are usually tagged so that the nurse is aware that further follow-up is needed. When forms are returned from parents records can be brought up to date with the data, appropriate staff can be notified, and records can be tagged for notification of parents to have the child reevaluated if needed. If reports are not returned, nurses may need to telephone parents to discuss the need for and importance of follow-up.

School nurses also need to plan time so that they are available at specific times during the school day for evaluating children referred by teachers. When children are referred, the nurse may send them back to class, have them rest in the nurse's office, or notify parents to pick up their child, depending upon the assessment.

In addition, school nurses must plan to work with teachers on integrating health concepts in the curriculum, to teach health concepts in certain classes, if appropriate, to schedule and carry out teacher–nurse conferences to evaluate each child in a classroom, and to work with teachers on assessing illnesses in the classroom. During teacher–nurse conferences the nurse helps teachers learn what to look for and adds to her knowledge of the home and community resources. A form may be provided for teachers to enter their observations on each student and these are compared with the nurse's records at the conference. Nurses should also inform teachers of any handicaps among their students and whether or not these require special considerations. Nurses may also alert teachers if there are increased incidences of diseases in the community, which may affect the school population. For example, if there is an increase in influenza the nurse would probably alert teachers and also review the signs and symptoms of the illness with them.

Health teaching is an important aspect of implementation in schools. In additon to working with teachers to integrate health concepts in the curriculum and to teach classes as needed, school nurses also teach in a variety of informal situations. When students come to the school nurse with injuries, the nurse can teach about prevention, or when students come with symptoms of illness the nurse can teach about prevention, treatment, and care of the body. In addition, school nurses may teach groups of students. For example, if a group of obese teenagers is interested in appearance, nurses may take the opportunity to work with them on nutrition, personal hygiene and grooming. Each contact with students allows the school nurse the opportunity for teaching about health.

Nurses also need to plan for emergencies in schools. Usually if children are injured during school hours a system is planned beforehand whereby the nurse may contact the parents for permission to obtain treatment or to have parents pick up the child and take them for treatment, or to bypass this procedure and notify the school or family physician directly.

EVALUATION IN THE SCHOOLS

Evaluation of nursing services may be difficult in the school setting because of the number of people involved in implementing health plans. For example, teachers may implement some of the health concepts integrated in the curriculum and they may supervise students in play areas, in the gymnasium, in shop courses, and in the classroom. They also are often responsible for assessing illnesses and defects in the classroom and, thus, may not recognize communicable diseases and defects among students depending upon their knowledge and other factors.

Certain aspects of the school nursing program can, however, be evaluated. Knowledge imparted as a part of health teaching in the curriculum can be tested by examinations. In addition, defects identified during physical examinations and screenings can be evaluated as to whether or not the children were referred for care, whether or not the care was received, and the results of care to be used in the school setting.

SCHOOL'S RELATIONSHIP WITH THE COMMUNITY

Because the school is an open system, there are various exchanges with the community. Although the impact of the economic, political, and other subsystems of the community are important, we focus here on the exchange with the family and health subsystems, as they influence the health of the school-aged child.

School-age children spend more time in the home than in the school and family beliefs and values are reinforced in that setting. Thus, unless parents are reached by the school nurse their goals may be at cross purposes. Families should be invited to participate in school examinations and any health problems discovered should be discussed with them. At the same time, the nurse has an opportunity to discuss growth and development, nutrition, rest and exercise patterns, community resources, and other aspects of prevention and treatment with them. When a child is sick when he reports to school, the nurse again has an opportunity to talk with parents about the need to keep sick children at home, aspects of nursing care for them, and means of preventing reoccurrences or the spread of the infection to others. At other times, the nurse may be interested in visiting the home of specific students to assess the home and discuss prevention and treatment with parents.

School nurses also work with the health system to provide care and obtain information on students in the school. In addition to working with the school physician, family physicians, sanitarians, and other members of the school health team, nurses may use various official and voluntary health agencies in providing care for students through their parents. Nurses may also interpret the school health program, its needs and purpose, to appropriate members of the health system, as a basis for the allocation of funding to the program. Likewise, when school nursing falls under the administrative direction of the health department, there is a need to report on nursing activities carried out in the school. Usually, these activities are reported on appropriate forms on a daily basis and are used in planning nursing services for particular schools.

Following is a guide that may be useful to student nurses during their school nursing experience for it organizes some of the factors in school nursing that have been discussed.

I. The School
   A. Level of education
   B. Enrollment ______ No. of classrooms regular ______ special ______
   C. General socioeconomic status of community
   D. Educational code and Health and Safety code
   E. Certification of health personnel
II. The Health Program in the School
   A. Organizational structure; philosophy
   B. Medical direction
      1. Type: ______ From whom: ______
   C. Health services offered to students and parents
      1. Kinds—purposes
      2. Physical facilities—(health unit)
      3. Safety provisions (*i.e.*, playground, physical ed.)
      4. Environmental health (*i.e.*, lighting, ventilation)
      5. Organized student or parent groups
      6. Special services (*i.e.*, psychologist, speech therapist, lunch program, dental health)
III. The Nurse's Participation in Health Program
   A. Organization position—to whom responsible
   B. Self-concept of role and functions
   C. Functions in available services
      1. Records and reports
      2. Kinds and purposes of health services (nurse's participation and role)
         a. Annual or periodic physical exam
         b. Safety
         c. Environmental sanitation
         d. First aid and emergency services
         e. Absenteeism and truancy
         f. Communicable disease control
         g. Detection of defects
         h. Screening programs
         i. Pupil-centered conferences

j. Curriculum consultation and program planning
k. Health counseling

IV. Relationship to Local Health Department and Community Agencies

THE NURSING PROCESS IN INDUSTRY

Nursing in industry is provided by various administrative patterns. Although the functions of nursing may be the same, there is a difference in the extent of the services provided. As a general rule there is one full-time physician for industries with 2000 to 3000 employees and one full-time nurse for each 300 to 750 employees. The full-time nurse would have access to a part-time physician. In industries with 100 employees, there is usually 2 to 3 hours of medical services and 6 to 9 hours of nursing service each week. According to the Bureau of Census approximately 75% of all employees work in industries with fewer than 500 employees; approximately 9% in settings with between 500 and 1000 employees; and 16% in settings with over 1000 employees.[33]

In smalll industries nursing services may be contracted from the local health department and nurses may be the major health representative in the organization. Thus, their assessment, which forms the basis for treatment (referring to a physician, or other aspects of health care) is extremely important.

ACCESSIBLE POPULATION IN INDUSTRY

A large proportion of the adult population is found in work settings where a significant amount of time is spent. The work environment can influence health and health can then influence productivity. Thus, industry, whose major goal is production, is interested in the health of its employees. From a community-health point of view, this population can be reached in the work setting for health matters and, as a result, services to this group will have a positive influence on community health.

According to the Labor Department there were 96 million people in the labor force in the United States in 1979.[34] Of these, about 60% were men and 40% women. Eighty-eight percent of this group was white.

INDUSTRIAL NURSING FUNCTIONS

Occupational or industrial nursing involves two kinds of programs. One program deals with the health of employees in relation to their work and the other deals with health care for nonoccupational illnesses and injuries. The two programs differ in relation to methods of financing and amounts and kinds of services provided, but both are important aspects of industrial nursing programs.

Various authors have outlined the objectives for industrial health programs differently although in essence they are basically the same. Since nursing functions evolve from the objectives of industrial health, some objectives are as follows:

- Physical and psychological assessment of workers to facilitate proper selection and placement
- Prevention of occupational and nonoccupational illnesses
- Provisions for treatment
- Fostering a high level of wellness for the workers.

Nursing functions that evolve from these objectives include the following:

- Participates in the health assessment program
- Provides nursing care to workers with occupational injuries and diseases
- Provides nursing care to workers with nonoccupational injuries and illnesses
- Counsels workers regarding personal and family health problems
- Plans and participates in health programs
- Advises on environmental sanitation and safety-education activities
- Carries out nursing administrative duties, which assures the efficient management of the industrial health service
- Works cooperatively with many professional and nonprofessional people at the local and state levels
- Compiles individual records for each employee, and compiles, evaluates, and interprets epidemiologic and statistical information concerning health and health services
- Evaluates health program and activities

DEFINITION OF OCCUPATIONAL HEALTH NURSING

Occupational health nursing is the "application of nursing and public health philosophy and skills to the relationship of people to their occupations for the purpose of prevention of disease and injury and the promotion of optimum health, productivity, and social adjustment."[35]

MAJOR HEALTH PROBLEMS OF THE INDUSTRIAL GROUP

The industrial group has the same distribution of nonoccupational-related diseases as the adult population. The four leading causes of death in this group, which accounts for 73% of all deaths, are diseases of the heart, malignant neoplasms, cerebrovascular disease, and accidents (see Table 6–1). In addition, all diseases in the top eleven are common among the industrial group, except number 9.

Death rates tell only part of the story in regard to nonoccupational health problems in the industrial group. According to vital statistics there were 314 million work-loss days for acute conditions in 1977, which accounted for a rate of 5.0 days per employed person for the year.[36] Although the majority of long-term illnesses are among individuals over the age of 65, a high proportion of these illnesses occur among individuals between the ages of 45 and 65.

According to Baetzer,

> studies of absenteeism due to disability have shown that over 90 percent of the cases and of the days of absence are due to nonoccupational illnesses and accidents as compared with about 0.1 percent due to industrial diseases and about 2 percent due to occupational injuries (except in the more hazardous occupations).[37]

Data from the National Health Survey showed that employed persons lost an average of 5.6 work days per person per year because of illness or injury and lost an average of 2.4 work days for each acute condition. Respiratory illnesses accounted for over one-half of all acute conditions. Other acute conditions accounting for loss of work included, wounds and lacerations, fractures, dislocations, contusions, and superficial injuries. The major chronic conditions causing loss of work included, heart conditions, arthritis, rheumatism, orthopedic impairments, conditions of the genitourinary system, mental and nervous disorders, hernia, peptic ulcers, asthma and hay fever.

The amount of absenteeism for all illnesses increases with age and is also higher in the lower income groups. In addition, women between the ages of 17 and 54 lose more time than men.

Table 6–1. Mortality Rates From Eleven Leading Causes of Death: United States, 1975

RANK ORDER	CAUSE OF DEATH	DEATH RATE PER 100,000 POPULATION
1	Diseases of the heart	336.2
2	Malignant neoplasms	171.7
3	Cerebrovascular disease	91.1
4	Accidents	48.4
5	Influenza and pneumonia	26.1
6	Diabetes mellitus	16.5
7	Cirrhosis of liver	14.8
8	Arteriosclerosis	13.6
9	Certain causes of mortality in early infancy	12.5
10	Suicide	12.0
11	Bronchitis, emphysema	12.7

(Vital Statistics of the United States, Vol. 2, 1976)

Table 6–2. Persons With Limitation of Activity Due to Chronic Conditions, by Degree of Limitation According to Age, United States, 1978

	AGE (YEARS)				
	ALL AGES	UNDER 17	17–44	45–64	65 AND OLDER
	Percent				
Persons with no limitation of activity	85.8	96.1	91.5	76.4	55.0
Persons with limitation of activities	14.2	3.9	8.5	23.6	45.0
Persons with limitations in major activities*	10.6	2.0	5.2	18.6	38.3

* Major activity refers to ability to work, keep house, engage in school or preschool activities

However, after age 54, they lose less time at work. It was also found that absenteeism because of illness is found among 15 or 20% of employees and there are many workers who do not lose time owing to illness.

The effect of long-term illnesses on activity can be seen in Table 6–2, which is adapted from the Health Survey Interview.[38] It should be noted that the proportion of the population with no chronic conditions decreases with age and conversely that the proportion with one or more chronic conditions increases with age. In addition, the degree of limitation associated with the chronic illness increases with age. A high proportion of the population in the 17 to 64 age group have chronic conditions. Almost one-half of the 17 to 44 age group have chronic conditions and 64% of the 45 to 64 age group have such conditions.

In addition to the nonoccupational-related illnesses and injuries, the working population also have occupational illnesses and injuries. According to the Public Health Service, in 1973, there were 2.2 million work-related disabling injuries.[39] Of these injuries, 14,500 resulted in death and about 90,000 resulted in permanent disability. As a result of these disabilities the loss was estimated at around $6.8 billion between liability compensation and work loss to industry.

In a study reported by Baetzer the incidence of occupational diseases in 28 states and for federal employees was noted.[40] The leading occupational disease was dermatitis which accounted for over one-half of all reported diseases. Other important occupational diseases include, diseases related to chemical agents and dust, diseases from repeated motion and pressure, and the untoward effects of heat and cold. The Bureau of Labor Statistics in 1979 also found skin diseases and disorders at the top of the list representing over 40% of all occupational illnesses in the United States and accounted for about 200,000 work days lost each year. This represented about one-fourth of the total time lost for all occupational diseases.[41]

INDUSTRY AS A SYSTEM

Like the school, industry is also a system made up of interrelated parts (workers, management) that function together to maintain the whole system. The goal of the system, which is production, determines the range of self-regulatory processes and any change in a part will affect the whole system. There is also input, output, retaining, and containing in the system. All of the characteristics elaborated upon in Chapter 1 and 4 pertain to industry as a system.

ASSESSMENT IN INDUSTRY

THE INDUSTRIAL POPULATION

The industrial nurse assesses workers for evidence of both occupational and nonoccupational injuries and illnesses. Often the initial screening is done by the plant foreman in an industry or a supervisor in another organization. These personnel are usually in close contact with the workers. After referral from these sources, the industrial nurse begins a more thorough assessment. A knowledge of industrial processes and their toxic effects as well as the chronic and acute diseases and injuries affecting this age group is helpful in this assessment. Occupational diseases may fall into any one of the following categories: "Diseases resulting from exposure to chemical substances such as dust and gases;. . . . Diseases resulting from the physical state of the environment such as temperature, radiant energy and noise . . . diseases resulting from mechanical factors such as pressure, physical strain, and movement; . . . and diseases due to infectious agents such as anthrax, brucellosis, and fungus diseases."[42] Nurses are interested in preventing diseases resulting from occupational hazards and in early diagnosis for workers showing signs and symptoms of deviations from the normal. In addition to a knowledge of industrial processes, the mode of entry for causative agents, and also the signs and symptoms of toxicity, nurses should know the Maximum Allowable Concentration (MAC) and Threshold Limit Values (TLV) of chemicals used in the organization as a basis for preventing toxicity in the workers. The **Maximum Allowable Concentration** refers to the maximum concentration of airborn chemicals a worker can tolerate without impairing health, and **Threshold Limits Values** are standards for allowable concentrations of chemicals in the air for daily exposure. These values are revised yearly by the American Conference of Governmental Industrial Hygienists and published in the Archives of Environmental Health, and they should be available in every industry using chemicals. Since respiratory-tract infections are the leading cause of illness for acute conditions, nurses should assess workers for these and other communicable diseases, which may spread to other workers and should also assess the immunization level of the work population. Chronic diseases are also common among this age group and assessment should include a consideration of the natural history of these diseases to prevent or identify early deviations within this population, which is at high risk because of age.

Periodic assessment is carried out by the physician in industry. Each employee is given a preplacement examination including an occupational history, personal and family history, physical examination, and laboratory testing. This is done to determine the health status of the workers and to provide suitable placement for them in the work situation. The physician may carry out the physical examination and the laboratory testing and the nurse may do the occupational history and personal and family history. After employment further periodic examinations are done to detect evidence of ill health and to determine if the employee's health is compatible with the work assigned.

INDUSTRIAL ENVIRONMENT

Industrial nurses also periodically assess the environment and all facilities in the organization to maintain a healthful working environment and to detect and appraise health hazards. In addition to the chemical substances, physical state of the environment, mechanical factors and infectious agents mentioned earlier, nurses are also interested in assessing the optimal conditions for work, such as, lighting, ventilation, temperature and humidity, and cleanliness of all areas in the organization to prevent contamination. This assessment in conjunction with the knowledge of plant processes, modes of transmission of causative agents, and conditions for optimal work output gives a baseline for recommendations to those in management for preventive and corrective measures.

PLANNING AND IMPLEMENTING IN INDUSTRY

Industrial nurses plan with the physician for periodic physicals and follow-up of exposed workers. During the implementation of these plans, they may obtain data on personal and family health and an occupational health history. They may also interpret the purpose and value of the examination, make routine tests, discuss the medical findings with the worker, plan with the worker for follow-up care, if needed, and discuss the findings with management as they relate to placement in the organization.

Nurses may also give emergency care based upon written orders for emergency nursing within their job description and limitations of professional nursing practice. Following this care, they will find placement for the workers as indicated in the standing orders and policies and will notify the appropriate people such as the physician and management. At the same time, they will use epidemiologic concepts in viewing this illness or injury as it relates to the worker and the environment to determine if injury and illness of other workers can be prevented.

Nurses also select, train, and supervise auxiliary nursing personnel to be used in selected aspects of the industrial nursing program. In addition, they work closely with plant foremen and supervisors, teaching them the knowledge they require to prevent diseases and injuries and to casefind.

An important aspect of the nurse's work in industry involves teaching workers. Teaching is most effectively done when workers come for periodic examinations of special problems. At these times, nurses may discuss oral hygiene, accident prevention, protective equipment, nutrition, or whatever is appropriate. They may also write articles for the industrial newspaper, place posters and educational materials on bulletin boards, and counsel groups of workers regarding health. In groups, nurses may interpret the safety program, teach signs and symptoms of occupational diseases and ways to prevent them, interpret workmens' compensation, discuss the use of protective equipment and other aspects of health.

Nurses also work closely with management. They may report unsafe and hazardous conditions, the health condition of employees necessitating a change in area of employment, or health conditions of workers requiring medical attention and a leave from work.

EVALUATION IN INDUSTRY

Evaluation in industrial nursing may be more difficult than in some less complex areas but certain aspects of the program can be evaluated. Over time, nurses can determine if there is a decrease in occupational diseases and injuries as a result of health promotional and preventive activities including, teaching of foremen, workers, and management. Nurses might also set as a goal the immunization of a large proportion of the workers and at a specified time evaluate whether or not the goal had been met. If hazards are noted, goals again can be set to reduce the hazards within a time frame and these can be evaluated.

INDUSTRIAL RELATIONSHIPS WITH THE COMMUNITY

Because industry is an open system there are exchanges between industry and the community. Workers bring their attitudes, knowledge, skills, and personal problems to the work setting and these may influence their work productivity. In addition, they bring their illnesses and some of these, such as acute communicable illnesses, may affect others in the organization. Thus, there is a need for nurses to use the nursing process in relation to home-and-work problems to improve the health and productivity of the workers.

In addition, there is an exchange between the organization (economic subsystem) and other community resources (social, health, or welfare subsystems).

Nurses establish relationships with the community. This may involve interpreting the health program and planning with community resources to meet the health needs of the workers. It may also involve setting up a referral system to arrange care for workers and their families or it may involve compiling data on absenteeism owing to illness to be used in calculating illness rates for the community. Nurses may also work closely with nursing programs and health agencies to provide learning experiences for students and others interested in industrial nursing.

RECORDING IN INDUSTRY

An important aspect of the nursing process in industry is recording. Individual records should be opened on each employee and should contain information on the preplacement and subsequent physical examinations, absenteeism, and treatments for illness or injury. Because the nurse is often the only full-time health worker in an organization, these records may be used in court cases dealing with workmens' compensation or where work-related disease or injury is suspected. Thus, records of such occurrences should include the time and place of injury or illness, cause, and a detailed description of the injury or illness and the condition of the worker. In addition, the immediate and follow-up care should be noted.

When defects are noted in workers, a system should be developed for referral and later follow-up by the nurse to determine whether care was sought, the defect corrected, and any special recommendations to be followed. Often nurses will tag records with different colored tags, which are coded for specific conditions. These records are then placed in order by weeks or months for follow-up by the nurse. After follow-up the records may be returned to the nurse's general file for worker's records.

In addition, nurses in industry usually complete administrative reports on a daily, monthly, and annual basis. These reports include work output and statistical data on injuries, illnesses, and so forth.

Records are a good source for detecting and eliminating occupational diseases and injuries,, for identifying areas of health teaching, for providing a system of follow-up, and for placement of workers in a job that is suited to their physical, mental, and emotional capabilities.

APPRAISING INDUSTRIAL NURSING

Student nurses are often given limited experiences in industrial nursing as part of their nursing program. This experience may occur during the wellness end of a wellness-illness integrated curriculum or may occur as part of the community health experience in a medical-model curriculum. The following Guide for Experience in Occupational Health is included to help students focus on important aspects of a limited industrial nursing experience:

- I. The Place of Employment
  - A. Type of plant, product, or services
  - B. Number of employees, sex, age range, socioeconomic and cultural factors
  - C. Job activities
  - D. Company organization and policy
  - E. Influence of organization in community
- II. The Health Program in the Place of Employment
  - A. Organizational structure; philosophy
  - B. Services offered to employees and families
    1. Kinds and purposes
    2. Title of unit
    3. Safety program
    4. Coordination within company
    5. Coordination with community agencies
  - C. Medical direction
    1. Type of medical direction
    2. Written, signed procedures for nurses
- III. The Nurse Participation in the Health Program
  - A. Organization position—to whom responsible
  - B. Self-concept of role and functions
  - C. Functions in available services
    1. Records and reports (confidential)
    2. Kinds and purpose of health services (and nurses participation)
       - a. preemployment physical exam (hearing and vision)
       - b. annual physical exam or periodic
       - c. safety
       - d. environmental safety
       - e. environmental health hazards
       - f. first-aid and emergency services
       - g. workmens' compensation and other insurance
       - h. absenteeism and return to work after illness
       - i. health counseling
       - j. other activities
- IV. Relationships to Local Health Departments and Community Agencies

MODEL FOR THE NURSING PROCESS

One model for the nursing process was developed by the author and colleagues at the University of California, School of Nursing in 1961.[43] The model in a modified form appears later in this section (see Fig. 6–5).

Community health nurses are committed to the philosophy of public health (see Chap. 5), they value health and have a thorough knowledge of it and are part of the health subsystem of the community. Thus, nurses can be viewed as intervening forces in the family system. Ideally, through the use of relationship-building models (see Chap. 7) and the use of the nursing process, these two subsystems (family and nurse) of the community can cooperate, and nurses can then assist families in maintaining, regaining, or obtaining a high level of wellness. In many instances, this assistance requires a change in behavior. However, before nurses know whether to reinforce observed behavior or to assist families in modifying their behavior, they must assess family health patterns and behaviors.

Assessment can be defined as the apperception and analysis of the forces and factors influencing behavior, which are conducive to healthful living.[44] As a process, then, assessment is composed of the two action-elements of assessing and relating, at a conscious level of awareness. The two actions occur simultaneously as assessing does not occur in a vacuum. It is an action in relation to or in response to someone, some phenomenon, something that must be or has been observed.

For example, while you are in a home or other setting with clients, you are observing, analyzing, and thinking, and at the same time you are focusing on the discussion and listening to particular health concerns.

Extra elements in a family or group situation are that you are responding to multiple individuals, or viewing the individual in relation to the total family, and considering the family as a group in relation to the community. Initial entry into the home is usually because of a health concern or specific health problem with one of the members, and the services may or may not have been requested.

Although the two actions—assessing and relating—are occurring simultaneously, for purposes of study, we view them separately. Methods of relating concepts are presented in Chapter 7.

As nurses are assessing in the home or other setting, they are observing and analyzing the family or group patterns of behavior. Our guide for this assessment is as follows:

ASSESSMENT FRAMEWORK

Indices For Determining Patterns of Health (essential elements):

- Physical status
- Emotional relations
- Values of Health
- Knowledge of Health
- Sex and reproductive patterns
- Source of help utilized for health concerns
- Hygiene and sanitation
- Authority distribution (in what areas or spheres for what kinds of decisions)

Determined to some degree by or affected by the following variables:

- Hereditary factors
- Agents of disease (community)
- Environment (resources such as geography and demography)
- Experience-past-present
- Values-cultural, religious, education
- Economic
- Mobility
- Law

Because there is no one ideal combination for all people of the factors influencing health status and behavior, we first look at the patterns in the family or group objectively. See Chapter 9 for the concept of interrelatedness and multicausation of diseases to enlarge upon the idea that no one combination of factors influences health and behavior.

Although we realize that we bring our own prejudices, values, past experiences, and biases into the family situation, we try to minimize these at this point and focus on what we see without making judgments.

We start with physical status, emotional relations, and so forth, and descend the list assessing the health status and behaviors related to these. For example, under health status we might be interested in observing the newborn or doing a complete inspection, using the Denver Developmental Screening Test, or other guide.

In addition to observing the elements of physical status, emotional relations of the group, and so forth, we must also determine which variables from the assessment framework affect these elements. For example, often the values of health index is influenced by the variables of culture, religion and education and, as we discussed earlier, various social-class groups with varying educational or cultural backgrounds have different concepts of and values in health. Or, we may find that a hereditary factor and past and present experiences have influenced the values of health. For example, if a child is born with a defect such as cerebral palsy, both the child and family may value health because of the numerous positive exposures to the health subsystem.

In addition to looking at the variables affecting these elements, we must also look at the strength of these forces or variables, which affect health status and health behavior (patterns), to determine in what way we can assist families to maintain healthful living patterns, or how we can assist family members to adjust to or to change their patterns. If the force that maintains the pattern is too strong, we may decide to wait until we have formed a better relationship with the family or group or that the force is too strong and that change would affect the family balance in a negative way and move them away from health. (This is where we use the concept of balance and risk to be presented shortly.)

For example, the family that has recently moved to our community from Mexico may be spending a large amount of their income for food that is familiar to them, at the expense of obtaining an adequate diet and meeting other basic needs. The nurse should question the importance of the eating pattern and its significance for the family. Here nurses may feel they can eventually help families plan more adequate diets based upon their financial resources, but should make this a long-range goal to be implemented after they have established a better relationship with the family, and the family has become acclimated to the American way of life.

Or a community health nurse may find a family whose religious convictions are against medical and health care and preventive services. Here the nurse might decide the force making the pattern what it is (religious convictions) is too strong to change, but could help the family adjust to illness and other changes as they happened.

At this point in our process, we are ready to make a judgment. We have looked at the family's health status and health patterns and the forces that make them what they are; we have also weighed the strength of these forces. We now look at the forces that seem detrimental to health and those that are conducive to health.

Our judgment here is based upon our knowledge of accepted standards for the elements previously discussed, based upon established norms for populations at various points in their life span. However, we realize that standards are only guideposts and not absolute. Standards may change as new knowledge evolves. For example, we in the health system have moved from the idea that infants should follow a rigid feeding schedule of every 4 hours to a more flexible schedule that is based upon demand and the infant's overall daily needs. In addition, we know there are individual variations within these standards. For example, some people need 8 hours of sleep nightly, whereas others consistently require less.

Some categories of standards we use in relation to the indices include the following:

- Hygiene—standards of general bodily cleanliness, sleep, exercise
- Sanitation—standards of general environmental sanitation, housing, refuse disposal, rodent control, accident hazards
- Knowledge of health—normal growth and development, various diseases and agents of illness, preventive services, community resources
- Physical status—height and weight within range for age, muscle tone, condition of mouth and gums, posture, condition of skin, hair, and so forth, as outlined in various physical assessment books
- Emotional relations—support for each other in family or group, sharing of experiences, allowing each member to live up to own capacity, meeting mutual respect and security needs
- Values of health—secures periodic health evaluation and preventive services appropriate for age, medical supervision, when indicated
- Sex and reproductive patterns—adjusted to family so as not to affect mother's physical health or emotional relations, and financial strain
- Source of help utilized—health facilities, private or free clinics, neighbors, community health nurse
- Authority distribution—joint parental decisions on childrearing; family spending. Joint family decisions among adult members on those things that affect the group.

NURSING PROCESS MODEL

Figure 6–5 is our model for the nursing process. Beginning with the Nurse and Family in the model, we plug in our various health patterns and the knowledge of the strength of the forces for the particular family, under assessment where health is listed. We next look at these in relation to the ones that are conducive to health and those which are detrimental. Our judgments are based upon the standards we have identified from a comparison of observed patterns with known standards from nursing textbooks.

Prior to setting priorities, we also add our knowledge of epidemiologic-alertness and balance-and-risk concepts. **Epidemiologic alertness** (epi-alertness) is defined as "awareness of health threats to groups is based on knowledge of the natural history of disease and injury process," and **balance and risk** is defined as the weighing of factors that are conducive to a degree of adjustment with those that are interfering.[45] For example, considering epi-alertness and the individual, family, and community relationships, a child in the home with questionable tuberculosis would influence our priority because of the possible implications for others.

Or considering balance and risk, we might see that a mother is jeopardizing her physical health by devoting all her time to a sick or retarded child. She may feel guilty and need to do this to meet her psychological needs. We might also see that she is not adequately meeting the needs of other family members, but they have adjusted to this. We know that this overprotectiveness is not healthy for the personality development of the child, but would consider what it would do to this mother and family if we were to try to change the situation (balance established by the family).

We weigh all of these factors (the health assessment, epi-alertness, and balance and risk) against autonomy (nurses, families, agency policy, community) and resources available (family and community) to determine our priorities at any point in time.

The process of assessing and setting priorities is a continuous process, and priorities may change as any one of the factors change—assessment of health including the strength of the forces, epi-alertness factors, balance-and-risk-factors, autonomy, or resources.

The arrows facing priority in Figure 6–5 show these changes, which influence priority setting. In addition, these arrows show the effect of relating (relationship) on priority setting. The basis of relating is to try to understand what the health patterns, forces influencing them, and so forth

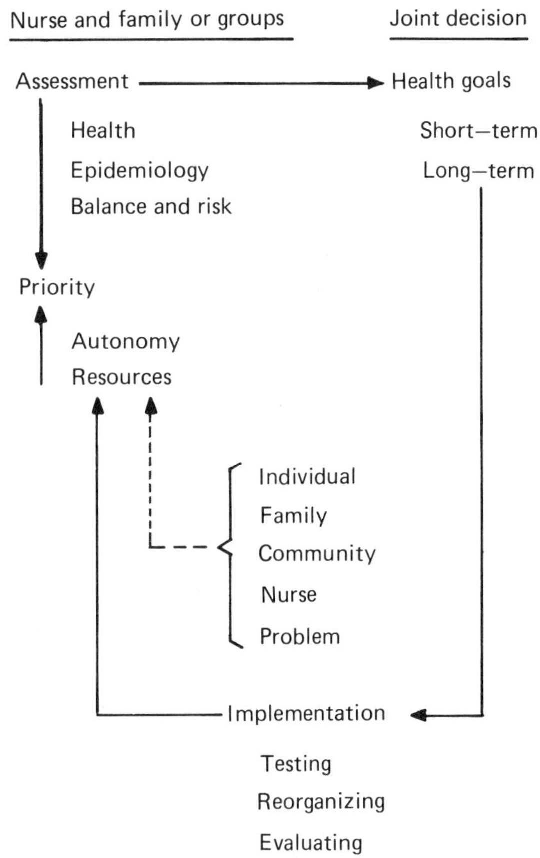

Figure 6–5
The nursing process. **Broken arrow** refers to the process of assessing and setting priorities.

mean to the family. In order to do this, it is necessary to use all our skills in interviewing, asking questions, creating an atmosphere that allows for expression of concern and so forth (see Chap. 7).

Here is also where, with the information we have, we plan to test areas where more information is needed to ascertain how the family views their health needs. For example, we may feel that the family is not eating an adequate diet and want to focus more on this during another visit to validate this hunch, before setting this as a priority. We may also test out cues we have previously received from the family in order to validate our hypothesis. This could include testing the accuracy of our understanding of the meaning (to the family) of the patterns and forces, testing cues regarding their resources (physical, emotional, financial) or the strength of the forces identified.

Only by understanding the particular family can we know in which areas we should attempt to support observed behavior, in which areas we should attempt to assist them to modify or change, and in which areas we should offer support during the process of change and adjustment.

It is essential that we always consider the family balance before supporting the behavior of family members by applying the balance-and-risk concept to this system. For example, if we support or assist the mother in changing her behavior, what will it do to the other family members? Will it disrupt the existing relationship balance and move the family away from health. What are some alternatives to modifying behavior while still maintaining some degree of balance necessary to meet the everyday life events or crises as seen by the family? Here we might think back to the mother who was meeting her psychological needs but abusing her physical health and to the family who seemed to have adjusted to this balance. What happens to the family situation if we try to change this behavior, that is, strip the mother of her psychological needs? Does this create new problems for the family to face and move them further away from a healthy balance?

Or, if the family believes that a piece of garlic around the child's neck is essential to his recovery, does that really hinder his health? And what happens to the family balance or our relationship if we try to change this behavior, which is based upon a strong belief system?

In our model, there is a broken arrow extending from a set of factors to the assessment-priority setting process. Any of these factors may affect priority setting.

For example, a problem identified during the assessment may set limitations on the role of the nurse, that is, the nurse may feel unprepared to deal with it and may turn it over to another such as a social worker (social problems) or to the hospital for acute care beyond the scope of community health nursing. The type of problem may also require facilities that are not available. For example, the nurse and family may go through the entire process of assessing and priority setting and decide a child should be placed in a foster home, but none may be available. Or, they may decide a mentally retarded child should be placed immediately in a sheltered home, but there is a long waiting list. Thus, priority setting would be affected.

The community may also affect the assessment- and priority-setting process. In a rural setting, families may be willing to go for health services, but transportation is inadequate, or facilities are not available to meet their needs. In an urban area, facilities may be available but not coordinated well enough for families to get to all their appointments in the time they have available. Thus, some priorities cannot be implemented.

The family may also affect this process. Different families perceive community health nurses in different ways based upon past experience. Some may see them as an authority from the health department and because of their attitudes about authority will reject health as a priority, others may appear interested in changing health patterns but will not put the plans into action. Some families may see nurses in the community as bedside nurses and thus refuse their teaching and counseling services.

Likewise, nurses may affect the process. They may identify with one member of the family without realizing it and this hampers the movement of the family as a whole. Or, they may not see themselves as members of a team and will try to work independently with the family giving them information that is conflicting with what other health team members have given. This may confuse the family and make them unwilling to carry out priorities. Or, if community health nurses are unclear as to their role, they may carry out functions that could best be handled by other community resources. In this way, they may consider something unimportant, when in reality it is very important and should be a priority.

Nurses' beliefs about their roles as helping persons may also affect the process. If they see themselves as individuals who relieve suffering by selfless personal service, they may distort their functions as helpers and continue to take care of individuals rather than allow them or the family to take over functions that would move them toward independent action. Or if nurses see themselves only as teachers, they may force the family into assuming the complete responsibility for care before they are ready or capable of doing this.

The process may also be affected by the amount of knowledge and degree of skill nurses have. If they have inadequate knowledge of nutrition, disease processes, and other concepts, they will be ineffective in assessing and setting priorities.

Once priorities are set, short- and long-term goals are planned jointly with the family. For example, we might see the need for personal care for an incapacitated member of the family. Our long-term goal might be independence or interdependence for the family member and a short-term goal would be to provide the necessary care to meet the basic needs of the family member. We would decide with the family the best way to meet these goals. Alternative ways might include the nurse giving the care, a home health aide providing care under the supervision of a community health nurse, a registered nurse who is not a community health nurse giving the care (without supervision), a family member giving the care, or a combination of these methods.

Once we pick a desired method, the actions to meet the goal must be programmed. These include the target group, the activity, and the time period to reach the goal. The target group in the above example is the incapacitated patient. Activities may include baths, feeding, mouth care, and so forth and would need to be specified, timing these activities around the daughter's schedule (if she is to give the care). We would also need to assess the daughter's resources and perhaps set goals and objectives for her, such as, teaching, bathing the patient in bed, nutrition, and so forth.

Once our plans are developed with the family we begin implementing them. If the plans do not prove adequate for the particular situation, the nurse and family reorganize and suggest other proposed alternatives to meet the goal. For example, if the daughter tried to give the necessary care but was unable to learn the needed skills, antagonized the sick family member, or is anxious about giving the care, the family and nurse may decide to use the R.N. to provide the care.

Evaluation is also a part of implementation in our model. Evaluation involves both the effectiveness of the services provided and the effectiveness of the nurse's skills and abilities.

Effectiveness is measured by the health and health-related changes in the family. For example, in the above example effectiveness could be measured by the care given and the patient's movement toward independence. Roberts and Hudson in *How to Study Patient Progress* provide one way of measuring patient progress by looking at the reduction of nursing needs in the course of care.[46] Another way of looking at this progress would be to look at the number of problems solved or eliminated on the Problem Oriented Record problem list.

Finally, we look at the excellence of our own professional practice as compared to that of our peers with similar education and experience. This is an ongoing process in which the individual nurse should take part. (See guide for self-evaluation in Appendix A.) Periodically nurses are also evaluated by their supervisors. In addition, some agencies use standards and guides such as the nursing audit to evaluate practice.

The process of implementation as the rest of the nursing process is an ongoing process. Nurses continually test, reorganize, and evaluate. As they continue to visit in homes they obtain further information about families, their own knowledge increases, they gain further understanding of the relationship of the family to the community, and further understanding of public health. They continually observe and test out these new observations in the light of new knowledge. They may readjust plans in the light of new information (assessment) or reorganize plans for accuracy in understanding family patterns and ways to assist them.

Nurses also continually evaluate the effects of movement or balance in the family toward achieving realistic and desirable health goals.

The entire nursing process may be started at any point but the process remains basically the same. For example, the nurse may use information from the client's record and begin setting goals and priorities, considering balance and risk and epi-alertness, before entering the home. Here, the nurse is starting with implementation from the model. However, we may see a different picture of the situation when we enter the home and move to the assessment area of the framework.

Or, nurses may focus on the community aspect such as with a referral on a tuberculosis contact. Here, they have only a referral with limited information and must enter the home to start the process under assessment. Interested readers are referred to an article by this author and co-workers, which narrates this process.[24]

RECORDING THE NURSING PROCESS

Recording is an important component of nursing practice in all settings. It allows nurses unfamiliar with systems (individuals, families, communities) to review a large amount of data and develop a realistic overview of the system. It also allows other nurses to know what has been done for systems and thus provides a basis for accountability. In many settings records are used to audit and improve nursing practice.

Problem-Oriented Medical Records. One of the most widely used methods of recording currently evolved from Weed's Problem-Oriented Medical Records.[47] During the initial assessment in Weed's method, the data base is collected from a patient profile, history, physical examination and laboratory reports. From this data, problems are identified and listed. This step is similar to the assessment step of the nursing process, which involves data collection, interpretation of data, validation of data and nursing diagnosis. Next, a plan is developed for each problem listed. Plans including the diagnostic, therapeutic, and patient education aspects of planning are related to each problem on the problem list by a number. This aspect of Weed's system is comparable to the planning step of the nursing process, which involves priority setting, goals and objectives, alternate methods to meet the goals, and actions to be taken. Weed's progress notes, which are written on each patient's contact, are related again to a specific problem on the problem list and include subjective data, objective data, assessment, and plans for each problem addressed. **Subjective data** involves symptoms and complaints that the patient or family verbalize and should be quoted where possible. **Objective data** includes the nurses observations and measurements, such as, temperature, blood pressure, pulse, and weight. In addition, objective data may include information from clinic and hospital records, laboratory reports, and other reliable data. **Assessment** is based upon the nurse's judgment about the problem, based upon the subjective and objective data. The **plan** includes a plan of action to resolve the problem identified in the assessment, and may include plans for additional data, plans for treatment or management, and plans for patient and family education. In some settings, plans refer to plans that were already implemented and plans for the future. Weed's progress notes also include flow sheets and discharge notes. **Flow sheets** are progress notes specifically designed for certain physiologic or mental parameters, such as, temperature, pulse, respirations, blood pressure, laboratory tests, and so forth, which are monitored on a regular basis. The discharge notes are the final progress notes and indicate the status of the patient and family in relation to each problem from the problem list. The progress notes can be related to the implementation and evaluation steps of nursing process.

Recording in Community Health Nursing. Currently, recording in community health is modeled after Weed's Problem-Oriented Records (just discussed). Nurses assess initially in the home, clinic, school, industry, or other settings and identify problems for the problem list. Assessment guides for the family and community are located in Appendices B and C. Problems identified may be physical, physiologic, demographic, or social. For example, one area of assessment in the family is the nutritional patterns. In one family, we might find that the diet is inadequate owing to a lack of knowledge about nutrition. Thus, our problem would be inadequate information related to balanced nutrition. This might be listed as problem #1 on the problem list. All other problems identified in the family would also be recorded in sequence on the problem list.

Next, we would record our initial plans to meet the problem. Plans may include those for additional data or diagnostic treatment or education. The goal for problem #1 could be to prevent poor nutrition in family members or to maintain adequate nutrition to all body cells. At the same time, because the family lacks knowledge of normal nutritional needs, another goal would be to increase learning regarding nutritional needs of family members. Planned actions to meet the goals of problem #1 might be to explain the danger of and to describe the specific effects of poor health habits and practice, to teach components of a balanced diet, to teach budgeting for food, and so forth, within a specified time period.

On a home visit, the nurse might hear the family say that they were trying to prepare more balanced meals, but were having some difficulty. The nurse would review the diet plans of the family and might discover that the only deficit in the diet was protein. Teaching sources of protein might follow this assessment. The nurse's progress notes then might read as follows:

Problem #1. Maintain adequate nutrition.
- S. Mother says, "I am having difficulty preparing balanced meals."
- O. Review of family meals for 24-hour period disclosed balanced diet, except for protein which was inadequate.
- A. Protein lacking in family meals.
- P. Discussed sources of protein with mother. Supported and reinforced progress made in other elements of meal planning. Asked mother to keep another 24-hour meal plan. Review meal plan on next home visit.

Some nurses use the subjective, objective, assessment, and plan format and include interventions and plans under the plan heading. Others use a more detailed format for progress notes. For example, Benson suggests SOAPIER for the progress notes.[48] In this format, S = subjective data, O = objective data, A = assessment, P = plan, I = intervention, E = evaluation, and R = revision or changing care plan as needed.

In either format subjective data includes all complaints or symptoms mentioned by the system and should be quoted whenever possible. Objective data includes all physiologic and psychological indicators such as temperature, pulse, blood pressure, mental status, and whatever other indicators are appropriate to the particular problem from the problem list. In addition, laboratory tests, reports from other nurses, hospitals or other social, health, or welfare subsystems of the community may be used as objective data. Under assessment, nurses make and record conclusions based on subjective and objective data.

If plans complete the progress note format, they include both the plans carried out, or interventions, and future plans. Plans may revolve around additional data needs, treatment, and educational needs.

Because families and communities are dynamic systems exchanging with their environment and because nurses continue to follow individual and family systems over time, new problems may be identified and old ones may be resolved. As a problem is resolved it is closed on the problem record and the particular number is not reused. For example, if inadequate diet in a family was problem number 1 and they were now maintaining their nutritional needs by eating balanced diets, this problem could be closed on the problem list, however, number one would not be reused on this family's problem list. If there were five problems recorded on the list and resolved, further problems identified on home visits would be numbered 6, 7, 8, and so forth.

Discharge Summary. The discharge summary should address each problem on the problem list and the individual's or family's status in relation to each problem. The summary should have information on the level of resolution of the problem and should justify discharge of the system from active nursing services. The record and discharge summary allows nurses to audit their performances and with proper feedback from an audit committee to learn their strengths and weaknesses, with a goal of improving nursing care. The record also allows nurses to evaluate performances in resolving problems by means of the nursing process.

Advantages of Problem-Oriented Medical Record's Method. Rakel compares problem-oriented recording with the traditional method and notes some differences.[49] All problems are recorded on one page and thus not forgotten in the problem-oriented approach. This was not the case with traditional recording where problems were forgotten or required an extensive search of the record for identification. When viewing particular problems, only those labeled by a number from the problem list had to be considered. Auditing was impossible in the traditional method because of sketchy unorganized notes with little assessment data, however, auditing can be easily done with the problem-oriented method because of the structure of the progress notes and the use of flow sheets. Continuity of care is much improved also because all agencies use the same method and problem lists in one agency can be duplicated and sent to another for follow-up when a patient moves (*e.g.*, one community to another or from home to hospital). In addition, laboratory reports are scattered throughout the chart in traditional records but are in one area of the chart in the problem-oriented record making it easier to review; other differences are listed in Rakel.[50]

REFERENCES

1. Yura H, Walsh M: The Nursing Process. New York, Appleton-Century-Crofts, 1978
2. Executive Committee and the Standards Committee of the Division on Community Health Nursing Practice. Standards for Community Health Nursing Practice. Kansas City, ANA, 1973
3. Liu B-C: Quality of Life Indicators in the U.S. Metropolitan Areas, 1970. Kansas City, Midwest Research Institute, 1975
4. Freeman R: Community Health Nursing Practice. Philadelphia, WB Saunders, 1970
5. Maslow AH: Motivation and Personality. New York, Harper & Row, 1954
6. Hanlon J: Public Health Administration and Practice, p 285. St Louis, CV Mosby, 1974
7. Ibid
8. Freeman R, op cit, p 65
9. Reinke W, Williams KN: Health Planning Qualitative Aspects and Quantitative Techniques, pp 236–239. Maryland, Johns Hopkins University, 1972
10. Ibid
11. Freeman R, op cit, p 66
12. Ibid
13. Ibid
14. Ibid
15. Byrne M, Thompson L: Key Concepts for the Study and Practice of Nursing, p 6. St Louis, CV Mosby, 1972
16. Bennis W, et al: The Planning of Changes, p 33. New York, Holt, Rinehart & Winston, 1969
17. Ibid
18. Ibid
19. Lewin K: Group discussion and social change. In Newcomb T, Hathey E (eds): Social Psychology, pp 197–211. New York, Holt, Rinehart & Winston, 1958
20. Bennis W, et al, op cit, pp 328–334
21. Ibid, p 222
22. Paul B: Health, Culture and Community. New York, Russell Sage, 1969
23. Davis MS: Variations in patient's compliance with doctors' advice. Am J Public Health, 58:274, 1968
24. Helvie C, et al: The setting and nursing practice. Nurs Outlook 16, No. 9:35, Sept 1968
25. Hanlon J, op cit, p 385
26. Freeman R: op cit, p 308
27. Ibid, p 308
28. Committee on School Nursing. Functions, Standards and Qualifications of School Nursing, A.N.A., 1965
29. Ibid
30. Report of the Committee on Terminology in School Health Education. Journal of the American Association of Health, Physical Education and Recreation 22:14, Sept 1971
31. Hanlon J, op cit
32. Sartwell P: Preventive Medicine and Public Health, p 736. New York, Appleton-Century-Crofts, 1973
33. U. S. Department of Commerce, Bureau of the Census, Social Indicators, 1976. Washington, DC, U. S. Government Printing Office, 1977
34. U. S. Department of Labor, Bureau of Statistics, Monthly Labor Review, p 57. 102, No. 7, July 1979
35. Fromer M: Community Health Care and the Nursing Process, p 413. St Louis, CV Mosby, 1979
36. U. S. Department of Health, Education, and Welfare. Estimates from the Health Interview Survey, 1977. Public Health Service, Series 10, No. 126. Sept 1978
37. Baetzer A: Health of the working population. In Sartwell P (ed): Preventive Medicine and Public Health, p 825. New York, Appleton-Century-Crofts, 1973
38. U. S. Department of Health, Education, and Welfare. Current Estimates from the Health Interview Survey, U.S. 1978, p 25. Public Health Service, Nov 1979
39. U. S. Department of Health, Education, and Welfare. Current Estimates from the Health Interview Survey, U.S. 1978, Public Health Service, 1979
40. Baetzer A, op cit, p 780
41. Wang CL: Occupational skin disease continues to plague industry. Monthly Labor Review Vol. 102, No. 2:17, Feb 1979
42. Baetzer A, op cit, p 780
43. Hill A, Helvie C, Bambino C: Model of Nursing Process. San Francisco, University of California, School of Nursing, 1962 (unpublished)

44. Ford L, et al: Defining Clinical Content Graduate Nursing Programs. Community Health Nursing. Boulder, Western Interstate Commission for Higher Education in Nursing, Feb 1967
45. Helvie C, et al, op cit
46. Roberts DE, Hudson H: How To Study Patient Progress. Washington, DC, Public Health Service, #1169, April 1964
47. Weed LL: Medical Records, Medical Education and Patient Care. Cleveland, Case Western Reserve University, 1971
48. Benson E, McDevitt J: Community Health and Nursing Practice, p 276. Englewood Cliffs, Prentice-Hall, 1976
49. Rakel RE: Principles of Family Medicine, Chapter 14. Philadelphia, WB Saunders, 1977
50. Ibid

7

Relating and Communicating: Processes Occurring Concurrently With the Nursing Process

Communicating and relating are processes that occur concurrently with the nursing process and can facilitate or hamper the comprehensive application of the nursing process. If nurses lack good interviewing and other communication skills, if they have negative attitudes and feelings about the client they are working with, or they lack knowledge about building relationships, they are not likely to collect adequate data during the assessment phase of the nursing process to meet the client's needs. In addition, these factors may interfere with the client's ability to carry out the planned interventions. On the other hand, if nurses have good communication skills and relate well with the client, they are more likely to collect adequate data during the assessment and to elicit compliance of the client in implementing planned interventions.

One model that is useful in evaluating the community health nurse's ability to use these three processes effectively has been presented by Dyer.[1] In Dyer's use of the Johari window, which is named after the inventor of the model, Joseph Luft and Harry Ingram, each part of a fourfold table represents an area of the nurse-client system relationship, as in Figure 7–1.

The upper left quadrant of the table represents the free interactional exchange between the nurse and client. As nurses begin working with client systems this area is usually small (Fig. 7–2). As they continue interacting with clients this area should become large as depicted in Figure 7–3, if the nurse is effective in applying the three concurrent processes. If this area of the window remains small, nurses should reevaluate their communication and relationship skills to improve their ability to be of assistance to the client.

The second quadrant represents data known to the client system but not to the nurse. This data includes pertinent aspects of health the client system has not shared with the nurse that is needed for a comprehensive assessment. It also includes the clients "feelings and unspoken reactions to the nurse."[2]

The third quadrant represents information known to the nurse, which has not been shared with the client system. This data may include confidential information or information that the nurse thinks the client is not ready to deal with or act upon.

The fourth area is the "unknown area of

feelings, attitudes, and reactions that people hold inside and often will not admit even to themselves."[3]

This model should assist community health nurses in evaluating their interaction with clients. Such ongoing evaluation is important if we are to effectively meet client needs.

Thus far, we have talked about the client system. Our client may be any of the systems discussed in Chapters 2, 3, and 4; that is, clients may be individuals, families, or community groups. As we work with any of these systems we become a part of the system and we can, thus, think in terms of the nurse-client system. This chapter looks at the nurse-client system, and ways we can facilitate the comprehensive application of the nursing process.

THE NURSE-CLIENT SYSTEM

As the community health nurse and client make contact, interact and work on the client's problems they form a system and will exhibit all of the characteristics of a system discussed in Chapters 1 through 4. The nurse represents a subsystem of the health subsystem of the community and the individual family, or group, represents a second subsystem of the community.

ENTRY

Initially, the nurse must gain entry into the system because systems allow input but they may also keep people and things outside their boundaries (containment). This was discussed in Chapters 2, 3, and 4. If nurses are visiting families at their homes for the first time, they should introduce themselves, explain their purpose for visiting, help families see the value of this service for meeting family needs, and begin building a therapeutic relationship to reduce the possibility of being kept outside (containment) the families' boundaries in later visits. Initially, some families may think the nurse is a social worker coming to check up on them or a bill collector who they wish to avoid. Thus, it is important for nurses to wear uniforms and carry a nursing bag to identify them as community health nurses. This may facilitate entry into the home.

	Known to client	Not known to client
Known to the nurse	Area of free communication 1	Hidden area 3
Not known to the nurse	"Blind" area (for the nurse) 2	Unknown area 4

Figure 7–1
(From Dyer WG: Working with Groups. In Reinhardt AM, Quinn MD (eds): Family-Centered Community Nursing, St. Louis, CV Mosby, 1973. Reproduced with permission)

Beginning relationships

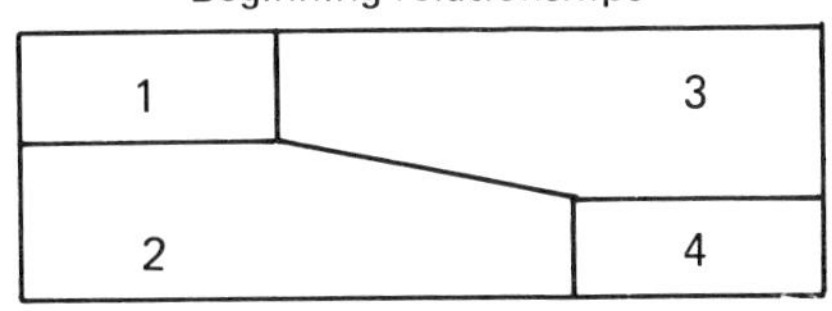

Figure 7–2
(From Dyer WG: Working with Groups. In Reinhardt AM, Quinn MD (eds): Family-Centered Community Nursing, St. Louis, CV Mosby, 1973. Reproduced with permission)

Ongoing effective relationship

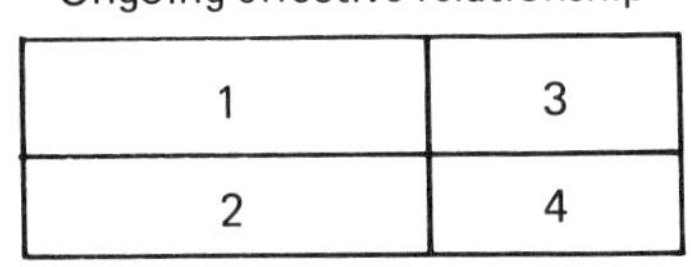

Figure 7–3
(From Dyer WG: Working with Groups. In Reinhardt AM, Quinn MD (eds): Family-Centered Community Nursing, St. Louis, CV Mosby, 1973. Reproduced with permission)

Families may wish to keep (contain) community health nurses from their boundaries for a variety of other reasons. For example, they may have had negative experiences with nurses in the past and fail to see any value in their services, or they may see the nurse as an authority figure who frightens them. Hall has suggested several techniques that may facilitate entry into the system.[4] "Professional hanging around may facilitate systems entry simply because the practitioner became part of the environment of the client system."[5] As clients become aware of the potential resources of the nurse, they may allow entry into the system. "Hustling is employed when the practitioner pushes his/her way into the proximal environment of the client system and actively sells resources."[6] In this technique, the client may allow entry of the nurse into the system as a result of pressure. "Demonstrating competence [which is another technique], facilitates entry because it takes place in the distal environment and affects the client system, although initially, it is beyond its awareness."[7] Most of these techniques seem feasible in a community meetinghouse or other community setting where families may be accessible, but they are not appropriate in the home setting for gaining entry.

NURSE-CLIENT SYSTEM DEVELOPMENT

Initially, when the nurse and client meet, they view each other in relation to how each fits preconceived ideas of the specific client or nurse role. If one or the other deviates too far from preconceived concepts of the "good nurse" or the "good client," they may be labeled "bad" and the relationship, the nurse-client system, may never begin. However, because nurses have a knowledge of how to build relationships and projects important helping characteristics, which are discussed later in this chapter, the relationship can go beyond this stage of stereotyping.

If the relationship continues, the nurse and client communicate with and relate to one another and establish their own roles in this specific interdependent system. At this time, they begin to see each other as individuals occupying specific roles, rather than as role stereotypes and develop complemental roles that fit together in a process similar to that used by the family or groups. Each learns what role behaviors to carry out and what role behaviors to expect of the other within the system. In community health nursing, the nurse's role behaviors may involve communicating concern, warmth, empathy, and the willingness to assist the client, providing emotional support, teaching prevention and treatment, assisting the client in identifying problems and resources needed to resolve the identified problems. On the other hand, client behaviors may include aspects such as sharing information and concerns with the nurse, considering alternative solutions to a problem, selecting the best course of action, and carrying out the actions to meet the mutually agreed upon goals.

Once the role behaviors of the nurse and client become somewhat patterned there may be rules about the roles and any deviation from roles will be censured overtly or covertly. However, these patterned behaviors are not fixed and must change as conditions within the system change. For example, as the client learns to carry out nursing and preventive procedures the nurse moves away from teaching in this area, or as the client becomes comfortable in the situation, the nurse reduces emotional support. This is similar to changes necessitated within a family system when one or more members arrive at new stages of growth and development (negentropy).

INPUT, OUTPUT, RETAINING, AND CONTAINING

There is input, output, retaining, and containing within the nurse-client system. Input involves the knowledge, skills, attitudes, and values brought to the system by the nurse and client. These are brought to bear on the client's problems. Some data are collected from clients, whereas other data are contained by clients, depending upon the purposes of the agency that the nurse represents and also the nurse's knowledge about and ability to communicate to and relate to clients. In addition, there may be input into the system about the nurse's or community's resources to assist the client. Community resources may be used directly by the client or may be used by the nurse with an indirect effect upon the client. For example, the nurse may invite the nutritionist to visit a family needing specialized nutritional counseling or may obtain consultation from the nutritionist and use this information to assist the family.

Information and energy are also retained within the system. Information pertinent to solving client problems and aspects of the relationship such as warmth, caring, trust, and empathy are retained by the system. In addition, growth (negentropy) that takes place within the system is retained by the client and nurse following the termination of the nurse-client system.

NEGENTROPY–ENTROPY

Over a period of time the nurse-client system grows and evolves (negentropy) or deteriorates and leads to the death of the nurse-client system (entropy). The choice between negentropy and entropy in the nurse-client system is primarily based upon the nurse's ability to build a therapeutic relationship and to effectively use the nursing process and communication skills to meet the client's needs.

There is also feedback in the nurse-client system in the process of communicating. When we interact with others, they in turn send verbal and nonverbal messages back to us that indicate whether or not we are understood, liked or disliked, and whether or not we are acting appropriately in the eyes of our clients. At times we may ask for feedback and at other times clients' feelings will be clear to us from their behavior (verbal or nonverbal). This is an important part of our interaction with clients if we are to be effective with them. Feedback should be an ongoing part of the communicating and relating processes and may be especially meaningful to us as a signal that the client has grown (negentropy) and that we must adjust our patterned behavior accordingly.

THERAPEUTIC NURSE-CLIENT RELATIONSHIPS

Leahy and co-workers define the therapeutic nurse-client relationship as "a bond between the nurse and patient that connotes mutual trust, respect, caring, sharing . . . it facilitates growth of the patient . . . it is made possible through the purposeful intervention of the assisting nurse."[8] Thus, the relationship is more than a social one, it has a purpose. The purpose is to help the system meet goals (equifinality) that they are unable to meet on their own because they lack the knowledge, attitudes, or skills to grow and move toward these goals. The goals may involve fulfillment of any of the needs discussed by Maslow in his hierarchy.[9] For example, Leitch says, "the client may be seeking greater physical comfort, psychological safety, belongingness, greater love and awareness of self and others, redefinition of a dysfunctional value system, or the knowledge and skills which are required in order to solve problems, achieve present goals or broaden the scope of future ones."[10]

Community health nurses assist clients in meeting their goals by using the following three processes: the nursing process, relating, and communicating. We now look at the characteristics needed by community health nurses to establish helping relationships and the process of building relationships using these characteristics.

NURSE CHARACTERISTICS FOR ESTABLISHING RELATIONSHIPS

Combs says that the characteristics of a helper are as important as the methods used in establishing relationships, and Rogers says that the helper's attitudes are more important than the theory and method used.[11,12] Thus, it is important for community health nurses to develop the necessary characteristics and attitudes if they are to be of help to clients. These characteristics include both personal characteristics or basic personality and the characteristics projected to clients as a result of the nurse's personality.

Self-Understanding. The basic personal characteristic of nurses in a helping relationship is an integrated personality. An integrated personality evolves from the ongoing process of analyzing so-called "difficult" situations encountered and our reactions to these situations to gain a better understanding of ourselves and our values. As we work through situations internally, the likelihood of experiencing conflict in future similar situations is less and we are thus better able to focus on clients and their problems. This facilitates an accepting attitude toward values that conflict with our own and we are less likely to project our own values onto clients. In Millon, Tannenbaum says, "The individual who has resolved most of his internal conflicts appears in a better position to direct energies to the understanding of others."[13]

As we gain self-understanding, we experience less conflict in interpersonal relationships and are

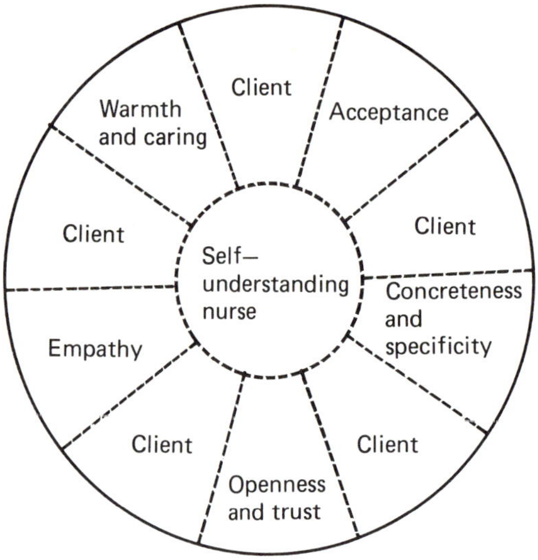

Figure 7–4
Necessary characteristics in a nurse to develop a therapeutic relationship.

better able to meet the needs of others, rather than use them to meet our own needs. This in turn leads to increased acceptance of others and a feeling of personal adequacy and fulfillment for nurses in the relationship. Without a sense of personal adequacy and a feeling of fulfillment, we are unable to help others. For example, Caplan says that the pregnant woman has increased dependency needs and must experience the fulfillment of these needs before she is able to meet the needs of the newborn.[14] Thus, she must feel fulfilled and adequate in order to help another. A similar process of self-fulfillment is necessary for nurses if they are to help others.

Combs and co-workers have identified five indicators of the adequate, self-fulfilled individual.[15] These include the following: identification with people rather than alienation; seeing oneself as adequate to deal with problems; seeing oneself as trustworthy; seeing oneself as being wanted because of one's basic personality; and seeing oneself as worthy. These indicators of the adequate self-fulfilled individual are also necessary in order to fully help another.

Self-understanding is a continual process of growth resulting from the analysis and understanding of our feelings and values in a variety of situations and with a variety of people. Techniques that may be useful in increasing self-understanding include, "participation in awareness group, sensitivity workshops, reflection, and meditation."

Nurses who have these personal characteristics are better able to effectively meet the needs of clients and to project to clients other necessary characteristics that will facilitate the relationship. Characteristics that have been found useful in facilitating a nurse-client relationship are discussed as follows (also see Fig. 7–4).

WARMTH AND CARING. One of the most important attributes for the community health nurse in facilitating the growth of relationships is the ability to demonstrate warmth and caring. **Warmth** involves consideration of and friendliness toward another person. This projects a personal kind of psychological closeness rather than apathy. **Caring** is similar to warmth although it is a more enduirng and intense emotion. When we care about others we demonstrate genuine concern about their welfare, which in turn makes them feel that they have worth as individuals. Warmth and caring can be demonstrated through both verbal and nonverbal communication. Smiling and eye contact are two methods for showing warmth. In addition, ordinary courtesy, such as, shaking hands, touching, offering a chair, and sitting close to someone while talking, demonstrates caring. Verbal behaviors that demonstrate caring include, calling a client by name, remembering details about the person or family, and recognizing and commenting on their strengths, such as, "You give such good care to Bobby," or "You really love Bobby, don't you?"

Caring and warmth are also demonstrated by being sensitive to the special needs of a particular client or to the changing needs over time. For example, caring is demonstrated by the nurse telephoning clients before visiting in the home to arrange a convenient time, responding to a client's needs for reassurance, and including them in goal setting to meet their needs. The demonstration and amount of caring and warmth may vary over time but it is especially helpful for the relationship during the early stages and at times when the client is experiencing stress.

EMPATHY. Another characteristic that facilitates the building of a relationship is empathy. **Empathy** is the "ability to enter into the life of another person, to accurately perceive his current feelings and their meaning."[17] When nurses empathize with clients they put themselves into the client's internal "frame of reference" and see the world in a similar way at that particular time. Thus, the nurse must see the experience as the client does and feel similar effects of the experience. This allows the nurse to understand the client and for the client to feel understood. In this process, nurses see and feel as the client does, but they do not lose their own identity and objectivity; they can perceive how clients are feeling and hear what they are saying and can respond accurately to both the feeling and content of the message.

When nurses empathize they take an internal rather than an external stance from the client's point of view. Thus, they question themselves about what their clients are feeling, how they are seeing the world and their problems, rather than asking "why" questions, which are external to the client (e.g., Why is the client anxious now?). Combs found that for perceiving client needs, the effective helper uses an internal rather than an external frame of reference.[18]

Nurses should employ empathy rather than **sympathy.** "Sympathetic understanding involves a process in which the helper loses his own separate identity and takes on the patients feelings and circumstances as if he were in his place."[19] When sympathy is felt by nurses they may lose their ability to perceive accurately and to assist the patient effectively because they are no longer separate from the client. They experience the world as the client does and consequently cannot understand and convey an objective understanding to the client who is no longer a separate individual.

Nurses may use both verbal and nonverbal communication techniques to convey empathy to clients. Verbally, the nurse may respond to a bedridden patient at home who is discouraged with a comment such as, "It seems as if you are discouraged by not being able to get up and do things as you did before." Or, the nurse may respond to a mother who is vacillating about having applied for welfare with a comment such as "It sounds as if you are not sure that you made the right decision." Any response made by the nurse must be based upon an accurate understanding of the feeling of the particular client at the particular point in time. These responses must carry the feeling tone of the client and be expressed in the client's language. If the client is sad, the nurse should respond with a sad feeling tone using terminology that is familiar to the client. Cameron says that the helper should "always adopt some of the client's own terms in their communication."[20]

At times, the nurse may ask for feedback from the client to clarify an empathic feeling tone that facilitates the relationship. An example of asking for feedback and clarification would be, "I feel you are sad about being unable to do things you've done before. Do I understand correctly how you're feeling?"

Kalisch has combined the works of several researchers into the Nurse-Patient Empathic Functioning Scale.[21] This scale is reproduced in Table 7–1. This scale has five points beginning with zero where no empathy is present. A nurse functioning at this level does not have a relationship with the client. The author defines conspicuous feelings as "the most evident and obvious ones—those that the patient is able to express himself." Hidden feelings are defined as "the deeper, below the surface emotions, which a patient cannot express or could not prior to the interaction with a nurse."[22] Other categories on the scale are also described in Table 7–1.

Openness and trustworthiness. Another characteristic that assists in building a relationship is openness and trustworthiness. Openness is especially important in the beginning of the relationship, but should continue to some degree throughout the relationship to help clients disclose their thoughts and feelings. **Openness** refers to the ability of nurses to disclose thoughts and feelings freely about themselves and where they are in relation to the client and the nurse-client experience. As nurses reveal themselves in a natural and spontaneous way, clients are more able to be open and honest. This facilitates a better understanding of the clients' perceived needs and allows the nurse to be of more assistance. Combs says that the effective helper uses self-revelations in building a constructive relationship and Brammer says that "trust is directly dependent on the extent to which helper and helpee are open to one another."[23,24]

There is a range of self-disclosure that is helpful to the client. Too much self-disclosure may confuse

Table 7–1. The Nurse-Patient Empathic Functioning Scale A Schematic Presentation

CATEGORIES OF NURSE EMPATHIC FUNCTIONING	LEVEL OF PATIENT FEELINGS	
	CONSPICUOUS CURRENT FEELINGS	HIDDEN CURRENT FEELINGS
Category 0	Ignores	Ignores
Category 1	Communicates an awareness which is accurate at times and inaccurate at other times.	Ignores
Category 2	Communicates a complete and accurate awareness of the essence and strength of feelings.	Communicates an awareness of the presence of hidden feelings but is not accurate in defining their essence or strength. An effort is being made to understand.
Category 3	Same as category 2	Communicates an accurate awareness of the hidden feelings slightly beyond what the patient expresses himself.
Category 4	Same as category 2	Communicates without uncertainty an accurate awareness of the deepest, most hidden feelings.

or threaten the client, whereas, too little self-disclosure does not facilitate openness on the part of the client. The amount of self-disclosure by the nurse should be only enough to facilitate client openness. Self-disclosure and trustworthiness means that the nurse must acknowledge and accept annoyance or other nonaccepting feelings felt in a relationship rather than to try to hide them. Such "hidden feelings" influence the relationship with clients, because there may be a lack of congruence between what is said and what is felt by the nurse. This lack of congruence may confuse clients or create a feeling of distrust in them. Thus, feelings must be expressed and in an unemotional way.

ACCEPTANCE. Heim says, "to accept means to receive willingly the hopes, sorrows, frustrations, and mistakes he [another] offers us. In return, we affirm through our communication his special one-of-a-kind self-different from others in the expression of his behavior, but similar in that his feelings, hopes, and dreams form a unifying bond with other human beings."[25]

Acceptance implies a nonjudgemental attitude that is communicated to clients despite the difference in values, attitudes, and behaviors from ours. In effect, we say, "You are free to be yourself no matter how different you are from me." We communicate this not only with words but with nonverbal actions such as being comfortable with the client at all times and by courtesy and receptiveness. We also communicate this with congruent verbal and nonverbal messages, such as, facial expression, body posture, and eye contact. This says to the client that "You are a unique individual and I accept you as you are. You do not need to conform to my wishes or need to please me. We are both unique with similarities and differences."

Acceptance of clients by the nurse follows self-acceptance, which is an on-going process. As nurses interact with and are open to other individuals and experiences, they "absorb, continually adjust to, and change their perceptions about people and events."[26] Identification of their reactions to these situations and further analysis of their thoughts and feelings help nurses accept themselves despite an incongruence between how they react and how they perceive they should react. As nurses accept themselves despite imperfections, they are able to accept the imperfections of others.

CONCRETENESS AND SPECIFICITY. Community health nurses should help clients to be specific and concrete rather than vague or general when discussing sensitive material or feelings. At times clients may think their feelings are unacceptable to the nurse and may discuss them in general terms. At such times, nurses should help clients be specific by asking them how they feel at that moment, asking them to focus directly on the concern, and to give examples, if necessary.

The nurse can model concreteness and specificity in the interaction. This is best done by clearly identifying with statements made to clients, that is, by saying, "I think" or "I feel" rather than using more vague terms such as, "Most people think" or "It is generally believed."

SELF-ASSESSMENT OF INTERPERSONAL SKILLS

Various authors have developed scales for measuring interpersonal functioning, which may be useful to community health nurses. Carkhuff's scale incorporates empathy, respect, genuineness, self-disclosure, concreteness or specificity, confrontation, immediacy and self-exploration by the helper.[27] Aiken incorporates empathetic understanding, positive regard, genuineness, concreteness, and self-explanation in her therapeutic relationship scale.[28] In Aiken's scale, five points are used on each aspect of the interpersonal-relationship scale and scoring of the dimension determines how well the nurse facilitates the relationship. Responses below three on an item indicates an inability of the nurse to facilitate the therapeutic relationship (three is a minimal level for facilitating interpersonal understanding). This scale is reproduced in Table 7–2 and an understanding of the categories on the scale should follow from the previous discussion of characteristics of the nurse in the helping relationship.

Rogers, on the other hand, developed certain questions upon which helpers can reflect to determine if they are creating a helping relationship.[29] These are the following:

1. Can I be in some way which will be perceived by the other person as trustworthy, as dependable or consistent in some deep sense?
2. Can I be expressive enough as a person that what I am will be communicated unambiguously?
3. Can I let myself experience positive attitudes toward this other person—attitudes of warmth, caring, liking, interest, respect?
4. Can I be strong enough as a person to be separate from the other?
5. Am I secure enough within myself to permit him his separateness?
6. Can I let myself enter fully into the world of his feelings and personal meanings and see them as he does?
7. Can I receive him as he is? Can I communicate this attitude? Or can I only receive him conditionally, acceptant of some aspects of his feelings and silently or openly disapproving of other aspects?
8. Can I act with sufficient sensitivity in the relationship that my behavior will not be perceived as a threat?
9. Can I free him from the threat of external evaluation?
10. Can I meet this other individual as a person who is in the process of becoming, or will I be bound by his past and by my past?

Each of Roger's questions for reflection relates to characteristics of the helper discussed earlier. Questions 1 and 2 relate to the characteristics of openness, and question 3 relates to warmth and caring. Questions 4, 5, and 6 relate to the concept of empathy, and questions 7, 8, 9, and 10 relate to the concept of acceptance.

Whether nurses reflect upon Roger's questions or evaluate their interpersonal skills using a model such as Aikens, they should continually be aware of the effect of their behavior upon clients and vice versa. Continuing evaluation and improving interpersonal skills on the part of nurses benefits the client because nurses will be better able to help them meet their needs. Such evaluation also helps nurses in both their professional and personal life as they grow in understanding of themselves and others.

Table 7–2. Facilitative Level of Therapeutic Relationship

SCORE	CORE DIMENSIONS
________	*Empathetic Understanding*
	1 = Significant detraction from patient responses due to failure of nurse to communicate that she is listening, is sensitive, or understands.
	2 = Nurse responds superficially or to stimuli other than what patient is actually expressing.
	3 = Nurse and patient expressions of feeling are interchangeable; nurse's responses neither add nor subtract but indicate willingness to be open.
	4 = Nurse's responses add deeper meaning to patient responses resulting in responses deeper than what he could express himself.
	5 = Full awareness responses which aid patient to express his deepest emotions.
________	*Positive Regard*
	1 = Total lack of concern for patient's feelings, experiences, and potentials is communicated.
	2 = Communicates superficial concern for the patient's feelings, experiences, and potentials of the patient.
	3 = Basic concern and regard are communicated to patient's overt responses.
	4 = Deep respect and concern for the patient is expressed in responses initiated by the nurse.
	5 = Communications express the very deepest respect for patient's worth as a person and his potential for individuality.
________	*Genuineness*
	1 = Responses clearly unrelated to nurse's feelings and/or the only genuine responses are negative ones with destructive effects.
	2 = Responses are slightly unrelated to what the nurse is feeling and/or her negative responses are not used constructively for expanding the basis of the relationship.
	3 = No positive or negative cues to indicate genuine responses, but no discrepancy between feelings and responses.
	4 = Gives positive and negative cues to indicate genuine responses.
	5 = Nurse is freely and deeply herself, spontaneous, open to all experiences both pleasant and hurtful.
________	*Concreteness*
	1 = Nurse's responses allow all discussion with patient to be only vague and anonymous.
	2 = Conversation is frequently characterized by vagueness and abstractness in relation to personally relevant material.
	3 = Nurse's responses neither hinder nor facilitate patient efforts to clarify concerns but communicate that she is open.
	4 = Nurse's responses enable patient to discuss personally relevant material in specific and concrete terminology.
	5 = Nurse's responses enable patient to express fully in concrete and specific terms almost all instances of concern.
________	*Self-Exploration*
	1 = Patient does not disclose personally relevant material.
	2 = Patient responds without affect to discussions lead by nurse.
	3 = Patient voluntarily discloses personally relevant material.
	4 = Voluntary self disclosures increase in number and are accompanied by congruent affect.
	5 = Patient's disclosures allow him to make discoveries about his feelings and his world.
________	*Total Score*
________	*Mean Score* = Practitioner's level of facilitation*

* Mean value of 3—minimum facilitative level

At times nurses may have values that clash with values found in clients. These situations and the resulting attitudes developed by the nurse may interfere with effective relationships.

VALUES AND ATTITUDES MAY INFLUENCE THE RELATIONSHIP

The nurse and client each bring values and attitudes to the relationship that influence the course of the nurse-client relationship. The following discussion on values and attitudes is presented to help nurses identify and resolve potential conflicts before interacting with clients. Resolution of internal conflicts from identified differences in values should facilitate the nurse-client relationship.

Values are "inner convictions of what is right and wrong, good and bad, desirable and undesirable."[30] They form the basis for evaluating the behavior of others and influence our reactions to the observed behavior.

Because people spend their early years of life in different social-cultural groups and have different experiences, they develop different values. When people with different values try to work together they may or may not be successful depending upon the self-understanding of the participants and their ability to facilitate the development of the relationship.

Conflicting values between the nurse and client in the nurse-client system may affect the ability of the nurse to help clients solve their problems. Ideally, nurses have encountered personal situations in which there were conflicting values in the process of growing to adulthood and have analyzed and resolved for themselves the conflicts experienced in these situations (see Philosophy, Chap. 5, and Characteristics of the Helper, in this chapter).

Although values vary from individual to individual, these may be grouped according to the values of the majority and some variations of these same values. Common values in our society and variations that may influence the nurse-client relationship follow.

VALUES REGARDING TIME. In our society we tend to think all people are future-oriented because that is the orientation of the middle- and upper-class majority. However, there is a variation of this value among the lower social class, which is present-oriented. As a result of their future orientation, middle- and upper-class Americans are more willing to act upon preventive health advice from the community health nurse because this will improve their health in the future. On the other hand, the lower class group often is so overwhelmed by meeting their day-to-day needs, that its members do not receive preventive care that will help maintain their health in the future. Irelan and Besner say that lower-class Americans feel powerless, meaningless, and isolated and as a result have an attitude of fatalism and resignation to what life has to offer and, therefore, an orientation to the present. Likewise Leininger says, "the present moment is the major concern to the people and determines how the people respond to questions about health and illness," and Leahy says the Indians "welcome the future but do not worry about it."[32,33]

If community health nurses are future-oriented and do not recognize the variations in time orientation among the lower social class or other cultural groups, they may become discouraged because families do not carry out a plan for preventive services. It is important, therefore, that nurses recognize the potential conflict in this value variation and attempt to look at the lower social-class family from a different time framework.

Many Americans also value time and feel it should not be wasted. The value that time is important is closely related to the value of individual achievement. If one is not making good use of their time, they will not succeed. Those who value time often see punctuality as an indication of caring and efficiency. Thus, it is important for the community health nurse to arrive promptly for prearranged appointments with families. Likewise, if community health nurses are giving bedside care in the home or doing catheter changes, dressing changes, and other procedures, these should be arranged for and carried out on schedule.

Punctuality is also important with American Indians, although they may not be punctual in their appointments. Polacca says, "If you say that you'll be at a certain place, at a certain time, every effort should be made to be there. Navajos do not set the same standards for themselves . . . you are educated, not they, and it is your culture that lives by the clock, not theirs."[34]

The lack of punctuality on the part of groups that are present-oriented may also create conflict for community health nurses. If nurses are running immunization, prenatal or other clinics, such behavior may disrupt the efficient functioning of the clinic, which is often run on a time schedule. Thus, it is important for nurses to identify the time orientation of the particular client system and to plan accordingly.

VALUE OF ACHIEVEMENT. Middle-class Americans who are future-oriented also value the individual who achieves success and accumulates material possessions. Achievement is often associated with higher education; thus, this group usually conceptualizes and is more verbal and abstract than individuals who do not achieve. Lower-class Americans place less emphasis on achievement and education and tend to value strength over intelligence as a source of authority. In addition, there is less emphasis on accumulating material possessions and on language development. Moles says that the language of the lower working class is simple.[35] They communicate with each other using short sentences without shades of meaning. These groups may be turned off by nurses who use abstract concepts.

If nurses come from middle-class homes, they may prefer working with middle-class clients who value achievement. They may also find it easier to communicate with these clients who are more verbal and able to conceptualize and grasp ideas easily. These nurses may find it difficult to visit homes where the clients respond only to concrete suggestions or their values are very different, therefore, interfering with the nurse-client relationship.

VALUE OF CLEANLINESS. Another American value is cleanliness. The nurse who values cleanliness of body and environment may have difficulty maintaining the nurse-patient relationship in homes that are dirty and insect-ridden. Leahy says, "For many nursing students, the actual experience of entering a dirty, insect-ridden, poverty-stricken home is a highly charged one. She may have intellectualized these conditions for some time, but coming upon the actual situations at a time when she may think she has seen all and is wise to the world and its ways can be shattering."[36]

RELIGIOUS VALUES. In our society we have a variety of religious beliefs that guide our decision making. If the nurse was brought up in one religious group with a specific religious orientation, the behavior of clients with different religious orientations may not make sense without careful study of the particular religion. Some religious groups accept the responsibility for their illness and the need to assist in the process of getting well, whereas others may see illness as an act of fate and will not be involved in the process of getting well. Some groups, such as Mormons, refrain from drinking tea or coffee. Others, such as the Christian Scientists, believe in spiritual healing and may refuse preventive and curative care. Some groups have various food restrictions.

The degree to which any specific client system follows his or her particular religious teachings from childhood can best be determined by asking the client for information. Thus, the nurse should be familiar with the background beliefs of various religious groups and the variations from those teachings in the particular client system.

ATTITUDES HAMPERING THE RELATIONSHIP

If nurses have not worked through conflicts from values that vary from their own, they may express attitudes that hamper the nurse-client relationship in either their verbal or their nonverbal communication. These negative attitudes may indicate to the client that we disapprove of their behavior. If we try to conceal our feelings we may convey a condescending attitude suggesting that our way is right. Such attitudes may convince clients that we are not truly interested in them and their problems. When we feel internal conflict and try to hide these feelings, we may not pay attention to what the client is saying and may appear unnatural in our interactions. This prevents the expression of warm, caring, empathic feelings that are important in building the relationship.

Stereotyping is usual when we believe that our way is right. If we interact with others whose ways are different, we may stereotype all people in that particular group (*e.g.*, all Blacks are uneducated or all Chicanos are lazy). Stereotyping prevents an objective assessment of client needs and interferes with the nurse-client relationship.

On the other hand we may see initial qualities in a client that complement our own and make snap judgments about how the client thinks; this may also influence later interactions. If we see similarities between the client's behavior and our own we may demonstrate interest, and if we see dissimilarities we may express a lack of interest. Since the nurse and client form a system, the client will respond to the behavior of the nurse in a way that facilitates or hampers the relationship. Hasty judgments tend to color our perceptions so we see only good or negative qualities in the client and, thus, are a failure in relating and assisting to meet the client's needs. As we open ourselves to others who are different and gain more information about them, we can begin learning more about ourselves and our clients, we will have more of a tendency to see them as they are and will develop attitudes that will facilitate the relationship.

Nurses who know and understand themselves and are able to project the characteristics discussed earlier are usually adept at building relationships with clients that go beyond a superficial level to a personally involved level in the relationship. The process for building this kind of relationship, which facilitates comprehensive nursing care, follows.

THE RELATIONSHIP-BUILDING PROCESS

The relationship between a community health nurse and an individual or group system ideally moves from an initial superficial level between strangers to a level where people care for, trust, and are personally involved with one another. The nurse and the client system bring attitudes, emotional reactions, and needs to the situation. These may influence the movement of the relationship so that it never progresses to the personally involved stage. For example, the client system may come into the interaction ready to change and may with a minimal amount of problem solving resolve the presenting problem. The relationship may terminate then as there is no further need for assistance. Or, the nurse may have attitudes and needs that get in the way of establishing a close relationship and assisting the system. At these times either the nurse or the client may terminate the relationship.

Usually, however, the relationship moves beyond the superficial level if nurses have a theoretical background and experience in relationship building with all kinds of people and have developed some or all of the characteristics of a helper in the helping relationship. The long-term personally involved relationship is especially useful in community health nursing because of the nature of this area of nursing (see Chap. 5).

INITIAL CONTACT

Initially nurses and clients react to each other with learned patterned behaviors based upon their concept of each others' roles. This is similar to patterned behaviors found in a family or group at any point in time and was discussed in Chapters 3 and 4. However, these patterned behaviors differ from family or group roles, which are learned in interaction with a specific group, because the initial nurse-client patterned behaviors are based on the individual concepts of the "good" nurse and the "good" client, which are learned outside the specific nurse-client system. In the initial interaction each evaluates the other in terms of how well they fit the expected behavior patterns of the other. Unless the nurse is adept at building the relationship, a lack of perceived fit between the parts of the nurse-client system can prevent the further development of the relationship and the ability of the nurse to help the system.

Certain nursing behaviors during the initial contact help move the relationship beyond the superficial stage where each sees the other as a stereotype of the good or bad nurse or patient. The nurse begins to gather data to clarify the system's needs for help, and at the same time clarifies the nursing role in relation to these needs. This helps the system begin to learn what to expect from this particular nurse. At the same time, the nurse is evaluating the client and learning what to expect. Thus, a new and specific interactional system (nurse-client) has begun in which each begins to see the other as an individual within a role rather than as stereotypes of the role they occupy.

The nurse establishes the nursing role with a client by verbal and nonverbal actions. Verbal actions that help clarify the nursing role including the types of data requested in the assessment, an explanation of how nursing can or cannot assist the client, the clarification of the client's needs, the elaboration of the specific responsibilities of each in reaching established goals, the process used for establishing goals, the discussion of planned times together in the future, and the purposes of the future times together. It is especially important during this contact for the nurse who is visiting a family or group system to include the whole system rather than a part. For example, on a first visit to a family with a newborn it is best not to say, "I have come to see how your new baby is doing" and to proceed to ask questions about the newborn only. This gives the family the impression that the nurse's role involves looking at the needs of the newborn only rather than the needs of the whole family. Nonverbal clues about the nursing role may be identified by such actions as taking a temperature, demonstrating a bath on a newborn, holding a small child while the mother attends to another child, or touching a mother on the shoulder as you tell her how well she is doing with her newborn. During this initial contact the nurse may also initiate a contract with the family. The contract between the nurse and system will be discussed shortly.

The system itself is also establishing a role as a result of this interaction. The nurse-client roles that evolve become patterned behaviors that fit together in a process similar to that used by the family or other group (see Chap. 3). However, as with the family, the patterned behaviors are not fixed and are subject to renegotiation as conditions within the system change. For example, as the client grows and becomes more organized (physical strength, mental knowledge, emotional stability), the nurse must be flexible and reduce the amount of physical care, teaching, emotional ventilation previously encouraged, or the emotional support given. The use of the nursing process and the establishment of goals discussed earlier should facilitate this dynamic change in the nurse-client system.

During the initial visit, nurses can also facilitate the movement of the relationship by being open and sharing parts of themselves that were previously hidden from the client. (This was discussed earlier.) As nurses are open and honest with clients, clients begin to trust them. Following the establishment of trust, the nurse and the client begin to see each other as individuals occupying roles. Feelings of warmth, caring, empathy, and acceptance on the part of the nurse facilitate this process.

As nurses are building relationships and expressing feelings with clients, they are also collecting data that is useful for identifying client needs. During the initial visit, the nurse uses broad questions in interviewing followed by more specific questions to help clients elaborate upon what they see as their needs. Broad questions, such as, "How are things going with you and the new baby?" can be followed with more specific questions such as "What is Johnnie eating now?"; "How often does he wake up at night?"; "How much sleep do you get at night?" and others depending upon the concerns expressed. This allows the nurse to clarify needs as perceived by the client. At the same time, the nurse may listen, clarify, paraphrase, and use other communication techniques to elicit exactly what clients perceive as their needs and problems.

During this initial contact some resistance may be encountered. This may be a result of the family or group not expecting or seeing a need for the community health nurse. For example, tuberculosis contacts of known cases or maternity patients discharged with their newborn may be unaware that they will be visited by the nurse and may not see a need for the service. On the other hand, some families may express a need for services and see a need for change in their behavior but express resistance or ambivalence about the effort needed to work through the change once plans are made jointly.

During this contact, beginning trust and empathy expressed by the nurse with the client tends to reduce resistance and assist in moving the nurse-client system away from perceived patterned behaviors. That is, as the nurse and client establish their respective nursing and client roles that fit together, and as rapport is developed between them, they will begin to see each other as individuals occupying certain roles based upon their interactions rather than upon their concept of what their roles should be.

Nurse-Client Contract. According to Sloan and Schommer a contract in community nursing is "any working agreement, continuously renegotiated, between nurse, patient and family."[37] Such a contract is similar to other legal contracts, except that it is less formal.

Although some nurses may object to the idea of a verbal or written contract with clients, a contract ensures that clients are involved in the planning of their care. When clients are involved in setting goals and selecting alternate ways of reaching goals, there is more likelihood that they will follow through on their part of the planning. As a result, the nurse may become less frustrated and the client's health needs will be more adequately met.

A contract, either written or verbal should be initiated on the first contact. At that time, the client should be aware of the purposes for the nurse-client interaction, the goals that are set jointly to meet their needs, and the responsibilities of the nurse and client in meeting goals.

Sloan and Schommer say that an operational definition of contracting in community nursing should include the following components: joint exploration of health, establishment of problems and needs of the client, setting mutually agreed upon goals, jointly exploring resources to meet the goals, developing a plan to meet goals, negotiating a division of responsibilities to meet goals, setting time limits to reach goals jointly, evaluating progress toward goals jointly, and modifying, renegotiating, or terminating the contract. This definition follows the steps in the nursing process closely, but major differences, which are important in community nursing, involve joint planning at each step with the client system, negotiation at various steps, and division of responsibility with clients.

Initially, the contract may be somewhat simple until the nurse has built a helping relationship with the client and has identified a variety of appropriate health problems to which nursing can make a contribution. An initial contract might involve the frequency of the nurse's visits for the purpose of talking with the client to identify ways in which nursing can assist. Later contracts may become much more specific and will be similar to the goals written on the nurse's care plan. For example, one goal might be that John and Mary receive the beginning series of immunizations within 1 month. If this is something the client and the nurse have agreed to work on, the division of responsibilities must be identified. Perhaps the nurse identifies resources that give immunizations within the family's financial means, help the family arrange for transportation, baby-sitting or whatever else is appropriate, and the client will agree to take the children to the identified resource. Following evaluation of the meeting of this goal the nurse and client may renegotiate, modify or terminate the goal depending upon a variety of factors such as the desire of the family to continue with the goal, the other pressures on them at the time and the importance of the immunizations from a health point of view.

ONGOING RELATIONSHIP

As nurses continue to work with clients, both the nurse and the client are better able to focus on the task at hand because they see each other as individuals in certain roles. During this phase of the relationship, the nurse continues to express caring, warmth, empathy, and acceptance as indicated. For example, empathy is especially indicated when clients are experiencing stress during the ongoing relationship. This stress may result from either the content being discussed or from pressures outside the interaction. During such times, caring, warmth, and acceptance on the part of the nurse will facilitate the client's ability to look at the problem and deal with it constructively.

TRUST MODEL

The ultimate outcome of our services should be a client who is more independent or interdependent in relation to health. Some of this interdependence is related to the increased knowledge clients have about prevention and treatment of illness, about community resources available for assistance, and other aspects of strengthening the system's resources (knowledge, attitudes, skills). In addition, the relationship developed with clients can also facilitate or hamper the building of interdependence in clients. Dyer, using Gibb's material, has presented a model which should guide our interactions with clients to facilitate interdependence for clients as a result of the relationship.[39]

In this model, the final condition of client interdependence is dependent upon successful completion of all previous steps in the nurse-client interaction (Table 7–3). The initial conditions are trust and acceptance upon which the whole model is built. This is so important to the establishment

Table 7–3. Gibbs Trust Model

CONDITION	DEPENDENCY BUILDING STRATEGY	INTERDEPENDENCY BUILDING STRATEGY
Step 4—Control	Imposed control, checking upon, following around, threatening	Self-control, interdependence
Step 3—Goal setting and decision making	Goals set by others; decisions made by others	Person sets own goals, participates in making decisions
Step 2—Data flow	Closed, restricted, one-way communications, little sharing of real feelings or sensitive information	Open, two-way communication, with wide sharing of important, sensitive information
Step 1—Acceptance or trust	Distrust of others, fears resistance, suspicion	Acceptance and trust of others, understanding empathy

(Dyer W G: The nurse-patient system relationship. In Reinhardt A M, Quinn M D (eds): Family-Centered Community Nursing, St Louis, C V Mosby, 1973. Reproduced with permission)

of interdependence that Gibbs named the model "the trust model." According to Gibbs the concerns of clients during the initial contact with a helper revolve around being accepted. From this acceptance, trust is built. Questions asked include, "Who is this person, what does she want, what is she going to do to me? Can I trust her? Will she tell me the truth? Should I tell her everything?"[40] Depending upon the relationship established, the client feels accepted and trusting or distrustful and fearful of the nurse. Gibbs says that the law of reciprocity operates in the development of trust, for as we are accepted and trusted we tend to accept and trust in return.[41] Many comments such as "I think I understand how you feel since I am trained to understand illness. I think I can help you and I will level with you at all times" and "I will keep my word with you," can facilitate the development of trust.[42]

In step two of the model, data flow is dependent upon the level of trust established in the relationship. If nurses do not accept clients, clients may be fearful of the consequences of freely giving data and will thus hold back.

Difficulty in collecting data and carrying on an open discussion should clue the nurse that the client may not feel accepted and secure in the relationship. This necessitates a movement back to step one to re-emphasize acceptance and trust building if we are to help clients move toward interdependence. During step 2 of the model openness on the part of the nurse which was discussed earlier, may facilitate client openness because openness is reciprocal. As we are open with clients, they will be open with us, if there is a basic trust.

Step 3 of the model involves goal setting and decision making. If there is a lack of trust and limited data flow between the nurse and client, decisions will be made and goals will be set by the nurse. However, these goals may not be carried out because the client has not been actively involved in decision making about reaching goals and, thus, lacks a commitment to the course of action.

If we are interested in obtaining a commitment by clients to actions that facilitate reaching these goals, clients must be involved in all aspects of decision making that involve them. This assists the client in moving toward interdependence. Involvement in decision making that affects individuals is also an important concept of change-theory and change is often a component of moving toward goals.

The last step in the model involves control and is a result of the previous three steps. An imposed control system, which keeps clients dependent, is the result of distrust, restricted communications, and one-sided goal setting. On the other hand, self-control and interdependence follows an accepting, trusting relationship in which clients feel free to communicate openly and to make decisions and set goals.

TERMINATING NURSE-CLIENT RELATIONSHIPS

Termination of the nurse-client relationship can create a deep sense of loss for either the nurse or client, unless clients are properly prepared in advance. The degree of loss felt will be dependent upon the depth of the relationship established, the effect of previous losses on the nurse or client, and the amount of preparation for the termination.

"Ideally, the nurse begins to prepare the patient for termination of their relationship even before it has been established."[43] During the initial visit with clients, nurses begin to set goals with them and also discuss the days and times they are available to them. Alterations in the schedule, such as holidays or days off, should be discussed with the client before they occur. In addition, if nurses know from the beginning what the length of the relationship will be, they should make this known to the client so that they can determine the degree of involvement that will be comfortable for the both of them. In community health nursing, the nurse-client relationship usually continues for a long period of time. However, during this time the nurse should prepare the client far in advance for any necessary terminations such as a transfer to another district, leaving the position, and so forth. Advanced notice of termination allows the client to work through the feelings of separation in the supportive environment of the nurse.

Ideally, the relationship is terminated when clients have grown to the point where they no longer need it. At such times, clients may have been strengthened by the relationship and have been able to form other significant relationships. Unfortunately, this is not always possible in community health nursing. Interruptions in the relationship before this point may occur because the nurse must move out of the relationship for the reasons given previously or because clients have not grown to a point where they can terminate although the nursing needs have been met.

Because of the feelings that may be aroused in both the nurse and client over termination of the relationship, the date of termination should be repeated for several visits prior to termination. If nurses have strong feelings about the loss of the relationship, these emotions may influence the clarity of the message to the client about termination. On the other hand, if clients have strong positive feelings toward the nurse and are denying termination, they may not hear the message in only one visit. Thus, it is important to reiterate the date of termination and to help clients work through the resulting feelings for several visits before the actual termination.

COMMUNICATING WITH CLIENTS

Communicating with clients is important in community health nursing for establishing a therapeutic nurse-client relationship and for identifying client problems or health needs and carrying out the nursing process. Communication is a process that involves verbal and nonverbal aspects. The process of communicating and the verbal and nonverbal aspects that are important to the community health nurse are now discussed.

COMMUNICATION AS A PROCESS

In Chapter 1, information was identified as one exchange between human systems and their environment, and the process of information input, transformation, and output was also discussed. This concept is enlarged upon at this time by looking at the process whereby two or more people are involved. During communication, the information output from one individual is received by another as input. This transformed input is responded to with output (verbal and nonverbal). From this output, the initial sender receives feedback about his message and may again go through the process of input, transformation, and output.

All communications start with "an idea—a reason for engaging in a verbal exchange."[44] The sender has a message, idea, or information that he or she wishes to convey to a specific person or group through the appropriate use of symbols.

This message may or may not be received, depending upon factors in the sender or receiver. Factors that influence the message may include, communication skills, attitudes, the level of knowledge, and the sociocultural systems of the sender and receiver.[45] Other factors include the needs and biopsychosocial condition of the receiver and sender and the setting in which the interaction takes place. These factors are continually changing in both senders and receivers and an awareness of these factors facilitates an understanding of the communication behavior between the nurse and client for community health nurses. Thus, the message may be received as input by the potential receiver or it may be contained in the environment and denied entry into the system.

If the message is received as input by the receiver it is transformed and retained or acted upon through output. Transformation includes interpreting the message in relation to the stored energy or information in the brain. Following transformation the message responded to as output will be different from the initial input. This output, in turn gives the sender feedback about the success or failure of the initial message. If such feedback is not clear to the sender, more feedback may be requested about the clarity of the message.

As the process of communication continues in a circular fashion, the response and feedback from the sender will influence further messages from the receiver. This in turn will influence the responses of the sender. Over time the patterns of communication between sender and receiver may become somewhat fixed in a way similar to the patterned role behaviors in a family or nurse-client system. However, these communication patterns will change as one or another part of the system or the whole system changes.

Feedback is an important concept in communication as it allows nurses to understand which messages are not understood and that it is necessary to make corrections. It also allows nurses to ask for clarification when clients are given unclear messages. As indicated in Chapter 1, there are both internal and external aspects of feedback. Internally, we have a self-concept about our identities and how we communicate. As we communicate, our voice and words give us feedback, which indicates whether or not we are in congruence with out internal self. For example, I may see myself as the warm, caring, empathetic person in all relationships. Yet, I may react to a loved one in an angry manner. This lack of congruence between how I see myself communicating and how I actually communicated creates tension for me, until I have either changed the internal concept or the external manifestation of the concept.

In addition to the congruence of perception of our internal concepts of communication and the external manifestations of behavior, we also receive feedback from the receiver in interactions. It is this external feedback that tells us whether or not we have been clear in the messages we have sent. If this input from the receiver indicates that we have been successful in communicating our message, we receive positive feedback. On the other hand, if our message has not been conveyed, we receive negative feedback. Positive feedback tends to reinforce the communication pattern because we know we are being understood. Negative feedback should lead to maneuvers by the community health nurse to communicate in a way that will produce positive feedback. This not only enhances the relationship but also gives the nurse accurate information that can be used to assist the client.

Verbal Communication. An imporant aspect of the nurse-client system is the verbal communication within the system. In addition to helping clients clarify the nurse's role, verbal communication can facilitate the relationship and the identification of health problems and needs where nurses can assist. Thus, verbal communication when used appropriately can facilitate comprehensive nursing care to client systems.

Verbal communication in community health nursing differs from communication in a social situation because it has a purpose. The overall purposes are to build a relationship and to identify client nursing needs that allow the nurse to assist the client. Verbal ways of meeting this purpose include, listening, leading, reflecting, summarizing, confronting, interpreting, and informing. These skills when used appropriately allow community health nurses to identify client needs as reflected in what they say, feel, and believe, and to help them plan for and resolve identified health problems and needs.

LISTENING. Listening is an active skill in community health nursing that gives us information about the client's needs, feelings, attitudes, and beliefs. It involves an analysis of the total message the client is giving and includes an awareness of the words, feeling tone, and body behavior. It is a faster process than talking. Murray says, "No matter how fast the speaker's mind is racing, he cannot articulate more than 200 words per minute, whereas the listener can take in words as quickly as he can think."[46] Listening may be difficult for many of us but it is necessary if we are to meet our purpose of communicating.

There are several nursing behaviors that facilitate the client's flow of speech as we listen and analyze. Nonverbal behaviors include eye contact, a relaxed natural posture in which the nurse leans slightly toward the client and sits appropriately in close proximity. Verbal behaviors include comments that indicate we are interested in the client and are listening without changing the direction of the conversation. These comments should relate to what the client is saying and may be general. "Some confirming, yet not too personal, comment such as 'I see what you mean,' or 'I can appreciate what you went through,' or 'That certainly seems to tie things together,' often helps to keep him [client] exploring and assures him that you are listening."[47] Other verbal behaviors such as paraphrasing and clarifying provide feedback to clients and allows them to continue if they have received positive feedback or to elaborate if there is negative feedback. **Paraphrasing** is a process of restating the client's basic message in fewer words and allows clients to know if they have been understood. **Clarifying** involves admitting confusion and asking for clarification if the material is vague or confusing or restating the meaning of the words during the conversation.

Silence is closely related to listening although during silence both the nurse and client may be thinking and analyzing. Silence may be used effectively or it may hamper the data collection and relationship. Often the nurse may use silence to encourage the client to break the ice and to continue talking. At such times clients may be problem solving or collecting their thoughts. This silence should not be interrupted unless it is prolonged; then nurses may ask clients to share their thoughts. If the silence is accompanied by non-verbal behaviors that indicate anger, the nurse should appear interested and undemanding. Following the silence, comments to get at the feeling state may be appropriate, such as, "I wonder what you are feeling now?" Often silence will be accompanied by behavior that reflects anxiety. At such times, clients may feel that they have nothing to say. In these situations nurses may initiate the communication process and structure it temporarily. Comments such as, "What are you thinking now?" or "What are you feeling now?" may help to initiate the communication process.

LEADING may be used by nurses in the nurse-client interaction to obtain basic information about clients, to clarify points they are making, to obtain additional information in important areas, and to evaluate nursing plans. Leading often takes the form of questions to elicit this information. These questions may be open-ended or close-ended depending upon our purpose at the particular time in the interaction.

Close-ended questions are used to elicit specific information from clients. When we interview clients we usually need specific data that allows us to formulate with them a nursing care plan. Such data may include age, sex, race, health history, current problems, use of community resources, and other data (elaborated upon in Chapter 6). For some data we may ask questions that elicit a limited response. Examples would include, "How old are you?"; "Are you married or single?" or "What church are you affiliated with?" Other limited-response questions may be answered with a "yes" or "no," such as, "Is it convenient for me to visit with you now?" or "Were you able to attend the immunization clinic this week?"

There are both advantages and disadvantages to using close-ended questions in interacting with clients. As indicated earlier, clients with limited education and vocabulary may be more comfortable with questions that require minimal response. Thus, close-ended questions assist nurses to collect data from this group. On the other hand, when used frequently they tend to block the free flow of communication between the nurse and the client. Although these questions cannot be eliminated completely from the nurse-client interaction, they should be used selectively to supplement open-ended questions.

Open-ended questions faciliate the free flow of communication between the nurse and the client because they do not restrict the client's responses or confine them to predetermined topics. In this approach clients are given the lead and so there is opportunity to determine something about their vocabulary, interests, attitudes, feelings, and beliefs. Thus, open-ended questions may be used effectively when initiating an interview to gain a better understanding of the client.

There are degrees of leading when we use open-ended questions. At times we may let the client take the lead, such as, "Tell me how things are going for you and your family?" During the discussion we might interject comments, such as, "tell me more about that," to gain additional information in specific pertinent areas. At other times, we may take a more direct lead to help the client elaborate upon an area with comments, such as, "Tell me more about your hysterectomy?"

Questions beginning with what and how, if used appropriately, can elicit information in open-ended questions, such as, "What is Brian eating now?" "What is he like with strangers?"; "What do you think?"; "What are you feeling now?"; "What are you doing about it?"; "How much does Brian do for himself?"; "How is he getting along?" and "How do you explain that?"

Open-ended questions also have advantages and disadvantages. Although they facilitate free-flow communication, they may also lead the interview into areas that are irrelevant. Overuse may also create confusion in the nurse and client by clouding the original topic and by giving a false impression of the nurse's and the client's role. Thus, they should be used appropriately along with close-ended questions.

REFLECTING. Reflecting is a method of encouraging clients to continue communicating and at the same time helping them to clarify and to accept their feelings. It gives clients feedback on their communication and allows them to feel understood. At any particular time, either feelings or the experience may be reflected. Subtle feelings of guilt, anxiety, pleasure, or hostility must be identified by the nurse and reflected back to the client with comments such as, "that made you feel bad" or "she made you feel angry" or "it makes you happy to be with him." When strong emotions are expressed, reflecting is unnecessary. Reflecting the experience involves both reading the verbal and nonverbal cues and reflecting the total experience with comments such as "you are smiling (behavioral description), but I sense you are really hurting inside."[48]

INTERVIEW SUMMARY. Following a long interview with clients it is usually helpful for the nurse to summarize the key points. Such summaries should focus on the major issues and feelings brought up by the client, any actions that are to be taken by the nurse or client before the next contact, teaching, and other interventions that the client will use, and plans for future visits with instructions for reaching the nurse if needed prior to the next contact.

INFORMATION-GIVING. After the nurse has identified problems and worked through the nursing process with clients, information may be needed by clients to fulfill their part of the contract. Much information-giving in community health nursing includes giving instructions on baby care, bedside care, nursing procedures, planning menus, location of community resources, and others listed under Interventions in Chapter 6. This is an important part of communications in community health nursing, but the timing of information-giving is important if it is to be used by the client. (See Interventions in Chapter 6 also for a more detailed discussion of the teaching-learning process.)

Many of the verbal communication skills have been summarized by Leiche from material in Brammer.[49,50] Because these skills are presented clearly in a chart and are fairly inclusive, they are reproduced in Table 7–4.

Nonverbal Communication. Handleman says, "one cannot not communicate."[51] In other words we are continually communicating to others whether with ideas and verbal messages or nonverbally with our behavior. The study of nonverbal body movements and their meaning is known as **kinesics.** In this section nonverbal communication includes kinesics as well as other aspects of nonverbal communication, such as, life-style and neighborhood of clients, which assists community health nurses in their assessment and relationship with clients.

Nonverbal clues can assist nurses in their work with clients only if these are used as one piece of data upon which a judgement is made. For example, laughter by a client may indicate either pleasure

(*Text continues on page 195*)

Table 7–4. Helping Skills for Understanding

BEHAVIOR	DEFINITION AND PURPOSE	GUIDELINES
Skill Cluster 1: Listening	*Definition*—An active process of attending to messages sent by the other that includes the observation of verbal and nonverbal behavior.	
1.1. Attending	*Definition*—A way of indicating intense interest that encourages the helpee to verbalize by its reinforcing effect. *Purpose*—Encourages helpee's verbalizing. Also provides a "fail safe" method of opening an interview as it furthers the goals of the helpee and minimizes the chances of making a destructive intervention. *Example*—"Um-m, I'd like to hear more about . . . ."	1. Establish eye contact. 2. Assume a natural, relaxed posture. 3. Use natural gestures. 4. Use verbal statements that relate directly to helpee's statements.
1.2. Paraphrasing	*Definition*—Restatement of helpee's basic messages in a more simple and precise form. *Purpose*—Allows helper to test understanding of helpee's messages and to communicate to the helpee that you are trying to understand and, if successful, demonstrates to the helpee that you have been with him during his verbal explorations. *Example*—"To put this another way, could you say that you are feeling a certain loss of hope, despair?"	1. Listen for basic message. 2. Restate simple summary of basic message. 3. Ask for a response to the accuracy of your restatement. 4. Guard against a stylized and distracting way of paraphrasing, such as consistently stating, "I hear you saying . . . ."
1.3. Clarifying	*Definition*—A statement of the supposition of the helpee's message for verification, clarification and interpretation. *Purpose*—Brings vague material into sharper focus. *Example*—"I lost track here. Let's go back to your major point which seemed to be . . . ."	1. Admit confusion about the helpee's meaning. 2. Try restatement or ask for clarification. 3. Avoid implications of criticism by acknowledging helpee's confusion.
1.4 Perception Checking	*Definition*—Requesting helpee verification of your perceptions of what was said over several statements. *Purpose*—Gives and receives feedback on the accuracy of communication. Effects the feeling of the helpee being understood. Clears up confusion in communications and corrects misperceptions. *Example*—"Essentially, you are confused then, by the demands of this situation: Is that right?"	1. Paraphrase what you think was said. 2. Ask for confirmation of the accuracy of your perception. 3. Allow the helpee to correct your perception if inaccurate.
Skill Cluster 2: Leading.	*Definition*—The act of anticipating where the helpee is going and the act of responding with an appropriately encouraging remark.	
2.1. Indirect Leading	*Definition*—Generally opening comments that allow the helpee to project his own ideas and directions in the interview.	1. Clearly determine the purpose of the lead. 2. Keep the lead general and vague.

(Continued)

Table 7–4. Helping Skills for Understanding *(Continued)*

BEHAVIOR	DEFINITION AND PURPOSE	GUIDELINES
	Purpose—Gets the helpee started and keeps the responsibility on the helpee for keeping the interview going. *Example*—"You were just talking about . . . ."	3. Pause, so the helpee can pick up the lead.
2.2. Direct Leading	*Definition*—A method of specifically focusing on a topic. *Purpose*—Encourages the helpee to elaborate, clarify, or illustrate. *Example*—"Tell me more about how you felt just now when you mentioned . . . ."	1. Determine the purpose of the lead. 2. Express the purpose in words that elicit specific elaboration. 3. Give the helpee the time and freedom to follow the lead.
2.3. Focusing	*Definition*—Pinpoints material that the helper thinks would be fruitful to explore. *Purpose*—Brings specific topics into focus when the helpee is vague and rambling. Reduces confusion and diffusion. *Example*—"Let's go back and talk more specifically about . . . ."	1. Use your own feelings of confusion as a guide to decide when to focus. 2. Be alert to feedback from the helpee about the priority of topics. 3. Assist the helpee to focus on feelings which he may be attempting to hide or avoid by confusion or diffusion.
2.4. Questioning	*Definition*—A method of obtaining information. *Purpose*—Assists the helper's understanding of the helpee. *Example*—"Tell me, what did you do after that and how did it feel?"	1. Ask open-ended questions which cannot be answered with a yes or no. 2. Ask questions that elicit feelings from what the helpee had said rather than information. 3. Ask questions that lead to clarification and not just for information.
Skill Cluster 3: Reflecting.	*Definition*—Demonstrates to the helpee that you are within his frame of reference and that you recognize his concerns.	
3.1. Reflecting Feelings	*Definition*—The expression in fresh words, essential feelings stated or implied by the helpee. *Purpose*—Focuses on feelings rather than content to bring vaguely expressed feelings into clearer awareness and to assist the helpee to "own" his feelings. *Example*—"You said you were feeling a certain tightness?"	1. Read the message of the total content, feelings, verbal and nonverbal messages. 2. Select a mix of content and feeling to promote the goal of understanding at this stage of the helping process. 3. Reflect upon the perceived experience. 4. Wait for the helpee's confirmation or challenge to your response. 5. Look for hidden feelings which may be disguised behind words. 6. Avoid stereotyping the response, such as "You think," "It seems that."
3.2. Reflecting Experience	*Definition*—The helper reads body language as well as verbal messages and responds to the total experience of the helpee. *Purpose*—Puts the helpee in touch with the totality of his or her experience. *Example*—"I notice your eyes have tears in them and yet you seem in a joking mood. What is it like to feel two things at once?"	

Table 7–4. Helping Skills for Understanding (*Continued*)

BEHAVIOR	DEFINITION AND PURPOSE	GUIDELINES
3.3. Reflecting Content	*Definition*—Repeating in fewer and fresher words the essential ideas of the helpee. *Purpose*—To clarify ideas that the helpee is expressing with difficulty and confusion. *Example*—"It is simply that you . . . ."	7. Timing is important. 8. Avoid a patterning of this response. 9. Avoid going beyond the depth of the helpee's experience. 10. Use appropriate language for the cultural and educational experience of the helpee.
Skill Cluster 4: Summarizing.	*Definition*—Attention to content, feelings, process, purpose, timing, and the effect of statements. *Purpose*—Serves to put together helpee's statements that may be intentionally diffuse for the purpose of avoiding discussion, keeping psychological distance, or to perpetuate the helping process. Also gives the helpee a feeling of movement in the exploration of feelings and ideas. Helps to finish an interview or process on a natural note. *Example*—"Let's take a look at where we've been and where we might be going."	1. Attend to the themes and overtones as the helpee speaks. 2. Make broad statements of basic meanings. 3. Do not add new ideas or meanings. 4. Ask helpee to summarize basic themes, agreements and plans, rather than assuming the full responsibility for such summaries based upon the following purposes: a. To warm up at beginning of interview. b. To focus on scattered thoughts and feelings. c. To terminate a particular discussion. d. To check understanding. e. To encourage exploration. f. To terminate the relationship. g. To assure the helpee that he is progressing.
Skill Cluster 5: Confronting.	*Definition*—A complex cluster of skills that consists of the recognition of feelings in one's self, the description of those feelings, and the sharing of them with the helpee. It includes the offering of opinions about the helpee's behavior; meditating, as a form of self-confrontation; repeating, as a form of emphasizing; and associating, as a method of getting in touch with feelings.	
5.1. Recognizing Feelings	*Definition*—The helper's awareness and expression of the feelings he is experiencing at what the helpee is saying or doing. *Purpose*—The recognition of the helper's feelings permits the helpee to let his own feelings into his awareness. *Example*—"I'm feeling suddenly tense and I realize it's because . . . ."	1. The judgment in the helper's expression of his feelings must be made on three conditions. They are: a. Is this feeling indicative of my own problems? b. Is this feeling a reasonable reaction to what the helpee is saying? c. Will the expression of these feelings enhance or retard the goal of the relationship?

(*Continued*)

Table 7–4. Helping Skills for Understanding *(Continued)*

BEHAVIOR	DEFINITION AND PURPOSE	GUIDELINES
5.2. Describing and Sharing	*Definition*—Clarifies and describes the helper's feelings. *Purpose*—Serves as a model for the helpee to recognize, clarify, and express his feelings, which serves to reduce tension. *Example*—"I feel angry when you attempt to blame others in this situation."	1. Caution should be taken in the expression of helper's feelings when the helpee is hysterical, extremely angry, under extreme duress, has a past history of instability, has strong resistance to the exploration of feelings, you are doubtful, your own life is unstable, time is not available to work through the defense, and support systems are lacking. 2. Otherwise, share feelings as a model. 3. Ask the helpee to share his feelings. 4. Be cautious in the extent and intensity of the sharing.
5.3 Feedback and Opinion	*Definition*—An honest reaction to the helpee on how you are affected. *Purpose*—Allows the helpee to understand his effect on others and, therefore, to change his behavior. *Example*—"The way you look away from me when you talk makes me feel that I am not very interesting to talk with. I wonder if you make others feel that way?"	1. Be sure the helpee is ready for feedback. 2. Describe the behavior first, your reaction second. 3. Describe the feedback in the form of opinions about behavior and not judgments about him as a person. 4. Give feedback in reference to those qualities only which the helpee has the capacity to change. 5. Give feedback in small, tolerable doses. 6. Give feedback promptly in response to current and specific behavior. 7. Ask for reactions to your feedback.
5.4. Meditating	*Definition*—A form of self-confrontation. *Purpose*—To stop the flow of action and ideas so the helpee can get in touch with himself, calm down, or prepare a new approach to problems. *Example*—"Why don't you stop talking now and take a few deep breaths, get in a comfortable position, and just be quiet for awhile."	1. Be familiar, through experience, of one or more style of meditating. 2. Explain the value of meditating. 3. Give specific directions for the process of meditation. 4. After a few minutes, ask the helpee to open his eyes and describe his experience, while encouraging other explorations. 5. Ask helpee to practice this procedure if it has been helpful.
5.5. Repeating	*Definition*—A method of helper-prompted self-confrontation out of the Gestalt tradition.	1. Note statements or gestures with feeling implications.

Table 7–4. Helping Skills for Understanding *(Continued)*

BEHAVIOR	DEFINITION AND PURPOSE	GUIDELINES
	Purpose—To generate and tap more feelings associated with particular words that may otherwise be obscured; opens possibilities for significant confrontation on attitudes which hinder effective functioning. *Example*—"Say that again—again—again—."	2. Ask the helpee to repeat key words, phrases, or short sentences until feelings are evoked. 3. Encourage the use of the present active tense. 4. Allow time for the impact to be realized and interpreted.
5.6. Associating	*Definition*—A more precise form of free association. *Purpose*—The freeing of feelings so they are more available for discussion. *Example*—"Say the word ________, and follow it with as many words as possible that it makes you think of."	1. Ask the helpee to say what comes into his awareness. 2. Explain that there is no need for logic or consistency. 3. Use the associations for the further exploration of feelings.
Skill Cluster 6: Interpreting.	*Definition*—A process of explaining the meaning of events to helpees to enable them to interpret their problems in new ways. The offering of a new frame of reference, adding the helper's meanings to the helpee's messages or offering hunches as to the underlying causes or motives of behavior.	
6.1. Interpretive Questions	*Definition*—Questions of a tentative quality about meanings or relationships. *Purpose*—A focusing effect when interpretations and discussions are being avoided. *Example*—"Did you notice a similarity in your feelings when you mentioned the death of your father and the discussion about your divorce?"	1. Look for and paraphrase the basic messages of the helpee. 2. Add your understanding of what the message means. 3. Keep the language simple and close to the helpee's meaning. 4. Qualify your ideas by stating that they are tentative. 5. Solicit the helpee's reaction to your ideas.
6.2. Fantasy and Metaphor Interpretations	*Definition*—A way of affecting interpretation that is less threatening to the helpee. *Purpose*—Broadened perceptions of the meaning of helpee behavior. Provides new and different ways of viewing problems and possible solutions. Facilitates insight. Teaches the helpee to interpret his own behavior. *Example*—"Let me see, is it like you were a small speck of sand on a great beach with everyone stepping all over you—and yet you know there is beauty somewhere and close?"	

(Leitch C, Tinker R: Primary Care, pp 475–480. Philadelphia, F A Davis, 1978, reprinted by permission)

or nervousness depending upon other factors in the setting. Likewise, a client may say "I am happy and relaxed" and at the same time be crossing and uncrossing his or her legs, grasping the arm of the chair, drying sweaty palms, fidgeting and tapping fingers and demonstrating other nonverbal clues of anxiety. Thus, it is extremely important that community health nurses look at nonverbal clues in the context of the total situation.

Nonverbal communication is a two-way process between client and nurse. In our interaction with clients we should strive for congruence between our verbal and nonverbal communication patterns and should also use nonverbal patterns and techniques to demonstrate warmth, caring, and empathy. In clients we should look for signs of incongruence between the verbal and nonverbal communication as a basis for our responses with them.

NONVERBAL HELPING BEHAVIORS. Eye contact can be used by community health nurses to indicate sincerity with clients. This is best used when listening to clients and the gaze should be varied occasionally because outright staring may be considered rude or a sign of seductiveness. Constantly looking away from clients, looking at a clock, or watch, or a notepad may indicate a lack of interest to clients. Thus, it is usually best not to take lengthy notes during an interview.

Touch may also be used effectively by nurses to communicate concern and compassion. Heim says, "touch is like a two-edged sword in communication. On the one side, it has cultural determinants steeped in traditions and strict forbidden social taboos; on the other, it has an important far reaching-out function that is needed (but not fully understood) within nurse-patient relationships."[52] Thus, touch must be used appropriately. In nurse-client interactions it should not be used excessively or earlier than permitted socially because it may be seen as an invasion of the client's private space. Nurses should be comfortable touching and being touched before using this nonverbal technique and should gauge touch by the client's response.

Body position may also assist community health nurses in demonstrating interest and concern to clients. The attentive position involves sitting forward in a chair with a slight sideward tilt of the head and with an attentive facial expression of interest. Interactions should always be carried out in a sitting position in which the nurse is relaxed and unhurried. If nurses see clients at a clinic, school, or other setting, they should invite the client to sit down with them. If clients in the home do not offer a seat, the nurse should ask if this is a convenient time to talk and, if so, ask if they can sit and talk for a while.

Seating arrangements may also assist the nurse in demonstrating caring for clients. If chairs are movable, facing a client will indicate openness and interest. Chairs should also be placed relatively close together.

OTHER NONVERBAL BEHAVIORS. Other nonverbal behaviors may be communicated by either the nurse or client and may indicate incongruence between the verbal and nonverbal communications or may give indications of feelings that are not being expressed. Community health nurses should be aware of this behavior as well as the verbal behavior of clients.

A variety of clues for later validation can be identified by observing the life-style of clients. As we enter the client's neighborhood we receive clues about the socioeconomic level of the family, the accessibility of community services, including health, the cultural makeup of the area, traffic patterns, industries and other potential health hazards. Inside the client's home we get additional clues about its facilities for personal hygiene, privacy, recreation, cooking, eating, and storage. We also get clues about parent-child interactions, discipline, family roles, and values as reflected in reading materials, plants, toys, and other household items. We also get clues about habits such as leaving medicine around on tables, keeping a tidy or untidy home, and leaving dishes piled in the sink. Depending upon the particular family constellation, these clues might be followed up for verification to assess the potential for accidents, inadequate space for privacy, lack of child stimulation, and so forth.

Clues about clients can also be obtained by their physical appearance. The height, weight, and any visible deformities may signal a need for verification of data. Likewise, the complexion, condition of hair, eyes, nail beds, lips, and other visible parts of the body may give us a clue that we should check further for cyanosis, fatigue, overexposure to the sun, or other potential health problems. In addition, the client's dress and appropriateness of dress at the particular time may give clues for further investigation. For example, if a client appears in a bathrobe with hair uncombed at 1 PM, we may need to verify whether they are physically sick, fatigued from being up late, working nights and sleeping days, or whatever, to determine if there is need for assistance.

The position of the client's head may also

provide clues about the client's feeling state. A head that is tilted forward may indicate anger, whereas, a head held rigidly upright may indicate anxiety, fear, or defiance. If a head is tilted to one side it usually indicates interest, and if it is down or bowed (eyes lowered), it may indicate sadness, shame, or guilt.

The face and eyes also communicate important clues. Gestures with the eyes, eyebrows, mouth, forehead, and chin can communicate information. Eyes are probably the most expressive part of the body and can often give clues to the feeling state of the client. This is so well accepted that religious literature often refer to the eyes as "the window of the soul." Rakel says that there are 40 different expressive positions for the eyebrows and 23 for eyelids. The eyes and its accessories often give away a sad heart on a smiling face.

Hands, arms, and their gestures may also provide clues about the client's feeling state. Because of the possible various positions of the extremities it would be difficult to catalog all possible positions and their meanings. However, some common positions with possible meanings (depending upon the situation) are as follows: Hands may be fidgety when anxious, droopy and flaccid when sad, or clenched when angry. If the hand is raised to pull on the earlobe or to touch the lips the client may wish to interject or to suppress a comment. Crossed arms may indicate defensiveness and distrust, insecurity, or comfort depending upon whether the client appears otherwise relaxed and open (sitting in a direction facing the nurse).

Legs may also give clues to a client's feeling state. Crossed legs may indicate a position of comfort or resistance by the client. Validation may be obtained verbally and by observing for other signs of resistance (a closed system) such as crossed arms, looking at the floor, or away, and showing anger or disinterest in the facial features. Fidgety feet as well as hands may also indicate anxiety. If these are seen in combination with feet in the ready-to-run position, and the client is sitting forward in the chair, the client may be very anxious. Feet placed far apart may indicate anger and feet moving in a slow circular pattern may indicate sadness. The walk of the client may also tell something of the client's feeling state. A slow shuffling gait with head bent forward is often associated with the depressed client, whereas, a brisk, skipping walk is associated with happiness.

Nonverbal behavior may assist community health nurses in clarifying with clients their particular needs and goals when viewed in relation to verbal communication and other factors in the setting. Thus, it provides another tool for assisting clients in meeting their needs and for building on the relationship.

REFERENCES

1. Dyer W: The nurse-patient system relationship. In Reinhart A, Quinn M (eds): Family Centered Community Nursing, p 148. St. Louis, C V Mosby, 1973
2. Ibid, p 149
3. Ibid p 149
4. Hall J E, Weaver B: Distributive Nursing Practice: A Systems Approach to Community Health, p 32. Philadelphia, J B Lippincott, 1977
5. Ibid
6. Ibid
7. Ibid
8. Leahy K, et al: Community Health Nursing, p. 62. New York, McGraw-Hill, 1977
9. Maslow A: Motivation and Personality. New York, Harper & Row, 1954
10. Leitch C: Helping and human relationships. In Leitch C, Tinker R (eds): Primary Care, p 453. Philadelphia, F A Davis, 1978
11. Combs A, et al: Florida Studies in the Helping Professions. Gainsville, University of Florida, 1969
12. Rogers C: On Becoming a Person. Boston, Houghton Miffin, 1961
13. Millon T: Medical Behavioral Science. Philadelphia, W B Saunders, 1975
14. Caplan G: An Approach to Community Mental Health. New York, Grune & Stratton, 1961
15. Combs A, et al: Helping Relationships: Basic Concepts for the Helping Professions. Boston, Allyn & Bacon, 1973
16. Leitch C, op cit, p 470
17. Kalisch B: What is empathy? Am J Nurs 73:1548, Sept 1973
18. Combs A, et al, op cit
19. Kalisch B, op cit
20. Cameron N: Personality Development and Psychopathology: A Dynamic Approach, p 769. Boston, Houghton Miffin, 1963
21. Kalisch B, op cit
22. Kalisch B, op cit
23. Combs A, et al, op cit

24. Brammer L: The Helping Relationship, Process and Skill. Englewood Cliffs, Prentice-Hall, 1973
25. Heim E: Communication in Nursing Practice. Boston, Little Brown, 1973
26. Ibid, p 71
27. Carkhuff R: Helping and Human Relations: Practice and Research. New York: Holt, Rinehart & Winston, 1969
28. Aikin L; Aikin J: A systematic approach to the evaluation of interpersonal relationships. Am J Nurs, 73: 863–867, May 1973
29. Rogers C: op cit, pp 50–55
30. Ujhely G: Determinants of the Nurse-Patient Relationship, p 3. New York; Springer Publishing Co., Inc., 1968
31. Irelan I (ed): Low-Income Life Styles. Washington, D C, U. S. Department of Health, Education, and Welfare, Welfare Administration Publication 14, 1968
32. Leininger M: Nursing and Anthropology: Two Worlds to Blend, p 121. New York, John Wiley & Sons, 1970
33. Leahy K, et al, op cit, p 155
34. Polacca K: Ways of working with the Navajos who have not learned the White man's ways. Journal of American Indian Education. Tempe, University of Arizona, Nov 1962
35. Moles O: Educational training in low income families. In Ireland I (ed): Low-Income Life Styles. Washington, D C, U. S. Department of Health, Education, and Welfare, Welfare Administration Publication 14, 1968
36. Leahy K, et al, op cit, p 148
37. Sloan M, and Schommer B: The process of contracting in community nursing. In Spradley (ed): Contemporary Community Nursing, p. 221. Boston, Little, Brown, 1975
38. Ibid
39. Dyer W: The nurse-patient system relationship. In Reinhart A, Quinn M (eds): Family Centered Community Nursing, pp. 139–144. St Louis, C V Mosby, 1973
40. Ibid
41. Ibid
42. Ibid
43. Hale S, Richardson J: Terminating the nurse-patient relationship. Am J Nurs, 63:116–119, Sept 1963
44. Heim E, op cit, p 6
45. Berlo D: The Process of Communicating, p 50. New York, Holt, Reinhart & Winston, 1960
46. Murray R, Zentner J: Nursing Concepts for Health Promotion, p 56. Englewood Cliffs, Prentice-Hall, 1975
47. Brammer L, op cit
48. Brammer L, op cit, p 91
49. Leiche C, op cit
50. Brammer L, op cit
51. Handleman B: Family Therapy Class Notes. San Francisco, University of California, School of Nursing, 1965
52. Heim E: op cit, p 193
53. Rakel R: Principles of Family Medicine, p 129. Philadelphia, W B Saunders, 1977

8

Community-Health Nursing Care Delivery: Methods and Process

Community health nursing must be dynamic and responsive to the needs of society to remain viable. As society and its nursing care needs change, nursing and health care delivery systems must also change. Community health nursing has traditionally used a combination of the case method and team method of nursing care delivery, depending upon the setting of care. For example, the case method was used in delivering nursing care to families at home, and the team method was used to provide care in well child centers and at times in the school and other settings. Currently, there is more emphasis on the team method of nursing care delivery and on primary care to some extent. These methods and the processes used in these methods are now discussed.

CASE METHOD

The traditional method for delivering community-health nursing services to the client system at home was the case method. **Case method** is the mode of nursing care delivery in which a member of the nursing staff provides total care for the client.[1] The pattern was to assign the nurse to a census tract, school and/or industry where the nurse had responsibility for the total care of the population under nursing care or at times selected parts of the population. For example, one pattern of care in the past was to have specialized nurses in tuberculosis, maternal-child care, and so forth, who visited families based upon their presenting problem. Another pattern was to have nurses from the voluntary nurses' organization provide bedside care and nurses from the official agency provide preventive nursing services. At other times, one nurse was responsible for the total population. Regardless of the varying patterns found, the community health nurse had total responsibility for assessing, planning, implementing, and evaluating the nursing care of those families assigned.

This method of care differs from the primary care method primarily in the degree of **accountability** and **responsibility.** In the case method approach, nurses are responsible for their assigned clients during working hours only. Although clients may be under nursing supervision for long periods of time, they are encouraged to use their own family or community resources during the evenings and weekends when nurses are off duty. Also, the assigned nurse is the only nurse who has responsibility for the client.

TEAM METHOD

The team method for delivering nursing care has also been used in the past and is increasingly being used in community health nursing. Community health nurses may be part of a so-called "nursing team" or part of a "health team." Douglas defines team nursing as the mode of nursing care delivery in "which a professional nurse [team leader] facilitates the efforts of a group of diversified health care personnel to provide for the health needs of an individual or a group of people in a hospital or community setting."[2] In this kind of team where the community health nurse may be leader, there is a diversification of talents and skills that are used to provide care. Care providers may include practical nurses, aides, volunteers, home health aides, and others. This approach to providing care has been used in clinics and in the home where there are clients with chronic illnesses needing bedside care.

Community health nurses have also been a part of health teams. Definitions by Rakel and Rubin are more appropriate to health teams because the nurse is not always the leader. Rakel says that the **health team** is "a group of individuals with different but complemental skills working together in the same facility or area toward a common goal" and Rubin says "a team is a group of people whose interdependence is necessary to accomplish a given task."[3,4] In some settings such as schools and industry, community health nurses have some independent and interdependent functions but work under the supervision of (or accept orders from) the physician, or they follow standard policies that are medically approved. Thus, although there may be team efforts when a crisis arises or during routine procedures such as physical examinations, the physician is always the team leader. Currently, there are some efforts to have community health teams made up of nurses, physicians, social workers, psychologists, ministers, and others who work with individuals and groups, with revolving leadership roles, depending upon the particular needs of the clients. The Student American Medical Association has several projects each year in Western Virginia and Tennessee, which involve such a team. In these projects students from medicine, nursing, social work, and other disciplines go into the communities and jointly assess needs, plan, implement, and evaluate a plan of care. In these projects the leadership role revolves. Two years ago, as a faculty member, I was also involved in working with an interdisciplinary team of medical, nursing, dental hygiene, nutrition, and psychology faculty who taught interdisciplinary teams of students from these disciplines. In addition to content on family dynamics; the process of assessing, planning, implementing, and evaluating; and the process of team development and maintenance, the student groups went into homes to do a group assessment. Following the assessment, the members developed plans and set priorities as a group and returned to the home to implement the plans. In later visits, they evaluated their plans. Although the approach of team health-care delivery, in which the leadership revolves, has long been a mode in rehabilitation, it is just beginning to be used in community health and has advantages in some settings.

THE NURSING TEAM

Families are at the center of the team in community health nursing because they retain the responsibility for the nursing care at times when other team members are not available. Other nursing team members may provide nursing care at certain times in the home, school, or industry, but in the evenings and on weekends, family members are at home and are responsible for the continuation of any care initiated.

Because care providers (all health personnel) on the community-health nursing team cannot be supervised constantly in the home, clinic, school, or nursing home, there must be a good match between the nursing needs of the particular client and the skills and knowledge of the nursing care provider. Initially, the community health nurse should do an assessment of the nursing needs of the client and if care is to be provided by the community health nurse, care can be planned jointly with the client. However, if care is to be provided by other nursing care providers, this care should be planned between the community health nurse, the client, and other care providers so that all members involved in implementing the care are aware of the total nursing care plan. In addition, any physicians involved in the client's care should be informed of the nursing care plan. Thereafter, the nurse may implement the care plan, or turn it over to other care providers with periodic care or supervision by the community health nurse.

The other nursing care providers on the nursing team have varying degrees of education and experience and must be supervised to ensure safe and effective implementation of the nursing care plan. In addition to periodic supervision of actual care given by the team members, nurses may request case conferences, practice sessions, teaching sessions, and record audits. Practice and teaching sessions are especially warranted if implementation involves techniques that have not been carried out for a long period of time. For example, an aide may have been taught to change dressings on clients at home, but she may not have performed this procedure for several months.

When members of the nursing team other than the community health nurse provide care to clients, periodic reassessment by the nurse is indicated. Unless warranted sooner by changes in the client's condition, these should be carried out within 3 months. At such times new nursing care plans may be developed necessitating changes in the pattern of implementing nursing care. For example, clients may improve and no longer need the services of the nursing team, or they may regress and require an extension of community-health nursing services for a period of time. If family members have been providing the bulk of the bedside care at home, there may be changes in the condition of the care provider necessitating an increase in the nursing-team care. Reassessment should involve the family, the physician, and all other involved members of the nursing team.

TEAM AS A SYSTEM

A nursing or interdisciplinary team meets all the requirements of a system. It has interdependent parts that function together to meet the goals of the whole system. For example, if a community health nurse, practical nurse, family member, and home health aide are all providing nursing care for a chronically ill member in the home, they must coordinate their efforts to provide effective care. All must know the goals of care, the nursing care plan, their particular roles within the complex of care providers, and how decisions about nursing care, which affect all team members, are made. On nursing teams, community health nurses are the leaders and they must be skilled in facilitating group decision making and in clarifying roles, goals, and communication channels to ensure effective and efficient delivery of nursing care by the team members.

Change in a part of the system affects the whole system. If the family member giving bedside care, the practical nurse giving medications and treatments, the home health aide preparing meals and cleaning, or the community health nurse who assesses, teaches and supervises in the home gets sick or leaves the team, then someone else must take over the vacated role. The new member must be oriented to the particular client and team members and must learn to fit (his or her role) into the (existing) intermeshing roles. New communication and relationship patterns within the team including the client and family members are set up, which affect the whole team.

As with the nurse-client system, the team members each have a self-concept and a concept of others in terms of "good" and "bad" roles. Through the process of communicating and relating, they may move from these patterns of stereotyping to patterned behaviors based upon seeing each member as an individual occupying a specific role.

Equifinality is present in the team system because there are different ways to meet the goals set up for the client. By using the nursing process the team considers alternate methods for meeting team goals and selects the best approach. This approach may vary from others that are used with clients with similar health and nursing care needs because of individual factors in the client's family, the community, or the team. Factors such as the family and team members' intellectual, physical, emotional, and financial resources, and the supplemental community resources must be considered in selecting an appropriate alternative.

Negentropy and entropy are also possible on nursing teams. If the team members work together and are allowed to grow individually and as a group to become more efficient and effective, negentropy is present. On the other hand, if excessive energy is used by the members in trying to fit together because the roles, goals, and group processes used for making decisions and communicating are unclear, entropy will be operating. Team development and maintenance are important to ensure negentropy on teams.

PROCESS OF TEAM DEVELOPMENT

Because the team is a system with interdependent parts that function together to meet the goals of the whole, the team members must work together and coordinate their activities if the team is to work efficiently and effectively. All members must pull together instead of pulling in opposite directions. From the beginning there should be a clear understanding of goals, roles, and the internal working of the group.

In a structured setting such as a hospital, goals of the team, roles of team members, and the internal mechanisms for working out group processes on a team may be relatively easy to define and to fit into for team members. For example, on a medical ward the purpose of the nursing team is to provide nursing care to a group of medical clients to facilitate recovery. The tasks to be done and the roles and functions of team members are relatively clear as they are usually assigned by the team leader. Internal processes for the team are also relatively clear. The team leader may receive orders and directions from a supervisor and a physician, but team members receive their orders from the team leader. Thus, the decision-making process is well established and resides with the team leader. Communication also operates largely as a one-way flow from the team leader to the members, although members may report on changes in the condition of clients. Although roles, goals, and mechanisms for resolving concerns of the group are relatively clear in this setting, the team may not be growing toward a more organized group (negentropy) because members are not involved in decision making and, thus, may lack a commitment to the externally imposed roles, functions, and so forth.

In a community setting, on the other hand, goals are broader and include all levels of prevention and all aspects of living that affect health. In addition, there is more likelihood of role overlap leading to role confusion in the many tasks to be accomplished.

There is also more opportunity for minor decision making by team members because of the various locations in which practice takes place usually without available supervision. Because different team members are involved in implementing the nursing care plan, group decision making and priority setting are also indicated to ensure a commitment to the plan. In these sessions, communication is not one-way but rather rotates among the members who solve problems in developing the nursing care plan. Because of the varying backgrounds of the team members, input from all members is important to generate the most alternatives from which to pick the best alternatives for the particular client. This group input on the nursing team or health care team (of which nursing is a part in the community) may lead to confusion and misunderstandings among team members. On the other hand, with appropriate team development and maintenance there is also the likelihood of greater growth (negentropy) within the team.

Team Goals. In the development of a team, goals should be identified by the team members because all will be affected by the goals established. Initially, the group should set an overall goal for their existence, unless this is established by the agency within which the members work. If the group prepares the overall goal, members should come to the group meeting with a written statement about what they see as the major goal. At the group meeting, all goals written by individual members should be presented and written (on a blackboard, for instance) so that the group can look at and think about them. Then the group should discuss and agree upon the overall goal from one of the individual member's goals or by picking the best of several statements. They should combine them into an overall goal. A recorder should summarize the group's discussion and final decision. A similar process should be used to develop goals for client care. However, these goals need to be specific and measurable as indicated in Chapter 6.

Goals for a particular client should be reviewed by the group to determine if they are clear, measurable, and meet other criteria for goals. After goals have been agreed upon for a particular client by the team, it is necessary to set priorities for the goals. Again, the total group should go through the process of reaching an agreement as to which goals are of highest priority, those that are in the middle, and those of low priority. One way to do this is to ask the group to verbally rank each goal as high, middle, and low priority, or undecided. Agreement can be reached by consensus or some other method of decision making. Following the initial ranking of the goals, the group can go through again and rank the undecided categories. Some disagreement may exist among group members about high and low priorities in categories such as primary versus secondary and tertiary prevention goals, or health versus social goals but an agreed upon method of making decisions beforehand ensures that the group will come up with a list of goal priorities. Some of the priority-setting models presented in Chapter 6 may be helpful to group members during this process. Once the group has set goal priorities, it has in effect developed a working contract similar to that in the nurse-client contract.

A critique after each goal-planning session is important in team development. Each member should write down what he or she likes best and least about the meeting and how the group could function better in the next meeting. Often such critiques will uncover areas within the group process that need correcting. For example, a member may identify a need to improve upon conflict resolution by confronting and compromising, rather than by avoiding or smoothing over issues. Another member may identify a need to improve upon group decision making so that there is consensus or unanimity rather than a monopoly of one or two people making decisions for the group. Individual comments should be shared and discussed within the group.

Patterned Team Role Behaviors. Any team should have a clear understanding among its members of what each team member's role involves. This is especially important on teams where there is role overlap among members, which may lead to role ambiguity, role conflict, or role overload. For example, community health nurses, registered nurses, practical nurses and aides on a nursing team may all have skills in doing certain procedures such as giving injections, changing dressings, and catheterizing patients. Unless these team members are clear as to their role responsibilities regarding clients, problems may occur for the individual members and the team as a whole.

On every team, members have certain expectations for themselves and for the other team members. If these expectations are not clearly defined and communicated, there is confusion and role ambiguity. **Role ambiguity** is the result of individual members being unsure of the specific job responsibilities included within their role. Likewise, if role expectations of team members are inconsistent, there is also **role conflict** within the group. In other instances the expectations for a particular member of the team may be too demanding and lead to **role overload.**

Role ambiguity, role conflict, and role overload all result from the expectations of each group member for himself or herself and for others on the team. Role ambiguity may be a result of team members being unsure of what they should be doing, what others on the team expect them to be doing, or what they expect others on the team to be doing. Likewise, role conflict may result from an inconsistency between what the individual member expects of himself and what other members expect of his performance, or it could be an inconsistency between what two or more team members expect of a team member's performance. For example, the community health nurse may expect to assess and to facilitate and evaluate the plan, whereas another member may expect her to do this as well as part of the implementation of the skills. Or the community health nurse may expect the aide to give bedside care as well as clean, and the practical nurse may expect the aide to clean and maintain supplies rather than give bedside care. Either situation results in conflict. In addition, there is the possibility that one member on the team will have role overload even though there is no conflict. In this situation, the individual will be unable to fulfill his or her role expectations, which in turn will affect the performance of other team members who are interdependent. For example, if the community health nurse has a backlog of initial assessments and also reassessments in the caseload, there may be little time left to meet with the team to plan and evaluate care. If this is an expectation of the nurse's role, the lack of time will interfere with the giving of care by other team members whose roles are dependent upon this input. If role conflict, ambiguity, and overload are not confronted and resolved, the team will be inefficient and will waste energy arguing and experiencing both intrapsychic and intragroup pressures. Thus, the developing group should learn how to deal with ambiguity and conflict in a constructive way.

These difficulties encountered by a team can be resolved through **role negotiation.** As the team begins to work together they must learn to identify role ambiguity, conflict, or overload and to resolve it through negotiation. This process can be diagramed as presented in Figure 8–1.

A process for doing this has been identified by Rubin and co-workers and is presented now.[5] Initially, team members write messages to each other asking for more of, less of, or the same amount of something that is needed. These messages should include what they want more of, less of, or the same amount of, and why it is important to them for carrying out their team functions. For example, a practical nurse might send a note to the community health nurse related to the community health nurse's overload (as in the example above), which reads as follows: "I need you to be *more* available for planning meetings (what) so that I can better prepare for giving nursing care to clients (why)." The messages are distributed to team members who read and think about them.

Two team members are selected to negotiate roles resulting from conflict or ambiguity noted in the messages. A third person is selected by the negotiators to act as a facilitator. The remainder of the team remain silent throughout the negotiation, but participates in the discussion afterwards.

The process of role negotiation involves the sending of the message, the clarification of the message by the receiver with the sender, the response of the receiver, the negotiations, and the contract between the sender and receiver; this is followed by a group critique. The sender must be specific about what behavior changes are needed, how this will help the sender, and may offer suggestions for changing the behavior of the receiver. The receiver must understand why the message is important and how it relates to team functioning. The receiver must also understand exactly what behavior changes are being asked for and attempt to respond in one of the ways that follows:

a. That is a good idea, I'll do it.
b. I can do that, if you (or some other team member) can do "something" to help me.
c. I can't do that, but I can do something else that will help solve your problem.[6]

Both receiver and sender must be sure that the final contract is one that they can abide by or at least try out. The third person (facilitator) must be

Figure 8–1
Process of increasing efficiency and effectiveness of teams regarding role behaviors.

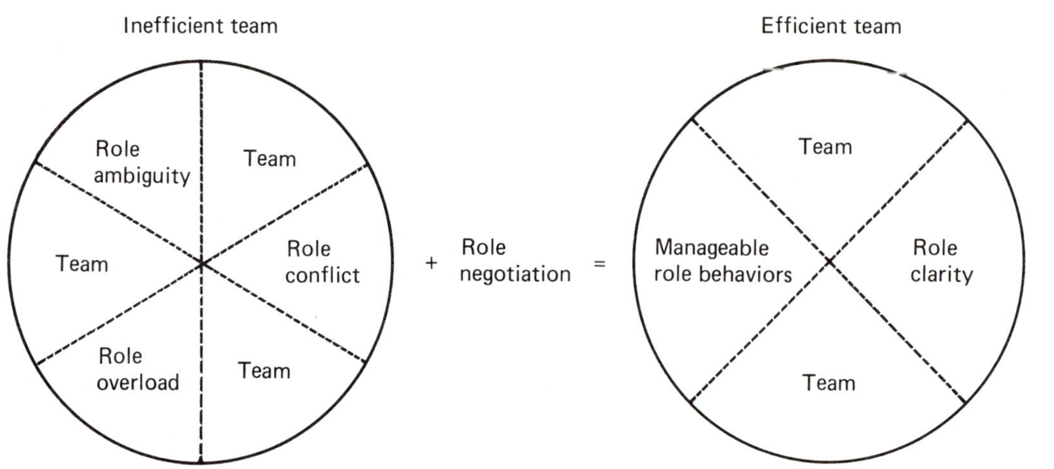

able to clarify throughout the process and help the receiver and sender to arrive at a point where they can develop a written contract. This person (facilitator) should also be knowledgeable about conflict resolution and help the team members confront and resolve rather than avoid or smooth over their problems.

The contract defines the problem, and what each person who is affected will do. It also includes a date for evaluating whether actual changes in behavior took place and the effect on the sender's and receiver's performance.

During the critique, input is encouraged from all team members to help everyone improve their skills in and their understanding of role negotiation. Observers are asked to evaluate if the sender and the receiver really listened to each other, how the third person (facilitator) was helpful, how the negotiators dealt with the conflict (avoiding, compromising, forcing, confronting, smoothing over), and ways to improve future sessions. In a way similar to role playing, the receiver, sender, and third party (facilitator) are also asked to share their feelings and thoughts.

Although time is usually not available to negotiate all of the conflicts and ambiguities with the team, additional methods may be used to resolve them. Rubins and co-workers suggest the following process:[7]

Members of the team review the messages at home and fit them into 1 of 5 categories presented in Table 8–1. All messages are placed into category 1 that are agreeable without negotiation. These messages can be put into a formal contract at the next team meeting. Ambiguous messages that are unclear are placed into category 2. Because the message is unclear, the receiver is unsure whether or not it can be accepted. Category 3 includes messages that are unacceptable and, thus, a role conflict is present; these must be negotiated. Category 4 includes contradictory messages from two or more members. Since there is not agreement between the senders, these messages must be negotiated among all involved members. Category 5 includes messages about expectations that are reasonable, but whould mean a role overload for the receiver. Therefore, negotiation is also necessary.

These messages should be written on large sheets of paper that can be posted at the team meeting. They can be arranged in a column for messages categorized as more of, same amount of, and less messages. In the second column the initials of the sender or senders are placed, and in the third column, the receiver lists his or her response using the five categories discussed previously.

Table 8–1. Categories of Messages by Team Members for Resolving Role Conflict and Ambiguity.

CATEGORY	MESSAGE
1	Agreeable—no negotiation necessary
2	Ambiguous messages—Clarification needed
3	Unacceptable messages—Role conflict present; negotiation necessary
4	Contradictory messages from two or more members—Negotiation necessary
5	Unreasonable messages—Role overload; negotiation necessary

At the scheduled team meeting each member shares the list with all other members. In addition, each member schedules a time and place for the needed negotiation sessions with other members. Following these negotiating sessions, formal contracts should also be written and should include a date for evaluation.

Renegotiation is a continuous process for the team members and should be encouraged to facilitate the efficient functioning of the team as a whole. The feedback process of individual members is a valuable indicator of the need to negotiate or renegotiate with other members. Following a role change that has been agreed upon, the member who has changed behavior must feel good about it. From a feedback point of view, the quality of work being produced as a result of the change must be congruent with the internal standards set by the team member. Otherwise, the individual will experience tensions that can only be relieved by changing internal standards or the external manifestation of the changed behavior.

Thus, the role behaviors of team members are tried out and become somewhat fixed patterns of behavior. However, as one member experiences incongruence between their internal and external standards (feedback), role conflict, ambiguity, and overload may result. This in turn leads to the need to negotiate and change fixed behaviors, which are tried, and if successful, again become somewhat fixed. This is a continuing process that facilitates the efficient and effective functioning of the team.

Team Decision Making. Decision making is another important aspect of team efficiency and effectiveness. Decisions are made at each step of the nursing process by a team. During the assessment phase decisions need to be made about who sees the client and who identifies problems for the problem list. During the planning phase decisions must be made about who discusses possible solutions and how the plans are selected from all possible alternatives. During the implementation phase decisions about who implements the plan, and during the evaluating phase, decisions must again be made about terminating nursing care or reassessing. Thus, numerous decisions must be made by a team that affect the functioning of all members.

Not all members of a team need to be involved in all decision making. However, there should be clarity among members about who should be involved and how they should be involved. "The issue is one of relevance and appropriateness: Who has the relevant information and who will have to implement the decision?"[8]

There are a variety of decision-making mechanisms that can be used by the team. There can be a decision by default when no one responds to a decision; there can be a forced unilateral decision made by one in authority; there can be consensus, majority rule, or unanimity.

Likewise, the same mechanisms for resolving role conflict can be used by a team to resolve conflict over decisions. The team can ignore the conflict, allow one person to force a decision, smooth it over, compromise, or confront and resolve the problem. A team must be aware of the decision-making processes used and their way of dealing with conflict.

Rubin has suggested the following processes to help a team develop awareness of decision making and conflict resolution regarding decisions.[9] The awareness and techniques should contribute to the efficiency and effectiveness of the team.

Prior to the team meeting, members should write out typical decisions the group has made in the past. At the meeting they should share the lists, discuss why each decision is important, select one to work on, and post the others for later team efforts.

Using the selected decision, the team places it on a sheet of paper or blackboard. Beside the decision, the names of all people who should be involved in making the decision are listed. These individuals may be placed into one of three categories for decision making. The first category includes members who should be directly involved, the second category is for people who should be consulted prior to decision making, and the third category includes individuals who should be informed about the decision. These categories may be marked by the persons' names on the chart with a 1, 2, or 3, or a D (directly), C (consulted) or I (informed). People who must implement the plan should be directly involved, whereas, advice, alternatives, and so forth may be collected from an individual who is an authority but is not involved in the implementation; these individuals are consulted.

In the team meeting one member should also be responsible for managing and seeing that the individuals identified as being directly involved are actually involved, that those identified as being consulted beforehand are consulted, and so forth. The manager also assures that a time is set for the actual decision. The manager may be either a directly involved member, a consulted member, an informed member, or not involved in the decision.

The process of assigning individuals and determining whether each individual is directly involved, consulted, or informed will give the team a feel for team decision making. In addition, the team should identify points in the nursing process where these individuals should be involved. From this process the team can answer questions such as: Was there agreement on the problem? Were all people involved in the discussion? How was disagreement handled? How was agreement reached? How can we do better next time? A discussion and evaluation of these processes should help the team begin to make more efficient and effective decisions.

Team Leadership. On a team the leadership role should be shared rather than allowing it to reside with one member. This is important because different members have different skills and knowledge and shared leadership allows everyone to contribute, which makes a more effective, efficient team. Some teams may use the method of leadership they know best from the hospital situation. In many instances, this will be to look to the physician for leadership. However, this is not always best.

In group meetings there are certain leadership behaviors that facilitate the movement of the team toward reaching goals and objectives. These include the task-oriented behaviors of initiating, seeking and giving information, clarifying and elaborating, summarizing and testing the consensus. In addition, there are maintenance-oriented behaviors, which include gatekeeping (time and record keeping), encouraging, harmonizing, and compromising.

Rubins suggests that teams look at these behaviors using the following process.[10] Initially team members identify members who perform each of these tasks well. This can be done at home prior to the team meeting. At the team meeting these lists are shared and combined. Thereafter, members may react to the feedback, which gives the team a picture of important leadership behaviors in the group, and allows members to see how they are received by the group.

Next the team should identify whether the task-oriented and maintenance functions in the group are being adequately fulfilled, under- or overrepresented. This discussion should be recorded. Following the discussion, the team members should negotiate to reduce the overrepresented functions and to increase the under represented functions. Following the discussion and agreement, an evaluation of the meeting should be done.

MAINTAINING TEAM FUNCTIONING

As teams continue to function, new members may be added and old ones may leave the team. This may lead to changes in team roles and relationships. In addition, there may be indicated changes in roles and relationships as clients and other conditions change. Thus, it is important that teams continually monitor their functioning. Their role behaviors, decision-making processes, leaderships behaviors, and goal-setting techniques should be evaluated periodically. The process discussed earlier can be used to improve any of these processes when needed.

A good diagnostic tool for identifying problems in a functioning team has been identified by Rubins and is reproduced in Table 8–2.[11]

Team members complete the scale at home and give it to the team recorder. The recorder prepares a summary for the group. Scale 1 refers to the goals and objectives of the team, Scale 2 and 3 refer to roles, Scales 4, 5, and 6 refer to decision making, and Scales 7 and 8 refer to team norms. A process for looking at team norms has not been discussed here but can be found in Rubins.[12]

If team members all have answers on the Individual Data Summary Sheet (see Table 8–2) that are near II, the team is functioning well and there is little need for going through processes to assist team functioning. However, if some or a majority of the members have answers near I, the team must work with the specific processes (roles, decision making) as discussed earlier.

If teams continue to have difficulties after going through these processes, they may need assistance from an outsider. Wise discusses consultation to help teams improve their effectiveness.[13] Initially, each team member was interviewed to determine the member's views on goals, roles, and so forth; team members were given feedback. From this, the team went through a process similar to the nursing process. Because they already had the data (assessment), they started with priorities from among the problems identified within the team. They also generated alternative solutions, set goals, allocated members to implement action, and developed methods for evaluation. During this process, the consultant helped members internalize the previous process approach and helped them to develop an attitude that would allow the change to evolve.

TEAM PROCESSES USEFUL IN FAMILIES

Both the team and family are systems made up of interrelated parts functioning together to meet the goals of the whole. Families may also have difficulty with role ambiguity, role overload or role conflict. They may also have difficulty with group decision making, leadership styles, and the other aspects of the team as discussed in this section. If these aspects are identified in the family assessment, community health nurses may also wish to use these processes or a modified version to help families improve their relationships and role functioning.

PRIMARY CARE

Nurses who work within the organized structure of agencies in community health nursing are not giving primary care unless they are on a primary care team. The primary care method differs from the case method in the degree of accountability for the primary care nurse is responsible for the nursing care of a patient on a 24-hour basis. The nurse may be on-call or may have an assistant who provides the care during certain hours, but the care plan and ultimate responsibility reside with the primary care nurse. In community health nursing agencies, the case method is used rather than primary care because responsibility does not include a 24-hour time period.

PRIMARY CARE TEAM

Rakel discusses the primary care team as a team made up of physicians, nurses, social workers, public health nurses, and others.[14] Tichy reviewed the composition of primary teams in 23 studies and found the most consistent team composition to be physicians, registered nurses, social workers, public health nurses, and family health workers.[15] Occasionally teams would include psychologists, dentists, nutritionists, psychiatric aides, lab technicians, and pharmacists.

Rakel says that most physicians think that they should continue to do the initial assessment and use allied health personnel for screening and continuing the management of problems.[16] Many of the clients who come to clinics can be screened by nonphysicians. Garfield classified patients into four categories: (1) well patients with no complaints and no abnormalities found on medical work up; (2) worried-well patients with complaints but no abnormalities found on medical work-up; (3) asymptomatic sick patients with no complaints but abnormalities found on medical work-up; and (4) sick patients who had complaints and abnormalities.[17] Garfield found that 3 out of every 4 patients seen in the clinic during the study could be classified as worried-well and could be adequately handled by nonphysicians. Others believe the nurse can work effectively with more of these clients in an independent or clinic setting (see discussion in next section).

Although Rakel discusses the team as a primary care team, the team is not available on a 24-hour basis and the physician remains legally responsible, and "for this reason he will to some extent always retain the leadership role."[18] Thus, this is more similar to the nursing team with a team leader than it is a primary care team.

INTRAORGANIZATION OR INDEPENDENT PRIMARY NURSING CARE

There has not been agreement among nurses about the best way to provide primary care in the community. Some believe this nursing care can be provided within the organized health-care system and others believe it must be provided outside the system. All agree that the current health care system is in trouble because it cannot or does not meet the needs of the population. These two approaches are discussed here.

Primary Nursing Within the Health Care System. In the late 1960s, physicians and others realized that physicians would not be able to continue to meet the total health-care needs of the U.S. population. This led to various approaches using nurses in the health care system to help fulfill this need. Nurses were used as primary care nurses in pediatrics, and in adult medical-surgical clinics. These studies have been reported by Ford and Silver, Ford, and co-workers, Steckle, and Lewis and Resnik.[19,20,21,22] Many of the studies have also been reported by Brown.[23]

These studies have led to the expanded role of the nurse. One expanded role that is appropriate in community health nursing is the family nurse practitioner. Conant says, "the family nurse practitioner is a practitioner who is prepared to make independent judgments and to assume principal responsibility for primary health care of individuals and families in organized services. She assumes major professional responsibility for decision making in relation to health needs. She works collaboratively with physicians and other members of the health team in the delivery of health services to individuals and families. Her practice is community oriented, related to needs, concerns, and priorities of the consumers."[24] Conant says that this nurse has responsibility for both wellness and illness. Wellness activities include health maintenance of all age groups including preventive techniques, screening, health teaching, and periodic examinations. Illness activities include an initial assessment of patients using all diagnostic procedures to determine whether the nurse should intervene or refer to a physician. In addition, the family nurse practitioners provides ongoing health maintenance and management of stable chronically ill patients.

Bowns describes a family nurse practitioner program that prepares nurses to give "nursing care to families needing (1) care of common illnesses, (2) care of chronic long–term illness, (3) preventive services, (4) family health counseling, and (5) health education."[25] Thus, she includes preventive and primary care concepts in her concept of the family nurse practitioner. The components of health maintenance and disease prevention and primary care of management of health care are reproduced in Figures 8–2 and 8–3.

Burnetto and Birk discuss the primary care nurse who is actually a generalist or family nurse practitioner on a health team.[26] The primary care nurse shares primary care with the physician and works with adults and children in ambulatory settings. He or she assesses problems, determines needs, implements plans, coordinates health action, evaluates outcomes, and teaches and performs preventive activities. Some of the functions are independent, whereas others are dependent and interdependent. **Independent fuctions** include coordinating and implementing plans with stable chronically ill clients, taking histories and doing physical examinations, providing preventive services, emergency triage, family planning, health education and patient counseling. **Interdependent functions** are carried out jointly with others and include such things as dietary planning and decisions regarding disposition. **Dependent functions** are performed under the physician's supervision and include such things as prescribing drugs, psychotherapy, and referral for diagnostic procedures outside the base of operation.

Burnetto and Birk developed a model for patient entry into the primary care team and the primary-care nurse's role (Fig. 8–4). Most of these efforts at primary care within an organized structure of community health do not fulfill the definition of primary care quoted earlier because the primary care members are not available on a 24-hour basis.

Primary Care Outside the Health Care System. Many nurses recognize the need to change the health care system or to move outside it to provide adequate community-health nursing services Leininger says, "we must substitute for our present closed, uniprofessional controlled system one that is open, flexible, diverse and oriented to the clients and to the community."[27] She continues to say that the current crisis is caused by inadequate use and distribution of health resources and a health care system that is operated and controlled by medicine. Kinlein says, "the whole health care system must be revised in order for the profession of nursing to be practiced in such a way that the benefit will accrue to the people of the community."[28] Ford also says that the current health care system is unable to meet minimum standards of quality health care.[29] This has resulted from poor use and distribution of health manpower and from the escalating costs of care.

Leininger has proposed an open health-care system to facilitate accessible, timely health care.[30] In her proposed system, clients would have a choice of services from various health professions and, if not needed, might not see a physician.

The Leininger model, which is reproduced in Figure 8–5, focuses upon clients coming from various backgrounds. This model evolves from Garfield's model, which was discussed earlier in the chapter, but Leininger's model includes cultural, social, and community data, and also includes the client in the process model. The client has a choice of health care providers and can expect health maintenance as part of the care.

Greenidge and co-workers describe their independent, group nursing practice, which evolved from an inability to provide quality and continuity of care within the present health-institution framework. These three community health nurses set up rules and policies that included 24-hour coverage

(*Text continues on page 213*)

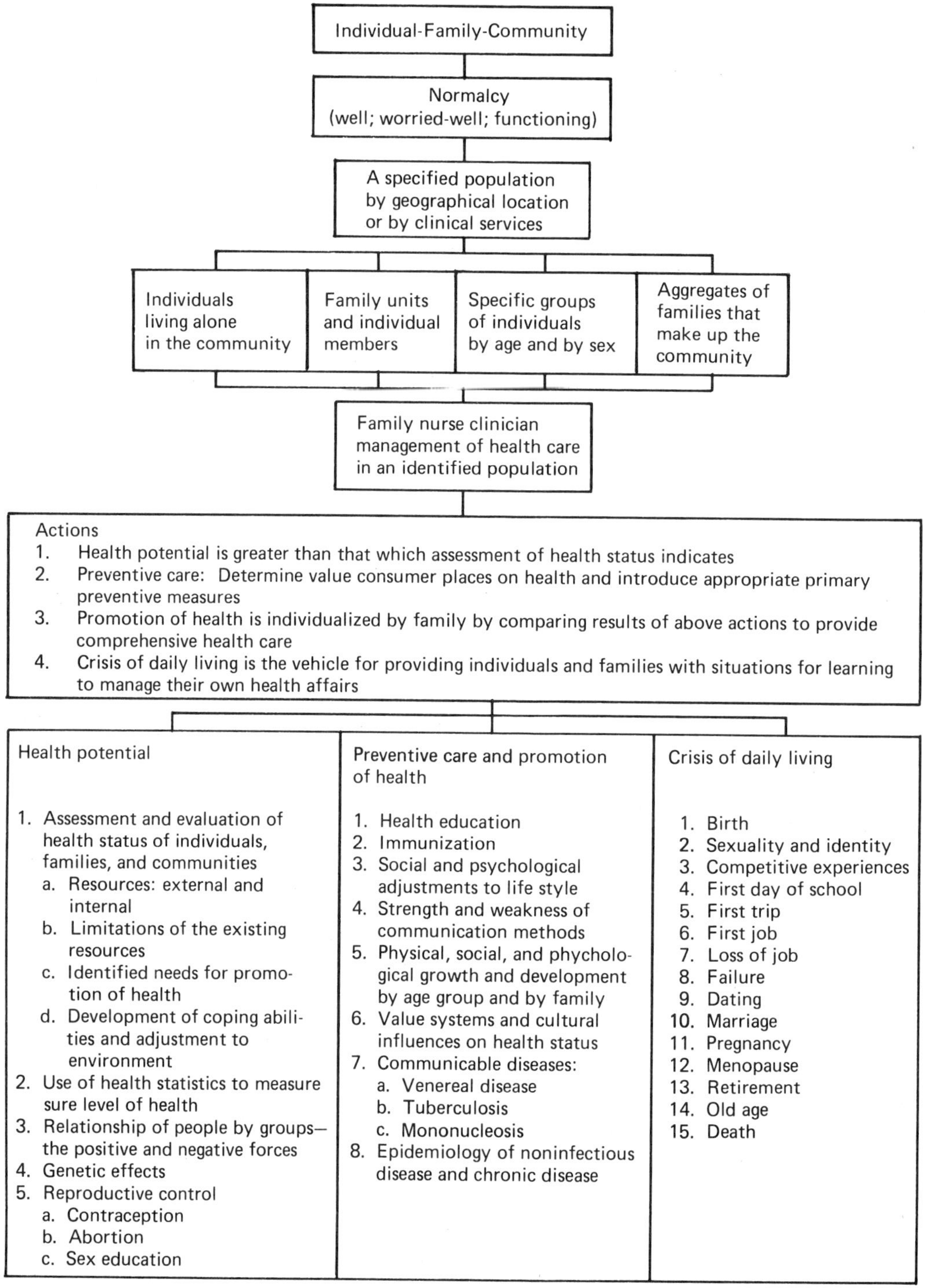

Figure 8–2

Health maintenance and disease prevention components in the health care management of individuals, families, and communities. (From Hymovich DP, Barnard MU: Family Health Care, New York, McGraw-Hill. Copyright © 1973 by McGraw-Hill, Inc. Used with permission of McGraw-Hill Book Company)

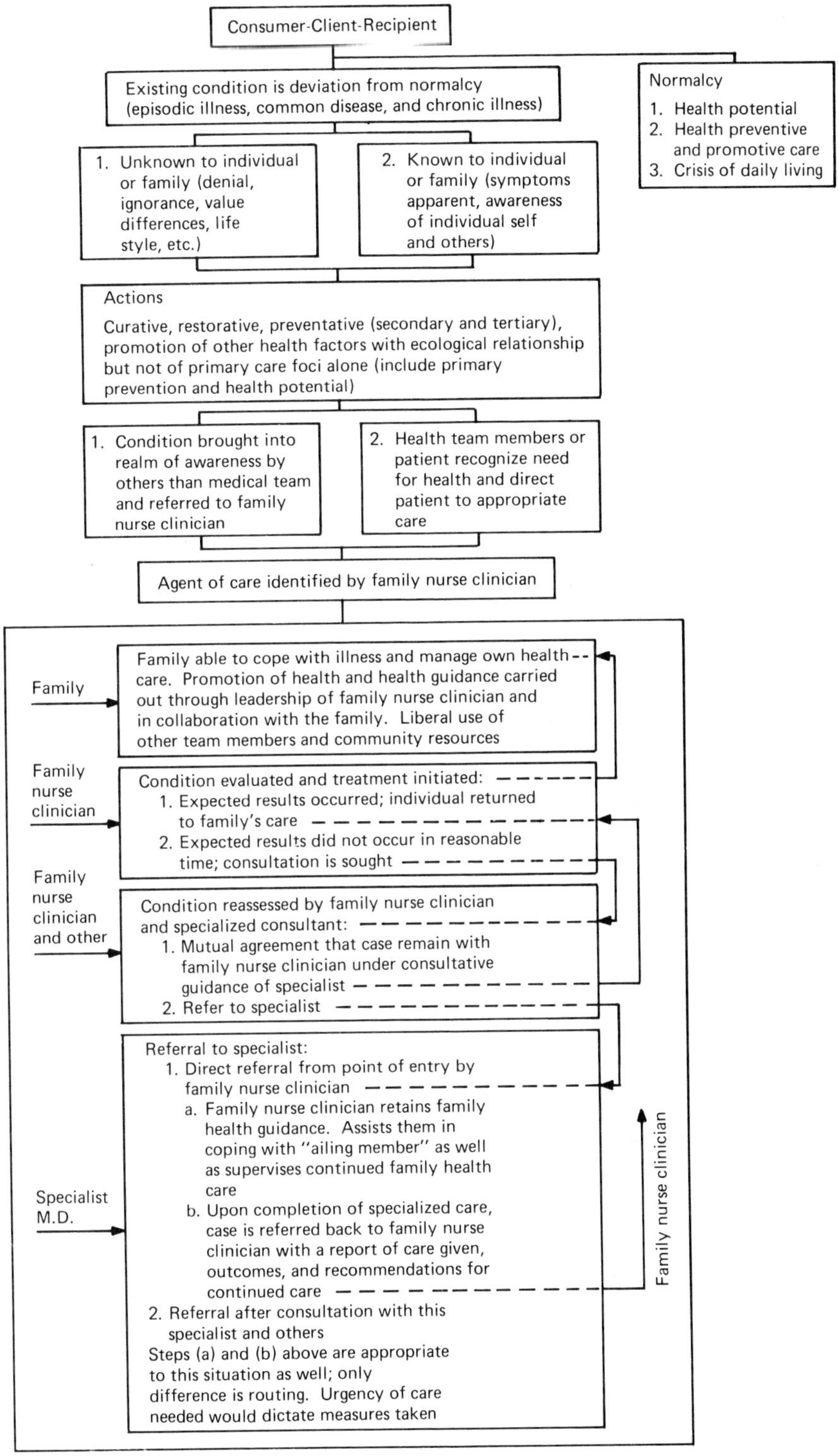

Figure 8–3

Primary care component of health care management of families and individuals. (From Hymovich DP, Barnard MU: Family Health Care, New York, McGraw-Hill. Copyright © 1973 by McGraw-Hill, Inc. Used with permission of McGraw-Hill Book Company)

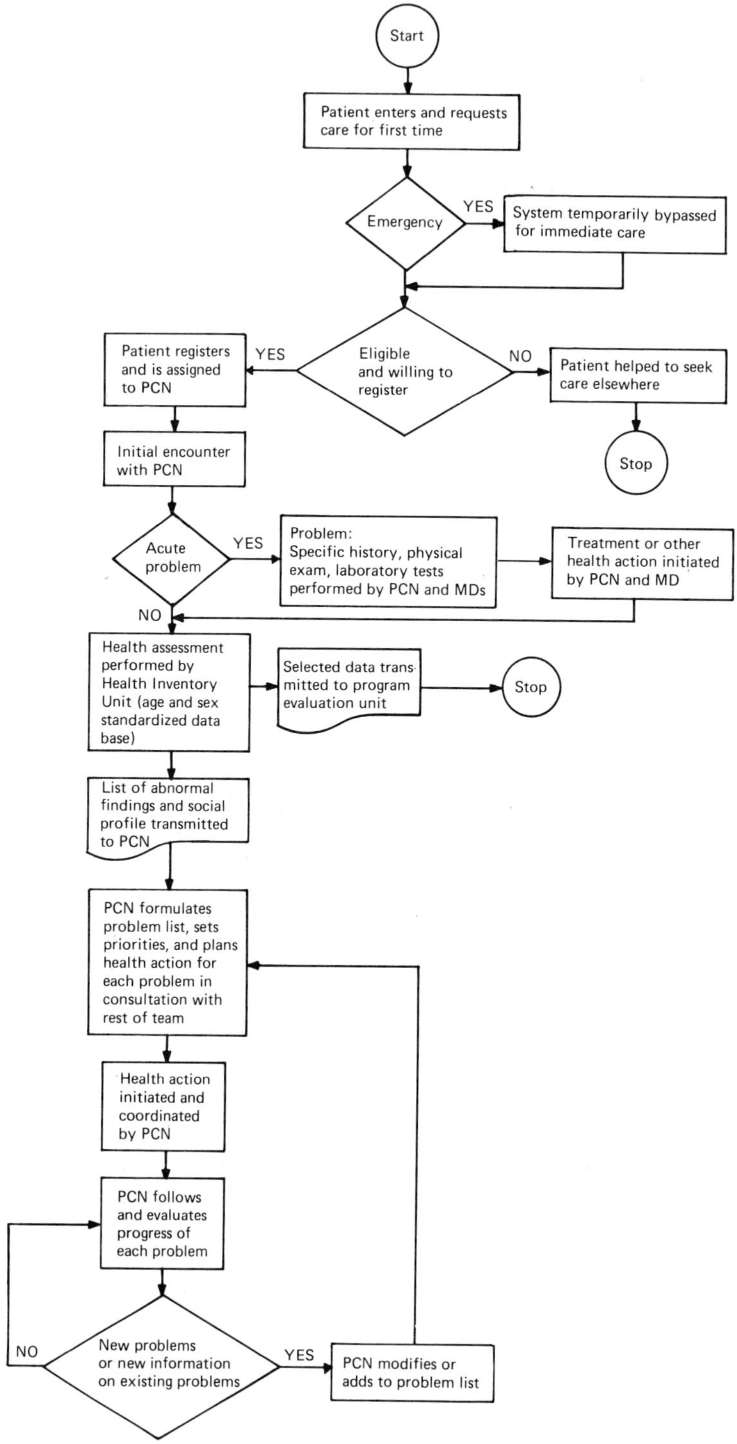

Figure 8–4

Patient entry into primary care team and the primary care nurse's (PCN) role in health action. (Bruno E, Birk P: The primary care nurse—The generalist in a structured health care team. In Spradley B (ed): Contemporary Community Nursing, p 132. Boston, Little Brown. Copyright 1975. Reprinted with permission)

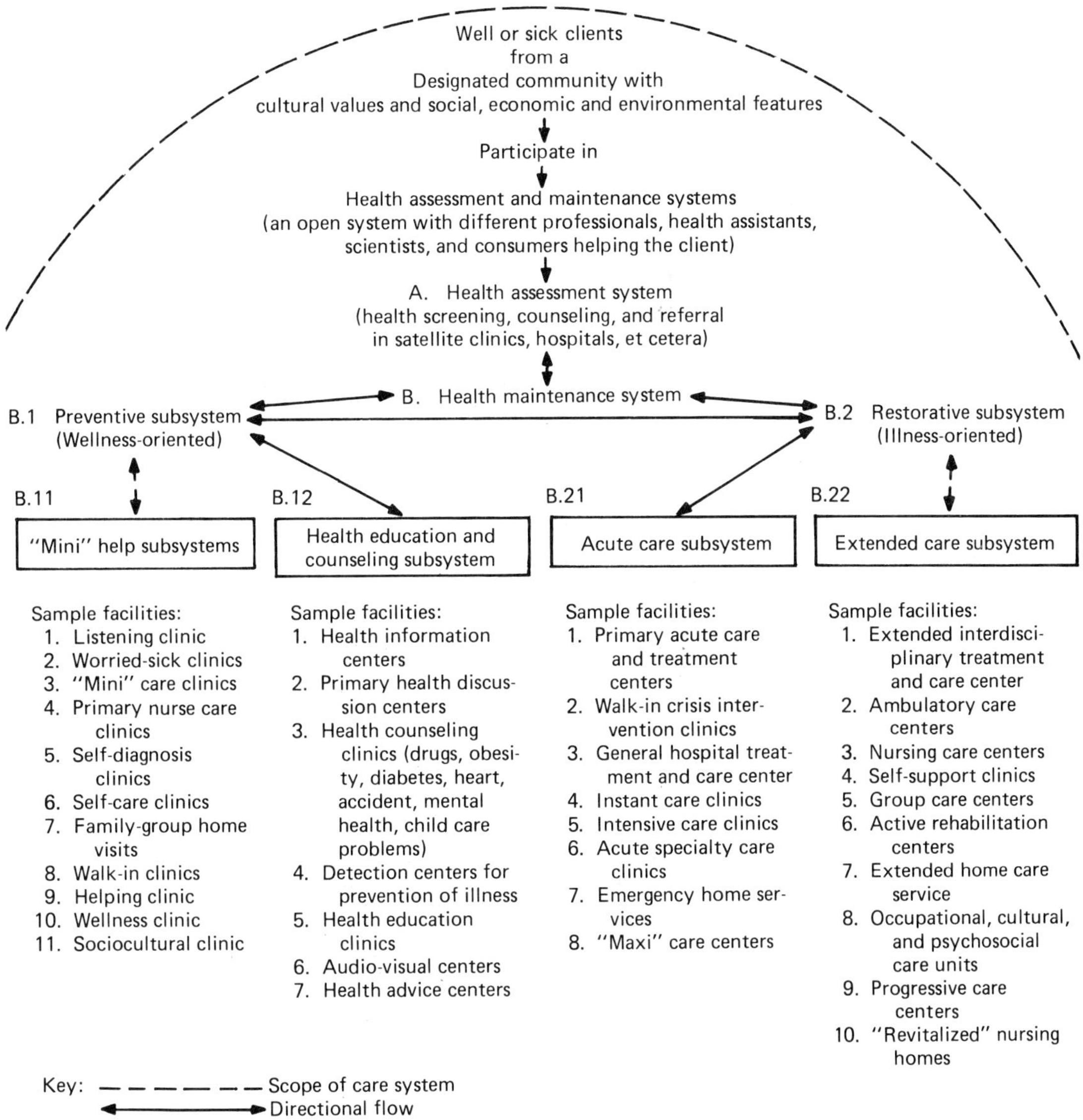

Figure 8–5

An open client-centered health care system model. Leininger; M: An open health care system model. In Spradley B (ed): Contemporary Community Health, p 16. Boston, Little Brown. Copyright 1975. Reprinted with permission.

of clients so they can be seen day or night, taking a complete history on all new clients, providing a fees-for-service basis, and setting up rules regarding patient medications. Clients are primarily self-referred although at the time of this writing one physician had referred a client for care. Nursing care has included physical care, psychological support, dietary and other teaching, assistance with medications, and activities of daily living.

Kinlein has also established an independent

(Text continues on p. 216)

Table 8–2. Team Effectiveness Diagnostic Instrument

Individual Preparation:

Directions: In the scales on the following pages, circle the letter that you think most accurately reflects where your own description of your team would fall between the two descriptive statements provided (I and II). Read both statements before deciding on your response. If your description is more like the top statement (I), then you should circle letter "a" or letter "b." If your description is more like the bottom statement (II), then you should circle "d" or "e." Your answer should represent how you think things actually are, not how they should be or how you wish they were. These responses will be summarized anonymously and discussed by the team.

In the spaces for examples below each scale, write down a real situation which describes your response on the numerical scales. These examples will not be collected or summarized. However, they will be useful in explaining to the others on the team what you meant by each of your responses. Therefore, you should share your examples during the discussions that will take place in the team meeting.

In answering the diagnostic questions, remember that the more open and honest you are in your responses, the more accurate and useful to you the assessment will be.

"Things about why we are here"

Scale 1

Statement I—I often wonder what is the basic reason for being here. It seems to me that there are people on the team (maybe even myself) who spend a lot of time and energy doing things that are not consistent with what I think is our main purpose in being here. They downplay or overlook important parts of our total objective or their time is directed at things I think aren't very important.

a. Just like I
b. More like I and II
(circle one) c. In between I and II
d. More like II than I
e. Just like II

Statement II—The team's basic overall objectives are very clear to me. All of my and everyone else's effort seems directly related to getting these key goals accomplished. Whenever a question arises over what things need to get done, we are able to set priorities by referring back to our basic objectives.

Example(s): In the space below describe one or more examples of situations in the team that illustrate your response on Scale I.

"Things about my job"

Scale 2

Statement I—Often situations arise on the job where I'm not certain what I am supposed to do. Frequently, I'm not even sure if a situation is my responsibility or someone else's. We never get together to discuss what each individual thinks he (she) and the others on the job can or should do to work together to do the best job.

a. Just like I
b. More like I than II
(circle one) c. In between I and II
d. More like II than I
e. Just like II

State II—In almost every situation I am very sure about what responsibilities I have and about what others on the job are supposed to be doing. These job responsibilities are often discussed by relevant members of the team, particularly when someone has a question about what he or someone else should be doing.

Example(s):

Scale 3

Statement I—Different people on the job are always asking me to do different things at the same time. Often these tasks get in the way of each other or there just isn't enough time to meet everyone's demands. My job makes me feel like a "juggler with too many balls."

a. Just like I
b. More like I than II
(circle one) c. In between I and II
d. More like II than I
e. Just like II

Statement II—I have no trouble in doing the different things that the job and other people on the team require of me. I understand why I'm supposed to do the things I do and it all semms to fit together. If I feel as though the demands people on the team make of me are getting too heavy or don't make sense, we resolve the problem with a discussion.

Example(s):

"How thing get done around here"

Table 8–2. Team Effectiveness Diagnostic Instrument *(Continued)*

Scale 4

Statement I—When some people try to participate in a discussion of job issues they often get cut off or their suggestions seem to die. People only seem to pay attention to some team members and not others. Some people seem to do most of the talking while otehrs don't participate very much.

	a. Just like I
	b. More like I than II
(circle one)	c. In between I and II
	d. More like II than I
	e. Just like II

Statement II—Everyone gets a chance to express himself and to influence the group in discussions about the job. We listen to every person's contributions and try to discuss the strong points in each. No one is ignored. Everyone is drawn into the discussion.

Example(s):

Scale 5

Statement I—When we sit down to discuss something I usually walk away wondering what we just did and what is suppoed to happen next. If, as a result of a discussion, I am assigned to do something, I often do not agree with the tasks assigned me. It seems like the same problems keep coming up for discussion even though we thought we had worked them through already.

	a. Just like I
	b. More like I than II
(circle one)	c. In between I and II
	d. More like II than I
	e. Just like II

Statement II—When we have a problem to discuss, I usually understand exactly what the issue is. By the end of the discussion, I usually understand what we have decided to do about it, and what my responsibilities are. Decisions made by this team are carried out effectively by the team members.

Example(s):

Directions: This scale is different from the previous ones. In this scale, read all the statements and circle the letter next to the one statement that most closely describes the general situation in your team.

Scale 6

When a disagreement arises in the team:

a. We assume it's probably best not to let it get personal, so we let it pass hoping it will cool down and eventually be forgotten. If it does start to ruffle feelings, we try to smooth the feelings and make the least of the disagreement (*e.g.*, ". . . well, there is really no point in fighting about it—so, let's forget it" or "we're all grown-ups, we shouldn't argue").

b. Often we end the disagreement when someone on the team takes charge and makes a decision, or decides not to discuss it any further.

c. We try to come to an agreement somewhere between the two disagreeing positions. In other words, we compromise. That way everyone gets a little and everyone gives a little and the disagreement is taken care of.

d. We get the disagreeing parties together and have them talk to each other about their points of view until each party can see some logic in the other's ideas. Then we try to come to an agreement that makes sense to everyone.

Example(s):

"What it's like to work around here"

Scale 7

Statement I—I often get the feeling that some people on the team don't think that some other people on the team have much of a contribution to make. Some people don't pay much attention to the problems or suggestions of others. People are often taken for granted.

	a. Just like I
	b. More like I than II
(circle one)	c. In between I and II
	d. More like II than I
	e. Just like II

Statement II—Everyone recognizes that the job could not be done without the cooperation and contribution of everyone else. Each person, including myself, is treated as an important part of the team. When you bring up an idea or a problem, people sit up and take notice. It makes you feel that you and your job are important.

Example(s):

Scale 8

Statement I—This job really gets me down. People do not seem concerned with helping each other get the job done. Everyone is pulling in opposite directions, everyone is out for himself. If you try to do something different, you get jumped on by people for being out-of-line, or if you make a mistake, you never hear the end of it.

(Continued)

Table 8–2. Team Effectiveness Diagnostic Instrument (*Continued*)

(circle one)
a. Just like I
b. More like I than II
c. In between I and II
d. More like II than I
e. Just like II

Statement II—I really like my job, and I like working with this team. The team encourages you to take responsibility. You feel really appreciated by the other members of the team when you do a good job. When things aren't going well, people really make an effort to help each other. We really pull together on this team.

Example(s):

INDIVIDUAL DATA SUMMARY SHEET

Scales	I					II
1. Goal clarity and conflict		a	b	c	d	e
2. Role ambiguity		a	b	c	d	e
3. Role conflict		a	b	c	d	e
4. Participation/ influence		a	b	c	d	e
5. Commitment/ understanding		a	b	c	d	e
6. Conflict management		a	b	c	d	e
7. Recognition/ involvement		a	b	c	d	e
8. Support cohesiveness		a	b	c	d	e

(Reprinted with permission from Improving the Coordination of Care: A Program for Health Team Development, Copyright 1975, Cambridge, Ballinger Publishing Company)

practice as a generalized nurse.[32] In her practice she implements a modified version of Orem's self-care concept as outlined in *Nursing: Concepts of Practice*.[33] Kinlein says that her method of nursing is defined as "assisting people in their self-care practices in regard to their state of health."[32] Examples of nursing care with clients are presented in the journal article. Kinlein says that nursing care in the future will involve "total control of judgments and decisions" regarding nursing care; a "legitimate nurse-client relationship" like other professional practice groups; identification of need in the relationship to be established by the client in the relationship; identification of self-care assets and deficits related to the need; identification of self-care demands resulting from the assets and deficits; nursing measures tailored to these demands; and assisting people in exercising their self-care practices.

Nursing in the community in the future will be different from today. As indicated, we currently have community nurses working within and outside the health care system to improve the quality of nursing care. Where nursing as a group moves is dependent upon how we can best meet community needs for nursing care. Whether this care is within or outside of the health care system, on nursing or health teams, uses the team approach, or individually uses a primary care method or a case method approach, nursing must continue to remain responsive to communities if it as a profession is to survive. Otherwise, the created gap will be filled by other health care disciplines.

REFERENCES

1. Douglass L, Bevis, E: Nursing Leadership in Action, p 118. St Louis, C V Mosby, 1974
2. Ibid, p 119
3. Rakel R: Principles of Family Medicine, p 78. Philadelphia, W B Saunders, 1977
4. Rubins I, Fry R, Povnick M: Making Health Teams Work: An Educational Program, p 2. Unpublished paper of The Alfred P. Sloan School of Management, Massachusetts Instituee of Technology, May 1974
5. Rubins I, et al: Improving the Coordination of Care: A Program for Health Team Development, p 105. Cambridge, Ballinger, 1975
6. Rubins I, ibid, p. 116
7. Rubins I, ibid, p 127
8. Wise H, et al: Making health teams work. Am J Dis Child, 124: p 540, April 1974
9. Rubins I, op cit
10. Rubins I, op cit, p 221
11. Rubins I, op cit, p 38
12. Rubins I, op cit
13. Wise H, op cit, pp 537–542
14. Rakel R, op cit, p 73
15. Tichy M: Health Care Teams: An Annotated Bibliography. New York, Praeger, 1974
16. Rakel R, op cit, p 75
17. Garfield S R: Prevention of dissipation of health services resources. Am J Public Health 61: 1499–1506, 1971
18. Rakel, op cit, p 90
19. Ford L C, Silver H K: The expanded role of the nurse in child care. Nurs Outlook 15: 43–45, 1967
20. Ford P A, et al: The relative roles of the public health nurse and the physician in prenatal and infant supervision. Am J Public Health 56: 1097–1103, 1966
21. Stoechkle J D, et al: Medical nursing clinics for chronically ill. Am J Nurs 63: 787–789, 1963
22. Lewis C E, Resnik B A: Nursing clinics and progressive ambulatory patient care. New Engl J Med 277: 1236–1241, 1967
23. Brown E L: Nursing Reconsidered: A Study of Change, Part 2. The Professional Role in Community Nursing. Philadelphia, J B Lippincott, 1971
24. Conant L B: The nature of nursing tomorrow. Image: Sigma Theta Tau National Honor Society of Nursing Vol. 4, No. 2, 1970–71, Reprinted with permission
25. Bowns B: The family nurse clinician. In Hymovich D, Barnard M (eds): Family Health Care, p 43. New York, McGraw-Hill, 1973
26. Brunetto E, Birk P: The primary care nurse—The generalist in a structured health care team. Am J Public Health Vol 62, No. 6: 785–794, 1972
27. Leininger M: An open health care system model. Nurs Outlook Vol 21, No. 3: 171–175, 1973
28. Kinlein L: Point of view. On the front: Nursing and family and community health. Family and Community Health Vol. 1, No. 2, 1978
29. Ford L: The development of family nursing. In Hymovich, Barnard M (eds): Family Health Care, p. 15. New York, McGraw-Hill, 1973
30. Leininger M, op cit
31. Greenidge J, et al: Community nurse practicitioners—A partnership. Nurs Outlook Vol. 21, No. 4: 228–231, 1973
32. Kinlein L, op cit
33. Orem D E: Nursing: Concepts of Practice. New York, McGraw-Hill, 1971

PART III
CONCEPTS, THEORIES, AND MODELS IN COMMUNITY HEALTH NURSING

9

Epidemiologic Concepts and Theory

Epidemiology is a body of knowledge and a method for obtaining knowledge. As a body of knowledge, epidemiology is the study of the distribution and determinants of diseases prevalent in humans. The purpose of this knowledge is to influence the health of populations in a positive way. From a systems point of view, epidemiology studies the imbalances in populations that are caused by excesses or deprivations of energy and information. In this chapter, a concept of health and the epidemiologic methods and knowledge that influence health are presented.

CONCEPTS OF HEALTH

STATIC CONCEPTS

Although the goal of all health care is the restoration or promotion of health, there is a great deal of uncertainty as to what this term means. For example, if the various organs in the body function well and humans are free from pain and discomfort, they usually believe that they are in good health. The criterion is then a subjective one. However, if an x-ray film shows strong evidence of tuberculosis, humans no longer consider themselves to be in good health. The criterion they now adopt is an extraneous one, that is, the assertion of illness is made by a physician who relies on objective or pathologic data. Because there are no measures of positive health, the usual medical model considers everyone healthy who is free from any evidence of disease or infirmity. This is a static concept of health based upon subjective and objective measures at a particular point in time.

There are several difficulties in any concept of health. First, health means different things to different people, dependent upon their social background, past experiences, and other related factors. Murray and Zentner discuss several variables that influence a client's concept of health and illness, and Koos presents research findings to substantiate social class differences in concepts of health and illness.[1,2] Second, because positive health cannot be reliably measured, health is often considered present when there is no evidence of disease or observable pathology, that is, a blood pressure within normal limits, a chest x-ray film that is clear, and so on. However, individuals free from observable disease and pathology have different capacities for dealing with environmental stress and for living up to an attainable health level. Consequently, there are levels of health beyond freedom from illness, even though these cannot be measured with current methods. Third, even tests for measuring health in the negative sense are evaluated on the basis of group norms and standards, which may or may not be relevant for any particular individual.

The World Health Organization defines health as a "state of complete physical, mental, and social well-being and not merely the absence of disease." Although this definition recognizes the social and mental components of health and recognizes health as more than the absence of disease it has limited value because it is too abstract, it lacks an appreciation of the varying degrees of healthfulness or wellness among those usually classified as well and it refers to a state of health. We know there is no such thing as a perfect or absolute state of health for the process of aging is always in flux bringing with it obvious physiologic changes. Likewise, social, cultural, economic, and other related forces are always affecting humans and may change the direction of health at any time. (See System Exchange with Environment and Adaptation, Chap. 2.)

DYNAMIC CONCEPTS

Many authors now think of health as an open-ended, dynamic, everchanging process.[4–8] This involves the acceptance of a dual concept of homeodynamics. First, the one most commonly accepted is the desirability of getting the total human (mentally, physically, emotionally, and spiritually) in tune or in balance in all dimensions to an end that allows their energy to be used for happy, productive living. Second, an equally vital concept of health is reflected in the idea that the health status of the individual, family, or community may be more than the absence of disease, includes at times some or all of the elements of well-being (mental, physical, emotional, social, or spiritual), yet the state is not static. A dynamic concept of health recognizes it as an everchanging continuum that is never static and never a passive state. A dynamic concept of health can be likened to the concept of behavioral adaptation. For example, Auger says, "behavioral adaptation refers to the dynamic adjustment to continually changing demands of both the internal and external environments designed to achieve a relatively stable condition of equilibrium between the two environments . . . equilibrium refers to a hypothetical fixed point of balance where opposing forces are cancelled out by one another."[9] This is a temporary steady state rather than entropy or negentropy, which is discussed in Chapters 1 through 4.

The evolving health status of humans is a result of their changing relationship with the environment. Humans are continually influencing and in turn are influenced by the environment of which they are a part. The relationship between them is in constant shifting states of equilibrium and disequilibrium, which requires that they continuously adapt. Health, then, is not a condition but a process, it is not static, but evolving. For example, Dubos says,

> It is clear that the real measure of health is not the utopian absence of all disease but the ability to function effectively within a given environment. And since the environment keeps changing, good health is a process of adaptation to the myriad microbes, irritants, pressures, and problems which daily challenge man. Thus health is viewed as the maintenance of a delicate balance between a disease agent, organism (man) and the environment and disease results when this balance is shattered.[10]

This balance has been diagramed by Leavell and Clark using the principle of the lever and fulcrum.[11] At equilibrium between the agent, host, and environment the fulcrum is balanced. Any change in this balance can be influenced by agent, host, or environmental factors. For example, if there is excessive noise, radiation, heat, toxins, or other agents affecting humans, the fulcrum tips in favor of the agent. Likewise, such host changes as immunizations, adequate sleep, exercise, personal habits, adequate nutrition, and recreation tips the fulcrum in favor of the host. Environmental changes may affect either the host or agent and tip the fulcrum in one or another direction. For example, poor aseptic measures, air pollution, or crowding may tip the balance in favor of the agent, whereas rat eradication, social harmony, and sunshine may tip the balance in favor of the host. Additional factors which influence the agent, host, or environment are identified later in this chapter.

Human adaptive mechanisms, which assist adaptation to a changing environment, may be physiologic, such as body heat regulations in changing physical environments; intellectual, such as the ability to learn new methods of coping or new social roles and skills; or mental, such as the ability to withstand a level of stress. These adaptive mechanisms may be a result of genetic and environmental factors and are influenced by factors such as age, social class, past experience, and others. For example, the process of aging has an effect upon the physiologic adaptive mechanisms of the body. Fitch says, "the ability of the body to resist stress of many different origins is reduced" and there is a "declining homeostatic capacity during aging."[12] In a similar vein Dunn says,

> Aging is a phenomenon of the physical body. When energy is bound into organization as it most certainly is in the complex human body, it tries to escape . . . Energy in large quantities is routed into the growing body. The energy tries to escape its confines. As the life cycle progresses, more and more energy goes into restoring what is worn away by attrition. The body loses its resilience. Fragility, brittleness, and rigidity are the order of the day. Finally the body as a topological structure breaks, which we have seen means death.[13]

Examples of genetic and environmental factors that decrease adaptation include the retarded person who lacks intellectual abilities to cope with changing environments, or the mental patient who has a long-term experience in institutions, which leads to a loss of social skills. Some of these adaptive mechanisms are fluid and can be influenced toward health by proper intervention, whereas, others cannot. For example, it is possible to resocialize the patient who has lost social skills owing to long-term confinement. However, factors such as age and mental ability cannot be influenced, and efforts toward helping the individual cope might involve manipulation of the environment.

Dynamic Concept of Health Classification System. Although positive health cannot be measured precisely for a given individual, family, or community at a particular point in time, it is possible to develop classification systems into which they may be theoretically placed. One such classification was developed by Rogers who sees health on a continuum ranging from optimum health to approaching death (Fig. 9–1). A spectrum theoretically allows for the placement of every individual *at any given time,* although there may not be agreement for differentiating the various levels of ill health. Theoretically, a person may move up and down the scale as their health improves or deteriorates, and the scale is applicable to social and mental as well as physical health. It should be noted, however, that scientific advancement such as the heart transplant may create difficulties over distinctions between life and death.

Dunn goes a step further with his health continuum and includes an environmental axis in his model (Fig. 9–2). The horizontal axis represents the health of the individual and extends from a point at the left marked Death to a point at the extreme

Figure 9–1

Health status scale: Theoretical classification of the level of health in a given individual at a given time. (Rogers ES: Human Ecology and Health, p 159. New York, Macmillan. Copyright 1960 by Edward S. Rogers. Reprinted with permission of Macmillan Publishing Co., Inc.)

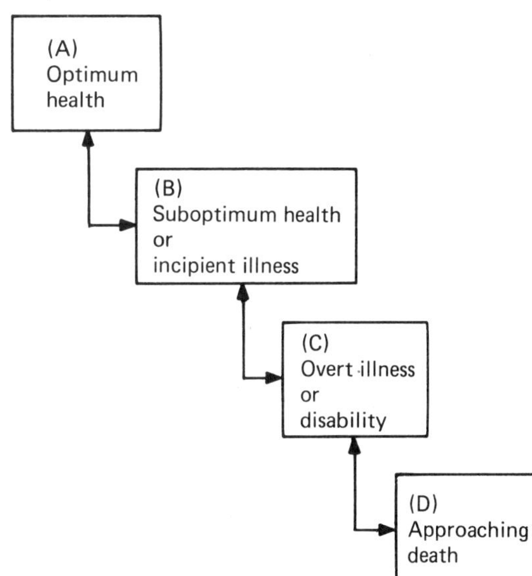

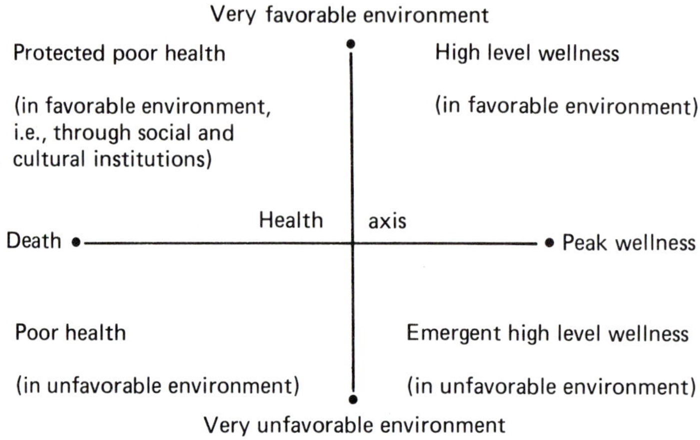

Figure 9–2

The health grid: Its axes and quadrants. (Dunn, H: High level wellness for man and society. Am J Public Health Vol. 49, No. 6: 788, June, 1959. Reprinted with permission)

right marked Peak Wellness. This horizontal axis represents degrees or levels of well-being as conceived by means of a stepladder symbol. Peak wellness should be thought of as a potential and as that condition that the individual arrives at when his capacities are used optimally, in one form or another.

The individual, regardless of physical condition, sex, age, or other factors, can be at any stage of health. As one moves on the projected health axis, Dunn conceptualizes him moving as a totality (as a body–mind–spirit). As we move from the point of illness area into the wellness area, we are affected by factors concerned with a high potential for living. One of these factors is thought by Dunn to be creative expression. This is an inner part of man, and release of this rational creativity brings purpose to one's life. Unless there is a reason for living, unless there is a purpose in our life, Dunn feels that we cannot possibly attain or experience high level wellness. Dunn defines high level wellness as, "an integrated method of functioning which is oriented toward maximizing the potential of which the individual is capable, within the environment where he is functioning."[16] High level wellness involves progression toward an ever-higher potential of functioning rather than the achievement of an optimum level of wellness. It also involves the human as a totality rather than as parts and is concerned with how the individual is functioning within the particular environment regardless of the degree of favorability or ability to manipulate it.

By conceptualizing levels of health on a continuum, the two preceding authors have attempted to go beyond the medical model of considering everyone healthy who is not hospitalized or suffering from obvious pathology.

I have also found another continuum useful for conceptualizing health, which is in Figure 9–3. I consider the right-hand side of the continuum as the population-at-large, not ill enough to be hospitalized and warrant the specialized attention offered by the institution. This end of the continuum encompasses those individuals in both favorable and unfavorable environments and the latter group falls closer to the barrier. Since everyone is well

Figure 9–3

Health continuum for individuals, families, and communities.

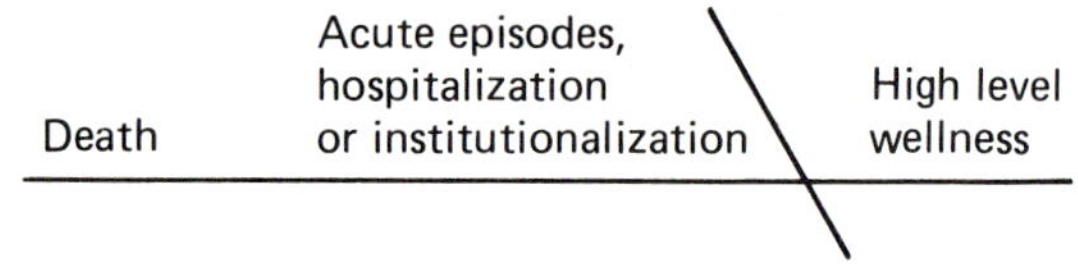

to some degree, the continuum encompasses all people. Individuals may fall between maximum health on the right side of the continuum to minimum health and death on the left. Man's location on the continuum is determined by his adaptation to his changing environment (biophysical, social-cultural), and because man and his environment are ever evolving, man will move up and down the continuum. For example, an individual with dental cavities may fall closer to the right than one with diabetes, and an individual with controlled diabetes (with no circulatory impairments) would fall closer to the right, than one in diabetic acidosis. The continuum encompasses mental and social as well as physical aspects of health as these are all interrelated. For example, an individual with an income inadequate to purchase food, clothing, medical care, and so on may be subjected to physiologic and emotional stress, and may be prevented from participating in social situations and consequently would fall lower on the continuum than one who could provide for these needs. However, even where adequate financial resources are available, a lack of knowledge of proper diet, improper attitudes toward food, lack of personal coping resources, and many related factors may move individuals toward the left end of the continuum.

Because individual health affects family health, which in turn affects community health, families and communities may likewise move up and down the continuum. The relationships between the individual, family, and community are discussed as exchanges of systems with their environment in Chapters 2 through 4.

Although community health nursing is concerned with the entire continuum, the primary focus is on the right side of the barrier (those outside the hospital or institution), and we are always striving to push the balance toward health (or toward putting humans in a favorable balance with their changing environment). Until recently, the care of sick individuals was delegated primarily to other health workers, but community health nurses are beginning to include more bedside care in their activities because of shortened hospital stays, more long-term illnesses requiring supervision in the home, and other related health and scientific factors. However, primary and secondary prevention remain an integral part of all such direct care.

DETERMINANTS OF HEALTH

Even though there are no measures or standards by which we can measure positive health or place individuals, families, or communities at a particular point on the health continuum, at any particular time, we do know some of the indices or determinants of health and can detect behavior that reflects signals of imbalance in health. In addition, there are measures that one can take to maintain health. An approach to assessing health and implementing health plans based upon these determinants and scientific concepts is presented in Chapters 6 and 7. However, an understanding of these determinants should contribute to an understanding of the concept of health and epidemiology.

Ordinarily, the complex causes of illness or injury are thought of as embracing three elements. These elements include (1) the disease or injury producing agent, (2) the resistance or susceptibility of the host, and (3) the environmental situation that brings the agent and host together.

It is now accepted that there is no direct cause-effect relationship between exposure to disease agents and diseases in humans. Rather there are interrelated factors that determine health and illness, that is, disease is a process that results from a breakdown of any one of a multiple of factors (failure to adapt), such as biologic, emotional, cultural, social, and economic. For example, tuberculosis involves, in addition to contact with The *Mycobacterium tuberculosis* organism, environmental factors such as crowding, temperature, ana humidity, and also such host factors as inherent physical constitution, habits, customs, occupation, fatigue, stress, and nutrition. If active tuberculosis is to occur in an individual, a combination of these various factors must favor the survival of the causative organism. In other words, the health status of humans equals their genetic base plus the total effects of their environment. Environment here is used in its broadest sense to include both past and present effects as well as the social-cultural, physical, and biologic environment.

If we look at auto accidents we would again see agent, host, and environmental factors. For example, agent factors such as the mechanical condition of the car, window visibility, available seat belts, condition of tires, and so forth; environmental factors, such as weather conditions and visibility, and type of roads; and host factors such as carelessness, fatigue, nervousness, worry, apathy, or foolhardiness all contribute to automobile accidents. According to Leavell and Clark, the environment and host factors provide the two fundamental reasons for accidents and some studies have estimated that 80% to 90% of accidents are due to host factors. A framework of factors that may influence illness or injury processes has been identified by Rogers and is presented in Figure 9–4.[17] He says that the agent may be weak or virulent, which will consequently influence the reaction of the exposed host. Some sources of variation in the agent, which accounts for its weakness or virulence, include genetic constitution, nutrition, favorable growth conditions, and dosage or intensity of impact. Conditions may also vary in the exposed host. The host may be resistant or suceptible to the disease agent. Sources of variation in the host accounting for the resistance or susceptibility at the time of exposure may be (1) genetic constitution (2) nutrition (3) balance of internal stresses and adaptation (4) age and sex (5) physical vigor or fatigue (6) specific immunity (7) knowledge and attitudes and (8) personality.

In addition, conditions may vary in the environment that bring the agent and host together. The environment may be favorable or unfavorable to a forceful impact. Some possible types of variation in the environment include (1) physical conditions, such as, temperature, humidity, heat, light and shelter, and traumatic hazards (2) biologic conditions, such as, sanitation, parasites, disease vectors, nutrient value of goods available, crowding and (3) nonmaterial conditions, such as, social and

Figure 9–4

Factors influencing the immediate and specific causation of illness and injury. (Rogers ES: Human Ecology and Health, p 166. New York, Macmillan. Copyright 1960 by Edward S. Rogers. Reprinted with permission of Macmillan Publishing Co., Inc.)

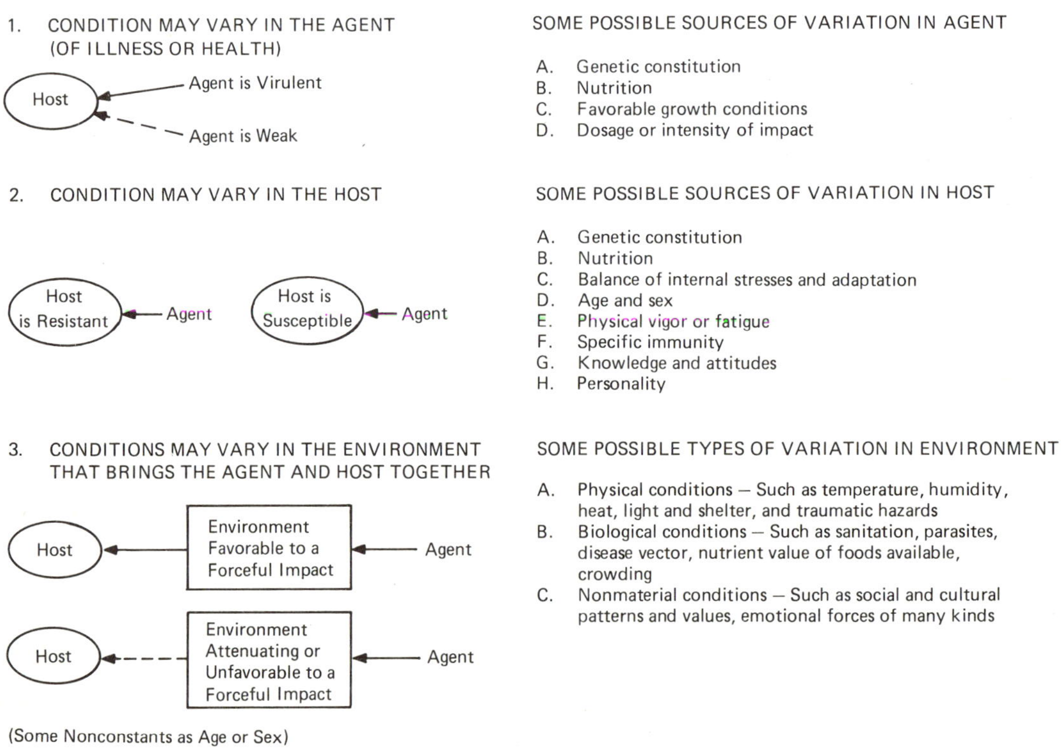

cultural patterns, and emotional forces of many kinds.

Using a host–agent–environment framework, Leavell and Clark have identified many of the factors that initiate specific disease processes.[18] Identification of these multiple related factors, which lead to the disease process, is a part of epidemiology and makes up the natural history of diseases. Knowledge of the natural history of diseases allows us to intervene to prevent or limit the effects of diseases. These and other aspects of intervention by using the knowledge gained from epidemiology is discussed later in this chapter.

Dynamic Interactions of Agent, Host, Environment. We live in a world populated with other forms of life, many of which threaten our existence. Dubos says,

> During the 18th and 19th centuries the American and Polynesian populations were decimated by epidemics of smallpox, measles, tuberculosis and other infections contracted from European explorers and invaders. However, after a few generations the mortality caused by these diseases began to fall spontaneously and progressively.[19]

A member of Cortez's group of invaders brought smallpox to the American continent during the Spanish conquest. The Indians were highly susceptible to the disease and many died. Later conquests of North America again reintroduced smallpox, which affected many American Indians.

> Repeated outbreaks decimated village after village, and at times whole tribes. Early in the seventeenth century, for example, the Massachusetts and Narragansett Indians were reduced in a short time from 30,000 and 9,000, respectively, to a few hundred. In the epidemic of 1837 the Mandan population fell from 1,600 to 31, the Assiniboins lost whole villages, the Crows one-third of their population, while the total deaths among plains tribes amounted to 10,000 in a few weeks. Similar outbreaks occurred in 1870–71 among the Blackfeet.[20]

Sartwell and Dubos have documented the influence of these forms of life (viruses, microbes, and so forth) on human groups.[21,22] Evidence now shows that two kinds of circumstances are most devastating to the existence of humans. The first is an isolated population such as an island from which the infection has been absent for many years. In such a population the usual balance of susceptible and immune humans is grossly disturbed. When introduced the infection usually sweeps through the entire population. Panun, Christensen, and Philips have discussed measles and mumps epidemics in isolated communities.[23,24,25] Conditions necessary for the absence of a common communicable disease over a long period include isolation, where the time required to travel to the place is longer than the incubation period of the disease, or where infected individuals rarely visit and there is a population too small to support the continued presence of the infectious organisms so that it dies out until reintroduced. The epidemic that follows is usually so intense that it affects all members and eliminates the reservoir of susceptibles and the disease is again extinguished until reintroduced. With modern means of transportation such communities are becoming increasingly rare. A second circumstance that may be devastating for humans exists when there is a constant or frequent influx of fresh groups into a closed or overcrowded community. This makes the epidemic potential high. An example is the usual practice of training military recruits. New recruits constantly arrive at basic training centers for a training period of several weeks to several months, and those who have completed their training are shipped out. In winter time, the result is frequently a sharp epidemic of upper respiratory diseases in each batch of recruits, which reaches its peak in 3 to 5 weeks after arrival and terminates in 7 to 10 weeks. Other such situations may be provided by the regular arrival of new susceptible children at an orphanage or school. The circumstances, then, which are necessary for this type of epidemic situation, are first, the steady recruitment of new susceptible subjects and, second, conditions of crowding or poor hygiene within the institution.

The severity of the threat to humans from other forms of life is influenced by their previous contact with these organisms. When a population is exposed to a pathogen with which it has had no past experience, exposure may bring about severe disease in many of its individuals. The generalized epidemic, however, calls into play adaptive changes in both the host population and the infective agent over time, which brings about an ecologic equilibrium between them. The infective agent may remain widely distributed in the community, but its presence need not be associated with injurious effects. Disease, when it occurs, is due to a change in the conditions under which the ecologic equilibrium has evolved. These changes may relate to agent, host, or environmental factors. In humans, the provocative cause of microbial disease may be a disturbance in any of the factors of their external or internal environment such as weather conditions, available food supply, working habits, economic status, or emotional stress.

Not all humans are affected the same by the introduction of a new microbe into the population. In addition to such factors as nutrition, rest, living conditions, personal hygiene, and emotional states, different humans are endowed with different hereditary backgrounds. Darwin long ago introduced the concept of "survival of the fittest," which showed that humans most resistant to the assault of microbes, before ecologic equilibrium is established, will survive and reproduce a more resistant group. Microbes also develop mutant strains through the same process. Mutant strains of the influenza virus accounted for the influenza pandemic of 1918 to 1919. Fear of mutant strains of organisms has also been of concern to those who see indiscriminant use of penicillin and some of the antibiotics.

EPIDEMIOLOGIC TERMS

Gradient of Infection. Differences in the response of humans whether caused by changes in humans, in the environment, or in the disease agent is seen in a gradient of infection. The term "gradient of infection" refers to the variety of host responses of infection.[26] On this gradient may be fatal illnesses at one end and inapparent infections at the other. In the middle are the illnesses that are severe to mild but are followed by recovery. **Inapparent infections,** which will be discussed in the next section, are infections that are so mild that they do not produce clinical illness or symptoms that are identifiable by way of current clinical means. They may be identified by recovery of the organism or by cutaneous hypersensitivity.

Some disease agents have a narrow gradient in populations. "Thus, measles infection is usually in the range of clinically apparent but non-fatal disease. Poliovirus infection, on the other hand, has a wide gradient."[27] Some individuals exposed to the poliovirus may have fatal diseases, others are mild with recovery, and there are about 200 inapparent cases for every clinically apparent case. "Few infectious agents (measles is one) fail to produce a significant proportion of infections which are inapparent."[28]

INAPPARENT INFECTIONS. Inapparent infections are disease processes that go through the evolution of a disease in the same period as a disease, but do not produce clinical symptoms. The term subclinical cases used by Leavell and Clark has essentially the same meaning as inapparent infection.[29] Inapparent infections are important in epidemiology in tracing the spread of a disease because often there are more cases of inapparent infections than of overt disease. Thus, the spread of disease can only be understood by identifying the inapparent infections. Most people who have a knowledge of epidemiology have heard of Typhoid Mary who was a carrier of typhoid in New York but did not have any overt symptoms. She was a classic inapparent case who infected many others.

CARRIER. A carrier in the broadest sense is an "individual who excretes an agent without having overt disease at the time."[30] Thus, there are various types of carriers including the incubatory carrier, convalescent carrier, chronic carrier and individuals with inapparent infections. **Incubatory carriers** excrete the agent prior to the onset of the disease and **convalescent carriers** excrete the agent during the convalescent period. **Chronic carriers** may continue to shed the agent over a period of months or years without further evidence of the disease. Lifetime carriers, however, are infrequent.

OTHER AGENTS OF DISEASE

Thus far we have focused on other forms of life (micro-organisms) as a threat to the life of humans. However, there are other agents in our environment that threaten our existence, and epidemiology takes into consideration these agents as well as the living disease agents. For example, accidents are a leading cause of death and disability in many age groups. In the instance of automobile accidents, the automobile is considered the agent of injury. The interaction of host, agent, and environment as influencing accidents was discussed earlier in this chapter. Other agents of disease that are important to community health nurses are the chemicals used in industry or in homes for cleaning purposes, the residuals of chemicals found on foods, unprescribed medications, and open fireplaces, among others. Many of these are in Chapter 2 as excesses in the exchange between the individual system and the environment.

EPIDEMIOLOGY: DEFINITIONS AND USES AS A SCIENCE

Epidemiology is the study of the distribution and determinants of diseases prevalent in humans. It is useful in looking at the relationships that make up the natural history of disease processes, as a basis for preventive interventions. Two main areas are indicated in the definition: These are the study of the distribution of disease, or descriptive epidemiology, and the search for the determinants of the noted distribution, or analytic epidemiology. The first type of epidemiology, **descriptive epidemiology,** is the study of individuals in the population selected for attack by a specific disease agent in relation to age, sex, race, occupation, susceptibility, place of residence, exposure to specific agents, or whatever other characteristics are pertinent. Descriptive epidemiology is also concerned with temporal distribution of diseases and includes trends, cyclic patterns, and the intervals between the inciting factor and the onset of disease.

This data may be combined with data obtained from analytic epidemiology to piece together the natural history of diseases, to plan the strategy for solving community health problems, or to determine gaps in knowledge and preventive measures. Descriptive epidemiology forms the basis for setting priorities on a local or federal level. For example, we are currently involved in preventive and treatment efforts in the areas of heart, cancer, and stroke disease, which are the three leading causes of death in this country. This does not mean that other areas such as communicable diseases are ignored. It means that a major emphasis in identifying the factors in the disease processes and in treating and preventing their occurrences, are of high priority because of the large numbers affected. Priorities based upon disease patterns vary in time and place. For example, if we compare the three leading causes of death in the U. S. at the turn of the century with those of the present, or compare an undeveloped country with a developed country, we get varying patterns. In the U. S., in the early 1900s, the three leading causes of death were pneumonia, tuberculosis, and diarrhea, which are all communicable diseases. Today, these have been replaced by diseases of the heart, malignant neoplasms, and vascular lesions affecting the central nervous system. Hanlon shows the extent of this shift when he says, "While at the beginning of the century 61% of all deaths were caused by infections and parasitic diseases and only 28% by degenerative diseases, the situation is now reversed with 80% of all deaths caused by degenerative diseases and only 7% by infections or parasitic diseases.[31]

There has also been a shift in the age patterns of diseases from the young to the old. This is partly due to a reduction in death rates among the younger age groups, which has allowed a higher percentage of the population to reach the age of greatest risk from chronic diseases. For example, Goerke says, "more than 60% of all deaths were among persons 65 years of age and over. The mortality rates for the broad category of major cardiovascular diseases were about 7 times as great for persons over age 65 as they were for those between the ages of 45 and 64."[32] If we compared a developing country with the U. S., the developing country would be similar to the U. S. in the 1900s, that is, the disease patterns in the developing country would tend to follow the communicable disease patterns that were present in the U. S. in the 1900s.

Epidemiology is an analytic science because through its methods it collects data to explain the causes for the occurrence and distribution of disease. At any point in time, epidemiologists look at groups exposed to harmful effects (such as children separated from their mothers) and will discover that some become sick and some remain healthy. Of the latter group, some will become sick as the harmful effects continue, but others will continue to be healthy. They are then interested not only in the causes of the sickness for some, but also the reasons for the health of the others with the hope that this understanding will allow for the development of interventions to improve the ratio of sick to well people in a population. Or they may observe a group of physically sick and well persons and look for similar factors in the two groups. They will go down a list of attributes such as age, sex, drinking and eating habits, living conditions, and whatever else is appropriate, to look for differences in the two groups. They then begin to hypothesize reasons for the differing rates in various populations. For example, mother-child separation will not affect all children in the same way. In particular, the result is influenced by the age of the child at separation, health, personality, and relationship with a mother substitute. This example shows that epidemiologists are concerned with the prevention of mental illnesses or the possible long-term effects of mother-child separations as well as physical illnesses. The relationships among host, agent, and environmental factors are pieced together into the natural history of specific disease processes.

Although descriptive and analytic epidemiology have been separated, epidemiologists may use both methods in their survey. They begin with questions such as "What kinds of diseases are present?" "Which occupational groups or aggregates of people are most affected?" "Are certain foods more common to the affected?" As they study the variables, they find relationships among the factors and the diseases in question. These may be hunches, which they will later examine using more elaborate research designs.

Epidemiology is also a constructive science in that the relationships between attributes and a disease (developed from analytic epidemiology) are pieced together into the natural history of a disease. The natural history of a disease is usually not complete because humans and their environment are continually evolving. In addition, disease patterns and health knowledge are evolving. However, we can often use the knowledge we have at any point in time to break the weakest link in the man–agent–environment triad to put humans in a favorable balance and thereby reduce the incidence and prevalence of specific diseases on a community basis. This is a goal of community health at the primary-prevention level. For example, we do not have all the factors leading to the inability of an individual to form close emotional relationships as an adult, but we know that mother-child separation and the thwarting of personality development at certain ages are important factors for a large proportion of a group, so we would be aware of this and plan our interventions accordingly in such situations encountered in the community. Nor do we know all factors in the causation of tuberculosis, but isolation of cases harboring the organism, proper diet, rest, personal hygiene, adequate living space and so forth are important contributing factors and attention to these factors and interventions when indicated while working with families in the community may reduce the incidence of this disease.

HEALTH SYSTEM INTERVENTIONS USING EPIDEMIOLOGIC KNOWLEDGE AND A DYNAMIC CONCEPT OF HEALTH

If we consider health and illness as processes involving various factors in humans, disease agents, and the environment, intervention is possible at several steps in the process. First, because every condition in health and disease has its origin in other processes even before humans are involved, it is possible to assist the health of humans by interrupting those processes before humans and disease agents are brought together. This is known as **primary prevention** and may involve efforts to increase the resistence of humans, decrease the resistance of disease agents, or make the environment less favorable for a human–agent interaction. Primary prevention on a community basis has the goal of reducing the incidence and prevalence of diseases in the population. Leavell and Clark have outlined a variety of activities that assist in reducing the incidence and prevalence of diseases in populations when applied before human interaction with a disease agent. These activities may be general health-promotional activities, which help humans maintain their health. These general activities include health education, good standards of nutrition adjusted to the developmental phase of life, attention to personality development, adequate housing, recreation, and agreeable working conditions, which may influence a variety of disease processes. In addition, specific protective measures may put humans in a favorable balance against specific diseases and include such activities as specific immunizations, personal hygiene, environmental sanitation, and protection from accidents and carcinogens.

If primary-prevention efforts fail to reach individuals, they may experience interaction with the disease-producing stimuli. This may lead to a change in the form and function of the body and ultimately result in disequilibrium, defects, disability, or death. Humans interact with a stimulus (an environmental situation, an infectious agent, physical force, a chemical substance, and so forth) and respond with tissue changes that are not demonstrable with present laboratory methods, such as might be found in mental disorders. These tissue changes or altered reactions are often followed by signs and symptoms and a more or less typical course of illness until terminated by time or treatment. Leavell says that the natural history of a disease includes both the periods before and after humans interact with disease agents.[33] The natural history of a disease comprises all the interrelationships of the agent, host, and environment affecting the complete process and its development from the first forces that create the disease stimulus in the environment or elsewhere, through the resulting response of man to the changes that take place, leading to defect, disability, recovery, or death.

Following the interaction of a disease agent and the host, there are two kinds of intervention. The first is **secondary prevention,** which involves early diagnosis and prompt treatment. The assumption at this level of preventive intervention is that early and prompt intervention in the disease process reduces the duration of the process. Thus, a goal of secondary prevention on the community level is to decrease the number of days of illness for a significant proportion of the population affected. Activities of intervention at this level include individual and mass casefinding measures, screening surveys, and selective examinations of the population. The objectives of the examination are to "cure and prevent disease processes, to prevent the spread of communicable diseases, to prevent complications and sequelae, and to shorten the period of disability."[34]

The last level of prevention or preventive intervention is **tertiary prevention** and occurs at a later stage in the disease process. The goal of tertiary prevention on a community basis is to reduce the number of disabilities in the population at risk. Activities at this level of prevention include,

> Adequate treatment to arrest the disease and to prevent the further complications and sequelae, provisions of facilities to limit disability and prevent death, and rehabilitation including provisions of hospitals and community facilities for retraining and education for maximum use of remaining capacities, education of the public and industry to utilize the rehabilitated, as full employment as possible, selective placement, work therapy in hospitals, and the use of sheltered colonies.[35]

Model For Primary-Prevention Interventions. Caplan has proposed a model for primary-prevention interventions that is useful to community health nurses and other members of the health subsystem.[36] This model is based upon concepts presented earlier in this book. Concepts appropriate to the model include the following:

1. Adaptation requires a continual supply of energy and information commensurate with an individual's stage of growth and development.
2. Maladaptation or crisis results from either qualitative or quantitative excesses or deprivations of energy.
3. Short-term crisis (Chap. 10) changes the energy and information needs of the system.
4. The level-of-coping skills following the resolution of a crisis may influence the later health of a human system.
5. The goals of organized community efforts are to ensure the energy needs of populations within a range to which they can adapt and to help them reduce energy loss during developmental and situational crises.
5. These energy needs and the range of adaptability to energies change over time because of changes in populations, disease agents, and environments.

Caplan says that the goals of ensuring energy needs of populations can be accomplished by two related approaches.[37] These include social action and interpersonal action. Social action produces changes in the community, whereas interpersonal actions attempt to assist human systems to change. Thus, these two approaches can be used to assist populations in meeting their long-term energy needs for such things as food, clean air, water and housing, and in meeting their short-term energy needs during crisis situations at any point. The activities that fall under these two approaches may change over time because of the dynamic interactions of populations and their environments including disease agents.

Social action involves efforts to modify political and social policies, and also legislative and regulatory actions in the various community subsystems such as health, education, and social services (Chap. 3) in the light of environmental changes in energies, which may be detrimental to populations. These efforts improve the provisions of energies within a range that the population can adapt on a community-wide basis. For example, in Chapter 2 it was mentioned that the chemical energy of food, which met qualitative and quantitative standards, was required by humans. Iodine deficiency in the past led to endemic cretinism, but this condition has been practically eliminated by a regulation that introduced iodine into table salt. Likewise, psychoses caused by pellagra have been greatly reduced by social policies and community education programs that have changed food supplies and habits to provide an adequate intake of vitamin B. Other social actions to protect community populations include such things as seat belts in automobiles, laws against drinking and driving or driving without a license, child safety-caps on medications, laws about air, food, and water pollution, and laws against lead in interior paints, which children can eat.

Social action is also concerned with improving the adaption of populations during life crises. This involves the following two focuses: (1) attenuation of hazardous circumstances and (2) services to foster healthy coping behaviors.

Although it is neither possible nor desirable to prevent all crises since psychological growth (negentropy) is experienced following such periods, it is possible to modify certain elements so that the impact is less severe (for large numbers of a population experiencing similar situations that produce crises). For example, a crisis may be provoked by the hospitalization of a young child and may lead to severe maternal deprivation comprising such short-term symptoms as retarded growth (physical, intellectual, emotional) and long-term symptoms such as the inability to form close relationships with other humans and an emotional distance or retardation. This hazardous circumstance would be lessened through social action if hospital stays for this age group were shortened, if visiting hours were extended and parents encouraged to visit daily, or if hospitalizations were delayed until an age where separation would be less traumatic. Allowing the child to build a relationship with a particular nurse (such as would be found in the primary-care pattern of nursing) rather than being cared for by many nurses would also lessen the impact of separation. In this instance, then, modifying staffing patterns and visiting policies would lessen the hazardous circumstances surrounding the crisis. This would qualify as social action if legislation or some other means of enforcement were initiated on a community basis.

In addition, social action may be necessary to provide services to foster healthy crisis-coping behaviors. Personnel, program emphasis, and other aspects of organized community efforts should be provided for by taxes and other legal measures. This might involve requiring 24-hour open-door service at mental health facilities for people in crisis.

Community health nurses are actively involved in processes leading to social action on a community basis. As they observe changes in energies affecting groups of families in the community or gaps in services created by changes in the relationships of the population and the environment, they report these changes to supervisors who channel this information to appropriate administrative personnel for action. As changes are made in energies affecting populations or the resources to deal with these energies, nurses reassess the effects of change and channel information on new resources to the appropriate families in the community.

The second approach of organized community efforts to assist humans to live within a range of energy to which they can adapt is **interpersonal action.** This involves face-to-face-interaction between the community health nurse or other health personnel and individuals, families, and small groups. Although the focus of these interventions is on individuals, families or small groups, the priority assessment of high-risk families and groups is based upon a community-wide assessment, which is discussed in Chapter 4.

Interpersonal action is directed toward ensuring a range of energy to which these humans in the community can adapt and also toward promoting healthy crisis-coping behaviors. These activities are a major thrust of community health nursing and are discussed further at the end of this chapter in the section on the Nursing Process and Epidemiology.

EPIDEMIOLOGY AS A METHOD

Sartwell says that epidemiology can be thought of as a body of knowledge that includes the inferences derived from this knowledge, or it can be seen as a method or discipline. Thus far we have considered epidemiology primarily as a body of knowledge. The epidemiologic method is not so much a unique method in itself but rather it uses all the available, pertinent methods and tools to determine the distribution and determinants of disease processes. These tools are threefold, and they comprise clinical, laboratory, and field observations. These tools are not uniquely epidemiologic; it is their employment in certain ways and with certain objectives that constitute the epidemiologic method. In epidemiology the concern is not with individual cases as in clinical medicine, but with all cases in a defined population. Furthermore, the entire range of manifestations of the particular conditions has to be considered in relation to the population from which the cases arise.

ELEMENTS OF EPIDEMIOLOGY AS A METHOD

When used as a method, there are some important elements to note in epidemiologic studies. The first is the definition of the population used. In descriptive epidemiology, the epidemiologist is usually interested in how much of the disease is present and among which groups. This may be at a local, state, or national level. Although this sounds straightforward, there may be problems in arriving at rates or the method usually used for expressing the amount of disease present. **Rate** usually is expressed as the number of cases exposed to a harmful situation over the population at risk. There may be problems in determining the rate if cases are not readily identified by available methods. For example, the epidemiologist cannot use only hospitalized mentally ill patients for his or her definition of a case, nor is there much agreement for using symptoms as a basis for defining cases when a total community is surveyed. Likewise, a specific hospital in a community could not be used when considering a physical illness because other hospitals in the specific community also care for physical illnesses. In addition to possible missed cases in the total community, there is always ongoing immigration and emigration of patients to and from other communities for health care. Also, hospitals are selective in admitting patients because of their own concerns, finances, and so forth. Immigration and emigration from communities may also influence the base population (denominator) in calculating the rates.

Two rates are commonly used in community assessments of diseases. The **prevalence rate** is the number of cases at any point in time over the population at risk expressed per 1000 cases. The **incidence rate** is the number of new cases of a particular disease over an interval of time over the population at risk expressed per 1000 cases. The first rate is useful in planning services and the second is useful in evaluating preventive efforts and in exploring the natural history of the disease. Other elements of the Epidemiologic Method are discussed by Sartwell.[39]

In analytic epidemiology, the epidemiologist may move from the stage of hunches based upon the exploration of attributes among a healthy and sick group to more sophisticated studies, such as the prospective or retrospective study. The **retrospective study** begins with a group of cases with a disease who are contrasted with a paralleled series of controls who do not have the disease. The proportion who have the specific attribute to be studied is calculated. An attribute refers to a special characteristic or behavior being compared in the sick and well group. For example, we might be interested in the proportion of a group of cases with lung cancer who had previously smoked (attribute) as compared with a group of controls without lung cancer who smoked. In this kind of study, it is important that the control group compare in age, sex, and other demographic variables to the cases with lung cancer, and that it is representative of the population in general. Sartwell discusses other biases that should be avoided.[40] In the **prospective study,** the epidemiologist starts with a healthy group, some of which have the attribute to be studied. For example, if the epidemiologist were interested in the relationship between smoking and lung cancer, he would start with a group of smokers and nonsmokers and follow them over time to determine the proportion of each group that develops lung cancer. The prospective study is usually considered more reliable than the retrospective study, because there is less chance for bias in classifying because the status of the disease is unknown when individuals are classified by the attribute; errors in classification regarding the attribute are less likely since subjects do not need to rely on memory to classify themselves according to the attribute; and there is less need for matching.

The relationship between a disease and an attribute is usually stated in a 2 × 2 table. An outline of this table is presented in Figure 9–5. In a prospective study an incidence rate is usually established; this is written as $(a + c)/(a + b + d + d)$. For those having the attribute, the attack rate (proportion becoming ill) is $a/a + b$ and for those not having it, $c/c + d$. Additional statistical methods would determine whether or not a significant difference occurred in the two groups, which was beyond chance variation. Sartwell discusses these statistical methods for readers who are interested in furthering their knowledge in the area.[41]

THE NURSING PROCESS AND EPIDEMIOLOGY

Community health nurses use epidemiology in their practice with human systems. Consistently, they should use epidemiologic knowledge in assessing, planning, and implementing to prevent or treat diseases and to help human systems attain, maintain, or regain a higher level of wellness. At times, nurses may also use part or all of the epidemiologic approach when they identify an imbalance in segments of the population. For example, school nurses may notice that an increased number of children are coming to their offices at certain times with injuries. By exploring the activities of and other factors in the well and injured group, they may identify one group of children who are unsupervised on the playground during one school period and could then initiate interventions to correct the problem.

ASSESSING

During the assessment phase of nursing process, community health nurses should use all the epidemiologic knowledge available to identify potential or actual health problems. This knowledge involves the natural history of disease processes and ways to intervene in the multiple man, agent, and environmental factors to help individuals, families, and groups attain, maintain, or regain a higher level of wellness. This knowledge should be applied to the specific human system involved based upon the host and environmental factors observed and identified from interviews. For example, if nurses observe a family member with measles in the home they use their knowledge of this disease process to help the sick individual regain wellness (or balance)

Figure 9–5
Relationship between a disease and attribute. (Modified from lecture notes in Epidemiology, Johns Hopkins University, School of Public Health)

		The Disease		
		Present	Absent	Total
The Attribute	Present	a	b	a & b
	Absent	c	d	c & d
		a & c	b & d	a&b&c&d

and purposeful direction. They also help other members maintain their wellness. In assisting well members, nurses assess factors present that make up the natural history of the specific disease such as crowding, nutritional status, personal habits, and rest patterns. They also assess specific preventive actions taken by the family such as immunizations against measles, isolation of the sick member, precautions taken when working with the sick person, adequate diet and rest patterns of the well individuals, and previous experience with measles. Based upon their assessment, nurses may teach about the signs and symptoms of measles, community resources, cautions in caring for the sick individual, isolation of the individual, and so forth.

PLANNING AND INTERVENING

Planning and interverning are based upon the specific information obtained for the specific human system. However, these interventions should be based upon knowledge of the natural history of disease. For example, it is known that smoking is one factor in the natural history of such disease processes as lung cancer, emphysema, and heart disease. Thus, working with an individual to help him reduce or eliminate the smoking pattern would be based upon this knowledge.

Many community-health nursing interventions involve health teaching, counseling, and direct physical or psychological care. These interventions can be conceptualized on a continuum such as identified in Figure 9–6.

This continuum is not absolute and varying combinations and degrees of activities may be carried out simultaneously or emphasis may be placed on one end of the continuum at one time and on the other end at another time. The nurse's emphasis on activities of intervention on the continuum is dependent upon the health–illness stresses encountered by the system (individual, family, group) and the adaptation to the stresses and the resultant behavior, which is a reflection of attitudes, values and knowledge, and resources of individuals, families, or groups who are coping with the actual or potential stress. For example, in one situation nurses may teach diabetics to take insulin and to regulate their diet, but at the same time continue to change dressings. Or, nurses may take vital signs on hypertensive patients at home, and at the same time teach diet and personal hygiene habits. Basic to such activities, however, is an adequate assessment of the particular situation based upon concepts that allow the individual, family, or group the greatest autonomy consistent with a positive level of health and health behavior.

Figure 9–6
Nursing interventions with human systems.

Direct physical care	Health teaching
Complete dependence of client system	Counseling

If we accept health and illness as dynamic processes and have a knowledge of the natural history of diseases, intervention is possible at various stages in these processes, that is, prior to, during, or following the health–illness stresses. This concept and the activities at the various levels of intervention are discussed earlier in this chapter. However, as a basis for nursing interventions, the nursing continuum presented in Figure 9–6 can be related to the health continuum presented in Figure 9–3. On the left side of the health continuum are individuals in hospitals and institutions who are acutely or chronically ill (failure to adapt to a stress). These individuals are usually dependent in a variety of areas (biologic, emotional) and, as a result, nursing care, which meets the immediate challenge to the individual, may be direct care. At the right end of the continuum are individuals and groups who are in the community and are approaching high level wellness, who are not currently challenged by an illness stress, and whose potential for high level wellness may be unrealized because of a lack of knowledge or improper attitudes and values in relation to health. Here the nurse's role may be primarily teaching and counseling, supporting and problem solving to help improve their level of wellness. Thus, this group may be maintaining or attaining a higher level of wellness and nurses may be working with the learned behaviors of clients, while in the previous group, nurses are putting to use their own learned behaviors.

This discussion does not negate the teaching role of the nurse with individuals on the left side of the barrier (on the health continuum) or direct physical care to individuals on the right. Some teaching is usual as clients move from the left side of the health continuum where they experience the greatest challenge to life. Likewise, with shorter hospital stays, medical and health advances, and increased numbers of individuals with chronic long-term illnesses, more individuals recovering from an acute illness or an exacerbation of a chronic illness are cared for in the home and consequently direct physical care may be given to some individuals just to the right of the health continuum barrier. In other words, depending upon the individual's or group's location on the health continuum at any point in time, nursing interventions will vary. Over time individuals and groups either move up or down the continuum and nursing care will also move up and down a continuum.

Other aspects of nursing such as interpersonal relationships, problem-solving skills, and communication skills also vary depending upon the client-system's location on the health continuum. For example, at the left side of the continuum, when the individual is challenged by a life–death crisis, the interpersonal relationship between the nurse and client may not be as important as good, direct nursing care (*e.g.*, a comatose client). As the individual moves away from this position, the interpersonal aspect of nursing care becomes exceedingly important. Likewise, at the left side of the health continuum, nurses may go through the problem-solving process as a basis for nursing care with clients, but as individuals move from this end of the continuum, nurses should assist them in solving problems.

REFERENCES

1. Murray R, Zentner J: Nursing Concepts for Health Promotion, pp. 5–15. Englewood Cliffs, Prentice-Hall, 1975
2. Koos E: The Health of Regionville. New York, Columbia University, 1951
3. Dunn L: High Level Wellness. Washington, D C, Mount Vernon, 1961
4. Dubos R: Man, Medicine and Environment, p. 67. New York, Praeger, 1968
5. Murray R, Zentner J, op cit
6. Jones D, et al: Medical-Surgical Nursing—A Conceptual Approach. New York, McGraw-Hill, 1978
7. Byrne M, Thompson L: Key Concepts for the Study and Practice of Nursing. St Louis, C V Mosby, 1972
8. Dunn H, op cit
9. Auger J: Behavioral Systems and Nursing, p. 10. Englewood Cliffs, Prentice-Hall, 1976
10. Dubos R: Mirage of Health. Garden City, Doubleday, 1969
11. Leavell H, Clark G: Preventive Medicine for the Doctor in his Community. New York, McGraw-Hill, 1965
12. Fitch C: Biological theories of aging. In Burnside I (ed): Nursing and the Aged Patient, p. 93. New York, McGraw-Hill, 1976
13. Dunn H, op cit
14. Rogers E: Human Ecology and Health: An Introduction for Administrators, p. 159. New York, 1960
15. Dunn H: High-Level wellness for man and society. Am J Public Health, Vol. 49, No. 6: 786–792, June 1959
16. Dunn H, High Level Wellness, p. 4
17. Rogers E, op cit, p. 166
18. Leavell H, Clark G, op cit
19. Dubos R, Mirage of Health, p. 74
20. Dubos R, Ibid, p. 74
21. Sartwell P: Preventive Medicine and Public Health. New York, Appleton-Century-Crofts, 1973
22. Dubos Rene: Man Adapting. New Haven, Yale University, 1967
23. Panun P L: Observations made during the epidemic of measles on the Faroe Islands in the year 1864. New York, Delta Omega Society. Distributed by The American Public Health Association, 1940
24. Christensen P E, et al: An epidemic of measles in South Greenland. Octa Med Scandinar, 144:313, 1952
25. Philips R N, et al: Observations on a mumps epidemic in a "virgin" population. Am J Hygiene, 69:91, 1959
26. Sartwell P, op cit, p 41
27. Sartwell P, op cit, p 41
28. Sartwell P, op cit, p 41
29. Leavell H, Clark G: op cit
30. Sartwell P, op cit, p 42
31. Hanlon H: Public Health Administration and Practice, p 393. St Louis, C V Mosby, 1973
32. Wilner D, et al: Mustards Introduction to Public Health, p 340. New York; Macmillan, 1973
33. Leavell H, Clark G: op cit
34. Leavell H, Clark G, op cit, p 22
35. Leavell H, Clark G, op cit, p 52
36. Caplan G: Support Systems and Mutual Help. New York, Grune & Stratton, 1976
37. Caplan G, op cit
38. Sartwell P, op cit
39. Sartwell P, op cit
40. Sartwell P, op cit
41. Sartwell P, op cit

10

Crisis Theory, Concepts, and Intervention

Any system may experience crisis at various times throughout its life span. As human systems move away from a steady state, stress and tension arise and may lead to crisis. Moving away from a steady state means that the system is experiencing negentropy, or excessive entropy. As the system moves toward increased growth and organization (negentropy) it experiences tension and stress until it reaches a new goal or redefines its goals through the process of feedback as discussed in Chapters 1 through 4. Depending upon the problem-solving abilities, the support system, and the perceptual field of the system during this stress period, it will resolve the conflict or it will experience crisis. Crises resulting from negentropy are referred to as maturational crises. On the other hand, excessive entropy in a system sub- or suprasystems leading to illness, loss of a body part, or death of a loved one may create stress and tension for a system and cause a situational crisis. Whether or not the system experiences crisis is again dependent upon the three factors identified (problem-solving abilities, support system, and perceptual field). Crises resulting from entropic processes are referred to as situational crises.

CRISIS DEFINITIONS AND OVERVIEW

Taber's Cyclopedic Medical Dictionary defines crisis as "a turning point, a very critical period."[1] Murray and Zentner define crisis as "any transient situation that necessitates reorganization of one's psychological structure and behavior, that causes a sudden alteration in the person's expectation of himself, and that cannot be handled with the person's usual coping mechanism."[2]

Because there is a breakdown in the system's coping mechanism, a **crisis** can be defined also as a period of disequilibrium overpowering the human system's (individual, group, organization) homeodynamic mechanisms. The crisis results from an inadequate repertoire of coping responses to bring about the resolution of a problem that is a threat to the system. Crises often are precipitated by an identifiable event, either within or outside of the system, and the processes of coping and resolution are longer than usual ranging from 4 to 6 weeks usually. The initiating problem is one that cannot be avoided because it is linked to fundamental needs of the human system and may involve "the loss of a source of satisfaction of basic needs, the danger of such a loss, or a challenge which overtakes a person's capacities."[3]

These problems may include situational problems such as the death of a loved one, a divorce, a role change, or a physical illness, and developmental or maturational crises during infancy, adolescence, and adulthood. Developmental crises may also affect families as they move from one developmental stage to another. Most maturational crises and some situational crises are predictable and thus allow community health nurses the opportunity to intervene with anticipatory guidance to prevent the crisis. **Anticipatory guidance** reduces the impact of the crisis and helps individuals or families to think through ways of solving the problem before they are in the situation where emotions may tax intellectual functioning. Families and organizations may also go through crises and it has been found that any human system going through a crisis revolving around a specific problem, such as grief following a significant death, will show characteristic patterns of behavior. Thus, a knowledge of these crisis situations and the behavioral patterns observed should assist nurses in identifying problems prior to crises more easily. It should also assist nurses in helping systems prevent or resolve crises in a healthy way. This knowledge is presented later in this chapter under individual, family, and organizational crises and is followed by aspects of the nursing process used to assist systems.

According to Caplan, this period of system disequilibrium should not be considered bad or harmful because it represents both a period of increased vulnerability and an opportunity for growth.[4] Thus, the system can develop new healthy problem-solving mechanisms and it can be better prepared for future crisis. Healthy resolution of a crisis moves the system to a higher level of wellness. On the other hand, without assistance, the system may resolve the crisis in an unhealthy way and move to a lower level of wellness. In addition, the periods of disequilibrium seen in maturational crises are necessary for the system to become increasingly ordered and complex (negentropy), which is compatible with life.

Crisis, thus, involves a mental–emotional imbalance in systems, which is relatively long term ranging from 4 to 6 weeks. Resolution of the crisis may leave the system at a higher or lower level on a wellness continuum.

CRISIS AS A PRIMARY-PREVENTION INTERVENTION

Crisis intervention with human systems in community health nursing is considered a primary-prevention intervention. It has the goal of reducing the incidence and prevalence of disorders on a community basis, which is a major focus of community health nursing. A crisis is considered at the primary-prevention level of intervention because it is not disordered behavior but can lead to disordered behavior if not handled adequately. Crisis is a period of disequilibrium causing acute changes in the system's pattern of behavior during which it tries to resolve a problem requiring new coping skills. The resolution of the problem, which usually occurs in 4 to 6 weeks, may leave the system at a higher, equal, or lower level of coping than before the crisis and thus may move the system up or down the health continuum in terms of dealing with future crises. It is believed that a series of crisis situations resolved in a way that continually decreases the coping ability of the system may lead to mental disorders. Thus, interventions geared toward assisting systems to identify and resolve crises in a healthy way increases their coping skills and moves them up the health continuum to prevent disorders.

A great deal of energy may be lost from the system from the emotions of fear, anxiety, helplessness, and so forth when a problem is not solved in the customary amount of time. In addition, this imbalance of the system owing to the excessive energy loss may tax the mind to solve the problem, and may affect eating and sleeping patterns, elimination, posture and a variety of other factors, which make the system more susceptible to physical illnesses. Thus, crises may reduce the energy level of the system and concurrently reduce its range of adaptability.

Beyond this consideration regarding prevention, nurses should also be concerned with how the system resolves the problem. Is it increasing the system's range of adaptability to future potential crisis situations or is it decreasing its range? It if decreases its range of adaptability and moves down the health continuum, is the system using excessive energy to repress unfulfilled needs of the unconscious mind, with less energy available for other adaptive processes such as heat regulation, defense against pathogens, and so forth?

INDIVIDUAL ADAPTATION TO CRISIS

There are four phases of an individual's adaptation to crisis. These include shock, defensive retreat, acknowledgment, and adaptation and growth.

SHOCK

Initially, during a crisis individuals feel stress, anxiety, helplessness, and at times panic. Their self-esteem is threatened and their thinking and behavior are disorganized. Confusion is always present and individuals may withdraw or become hyperactive. This phase may last from a few hours to a couple of days.

DEFENSIVE RETREAT

During this stage, individuals attempt to control the intense anxiety with a fight–flight pattern. They avoid or deny reality and indulge in wishful thinking. They also refuse to recognize that things are different than they were in the past. Anyone who points out reality is perceived as a threat and reacted to with anger. Reality with its accompanying anxiety is too painful at this time. Thinking is rigid and there is resistance to any suggestions of change.

ACKNOWLEDGMENT

When the reality of the situation can no longer be denied and the defensive behavior of stage two breaks down, there is a renewed encounter with reality and the stressor. Depression, agitation, and bitterness may be present. On the cognitive level disorganized thinking and confusion are later followed by appropriate planning and problem solving.

ADAPTATION AND CHANGE

During this phase individuals see the crisis situation in a positive way and integrate the painful event into their new self-concept. There is a modified self-image and they develop a renewed sense of worth. This leads to successful problem solving and expressing feelings about the event. There is an accompanying reduction of anxiety and a new ability to look at their present resources and future potentials and goals. At this time, the individual should be at a higher level of functioning from the pre-crisis period because of the new coping skills incorporated into their behavior.

CRISIS THEORY AND COMMUNITY HEALTH NURSES

There are several reasons why crisis concepts, theory, and techniques should be part of the community health nurse's knowledge and skills. First, crisis intervention with any open system may prevent disorders and, thus, falls within the goal of elevating community health by working with families and groups to promote health and to reduce disorders on a community basis. Second, nurses carry a caseload of families and other groups who are considered high risk and, thus, are more susceptible to stresses of all kinds, including crises. Because they carry this group over a long period of time nurses are likely to be available to a high percentage of clients during an actual or potential crisis. Third, nurses have established relationships with the families in their caseload that should facilitate a helping-person role during the crisis. Fourth, nurses know the nursing process (assessing, planning, implementing, evaluating) and can apply this in all aspects of their practice. This process is also indicated in assisting those in a crisis. The nurse assesses the situation by using observational and interviewing skills, looking for signs of increased anxiety and tension (whole man), and by assessing the verbal and nonverbal clues given by the patient. From this they identify the problem. Nurses then proceed to relate the assessment to their theoretical base on crisis to explain why the problem exists and what they can do about it. Next, they determine ways they can intervene to solve the problem. This approach will be elaborated upon later in this chapter.

It should be reemphasized that nurses need the theoretical knowledge of crises and techniques of intervention because without this base they can hamper rather than help individuals during such periods. For example, the nurse who is unfamiliar with the literature may not identify the birth of a premature child as a crisis for the mother and may thus reassure the mother who says she feels inadequate in caring for the child. Such blanket reassurance may hamper the mother's healthy resolution of the crisis by supporting her evasion of the crisis in an unhealthy way.

A final reason for including crisis concepts, theory, and techniques in community health nursing involves the nursing effort put forth for the results. Caplan says that individuals in crisis will use assistance better than at other times. Thus, with minimal assistance the system may regain equilibrium. The concept of doing the most good for the greatest number with a minimal amount of time, effort, and money is consistent with community health philosophy.

CRISIS THEORY

NORMAL PROBLEM SOLVING

Individuals, families, and communities are constantly faced with internal or external demands characterized as problems that require a solution. These problems are usually resolved with minimal time and effort using habitual mechanisms and reactions (patterned behaviors) acquired through the process of living and solving the problems of life. These responses, which require little self-awareness or strain to the system, help it to maintain equilibrium.

The characteristic process, then, involved in maintaining equilibrium when one is faced with internal or external demands involves a force or situation (the problem) that upsets the equilibrium.

> The problem calls forth a variety of habitual problem solving mechanisms, one of which solves the problem similarily and in a similar length of time to the way in which it has happened on previous occasions. During the short period before the solution, the organism is in a state of tension, but this is not excessive because the period is not longer than in previous experiences, and the individual or group has in that previous experience, in dealing with such problems by similar methods, developed the expectation of a successful outcome and an ability to bear that degree of tension, as well as a series of techniques for keeping the tension within certain limits by means of discharge mechanisms.[6]

Equilibrium is maintained by the feedback process which calls into play opposing forces when needed to maintain a steady state. The feedback process operates on the intrapsychic and interpersonal levels and is discussed in Chapters 1 through 4.

Aguilera says that Freud was the first to demonstrate the antecedents of solving problems (coping skills). In his principle of causality he stated that "every act of human behavior has its cause, or source in the history and experience of the individual." As a result of this principle he constructed a developmental psychology.

> Present behavior is understandable in terms of the life history or experience of the individual and the crucial foundations for all future behavior are laid down in infancy and early childhood. The most significant determinants of present behavior are the "residues" of past experience (learned responses) particularily those developed during the early years to reduce biological tension.[8]

Psychologists now realize that the current situation must also be considered. Thus, past behavior must be related to the current context by the system to determine its usefulness in adapting.

Thus, in a crisis, the process discussed is exaggerated because the problem is larger and outside the repertoire of habitual mechanisms and responses (learned behaviors) of the system and so tensions mount, the period of solving the problem is lengthened, and the accompanying behavioral manifestations of disequilibrium are more obvious. When equilibrium is reestablished, the new pattern may be different from the previous one and may move the individual up or down the health continuum.

CHARACTERISTICS OF CRISIS

When the system is confronted with a problem that requires a solution there is an initial rise in tension, which calls forth a habitual problem-solving response to the stimuli in an effort to maintain a steady state. If the habitual response is unsuccessful and the stimuli remain there is a further rise in tension, which may lead to a narrowing of perceptual awareness because all resources are focused on the problem. If a solution is not found by narrowing the perceptual field and using available resources, tension may rise further and anxiety becomes severe. Feelings of anxiety, fear, guilt, or shame may become intensified and the perceptual field becomes so narrow that the system loses the ability to reason. At such times the system's problem-solving or coping abilities are lost because of the extreme discomfort experienced by the system. Because the system is so focused on the discomfort, it is unable to identify the initiating problem, coping and supporting resources, or feelings experienced.

CRISIS CONCEPTS USEFUL TO COMMUNITY HEALTH NURSES

Studies of the behavior patterns of individuals, families, and organizations going through comparable crisis situations have shown consistent response patterns among these systems prior to the restoration of equilibrium. For example, Lindemann studied bereavement and found a well-defined process individuals go through in adjusting to the death of someone close.[9] Caplan found a similar well-defined process of adaptation to a premature child, and Janis identified this process with individuals undergoing surgery.[10,11] These and other studies that identify the characteristic course of particular crises and which form the theoretical basis for planning intervention are now discussed.

This section begins with crises affecting individuals and is divided into situational and maturational crises. Following this presentation, we will look at Family and Organizational Crises.

CRISES AFFECTING INDIVIDUALS

SITUATIONAL CRISES

Community health nurses may encounter various situational crises in families they visit. Thus, many of the more common situational crises are discussed. A **situational crisis** has been defined by Murray and Zentner as "an external event or situation, one not necessarily a part of normal living, often sudden, unexpected, and unfortunate, which looms larger than the persons immediate resources or ability to cope and which demands a change in behavior."[12]

Some individuals face stress situations with no ill effects, whereas others experience a crisis. The difference between those who have a crisis and those who do not is determined by the individual's perception of the event, his available coping mechanisms, and the support available to him in his environment. Where one or more of these factors is faulty, the individual experiences a crisis.

Prematurity. Any family experiences stress when confronted with a premature child. If this is a new situation for the family, it may engender feelings of inadequacy in caring for the child, anxiety about its possibility of survival, and possibly fears of the mother that she has been responsible for the premature delivery. Evidence shows that certain prenatal factors related to the mother may be instrumental in premature births and it is possible that the mother is aware of this data. It has also been found that mothers who attempt abortion unsuccessfully may later have guilt feelings and may seek constant reassurance about the child's condition. It is likely that a premature birth would exaggerate these feelings.

Mason and Kaplan have identified four tasks the mother must work through if she is to resolve the stress of having a premature child. She must acknowledge the fact that the child may die and must therefore go through an anticipatory grief process of withdrawing from the relationship established with the child during pregnancy. The mother must also acknowledge failure as a mother for not delivering a full-term baby. She must also break the relationship with the child during its hospital stay and resume the relationship at the time of hospital discharge. In addition, she must prepare herself for care of a child who has special needs and growth patterns.

Following the delivery of a premature child there is a great deal of stress faced by the family. Because of the decreased range of adaptability created by a premature condition, the child is shielded from a variety of external stimuli, including parents. Thus, they are unable to see and be with the child to reduce their anxiety about his physical condition and possibility of survival.

The behavior of the family during this stressful period will determine whether a crisis occurs or not. Mason found that in families where a crisis did not occur the parents expressed negative feelings related to their perception of the threat to the baby and actively sought and benefited from information about the premature infant from professional personnel.[15] They used this information to plan for the infant's future. In addition, he found the husband supportive of the mother. Thus, this group of families had a realistic perception of the event and were able to express their feelings; there was adequate situational support, and they sought information to allay their fears and to increase their skills (coping skills) in caring for the child in anticipation of the infant's discharge from the hospital. Indications that these families had coped well with the stress situation were found on follow-up studies where mothers were trying to meet the baby's physical and emotional needs with moderate success; the baby was gaining weight, and the family seemed proud. On the other hand, families who were unable to cope with the stress and showed symptoms of a crisis were those who denied their feelings of fear, guilt, and anxiety and seemed to deny the existence of danger to the child. They did not seek information about the child or accept help from professional personnel at the hospital. There also seemed to be a lack of situational support for the mother. Indications that this group of families had not coped well with the stress and had thus experienced crisis was found on follow-up studies following the discharge of the children, where mothers were found to neglect the children, showed unusual hostility, irritability, impatience, and lack of warmth; the baby was lethargic or ill, and there was a disruption in the cohesiveness of family relationships.

Thus, the behaviors that signal the families ability to cope with the stress of a premature child include the following:

1. The mother acknowledges a moderate-to-high level of anxiety about the child's chances for survival, its normality, and her competence.
2. The mother actively seeks information about the child's condition and its prognosis.
3. The mother is warm, objects to the separation from the child, has devotion to the family and expresses other strong maternal feelings even though the child has not been cared for.
4. The support system including husbands and other family members was strong.

Physical Illness. A chronic or degenerative physical illness is a stressful period for all individuals and may produce a crisis. During such periods the individual ceases to be a useful productive member of society, is usually excluded from his social group, and takes on the sick role. The sick role as identified by Parsons includes the following expectations: (1) the person is not held responsible for his incapacities, (2), he is released to varying degrees from normal role obligations, (3) he must recognize that illness is undesirable and have an expressed desire to get well, and (4) he must seek competent help, cooperate with treatment, and relinquish the right to make decisions to the physician and to other health care personnel.[16] In addition to his loss of freedom and autonomy, there may be fear related to symbolic or real losses. Hall and Weaver states that this fear can relate to loss of a body function and image, social roles, goals, persons, ideals—all the things that constitute the basis of one's self-concept and are necessary for effective ego-functioning.[17] In addition, pain and loss of a body part are often feared. Because of these potential changes in the individual's life and the required adjustment to be made, anxiety, tension, and feelings of guilt or helplessness may be present.

Janis studied patients waiting for surgery and identified groups that coped adequately and those that experienced crisis.[18] His findings, which are closely related to the findings of parents with premature children, have application for individuals facing any chronic illness. Janis found that pre-operative patients who experienced crisis were those who displayed an extremely low degree or high degree of anticipatory fear or anxiety before surgery. Those individuals who were best able to cope with surgery were those who displayed a moderate degree of anticipatory fear beforehand. He also found that crises could be prevented in the low-anxiety group by stimulating their fear and anxiety to a moderate degree. This group should be encouraged to express feelings and to seek information about the surgery. Patients in the high anxiety group must be assisted in reducing their anxiety to a moderate degree. If anxiety is based on misinformation, correcting the information may be helpful. If it is based on psychoneurotic reactions, brief psychotherapy may be indicated.

Crate says that individuals adapt to chronic diseases using a process similar to the grieving process. Clients with a chronic illness will adapt using a pattern of "disbelief, developing awareness, reorganization of relationships with others, resolution of the loss, and identity change."[20] Initially, the patient who learns of a chronic illness **denies the threat** of the disease for self-protection. During this phase nurses should allow the client to deny the illness by listening to feelings and helping to clarify them, while not reinforcing the denial with their own comments. During the second phase of adaptation, **developing awareness,** the client is no longer able to deny the illness and begins to develop awareness of the condition and its implications. Anger is a common reaction of clients during this phase and it may be diffuse initially. This diffuse anger is directed outward against numerous people or directed inward and manifested as depression. As the client begins accepting the illness, the anger becomes directed more specifically toward the illness. Throughout the process the nurse should allow the client to express his feelings, but should not enter into the process. The client may also move to a dependency phase following acceptance of the illness. Dependency is necessary for the client to move toward a more independent role. During the third phase, **reorganization,** the client begins reorganizing relationships with family and friends to allow them to accommodate to the illness. At this time the nurse may need to work with family members and friends to help them express feelings so that they can accommodate to the change in the family or interpersonal system. During the last phase, **resolution and identity change,** the client acknowledges changes in his self-perception and begins to identify with others having a similar problem. This process of adaptation is similar to the process outlined earlier.

Death and the Grief Process. After the death of a loved one, the remaining survivors typically experience certain feelings and exhibit behaviors, which are referred to as grief and mourning. Although these feelings and behaviors reflect acute and widespread disequilibrium, they are a part of the normal adjustment to the loss of a significant other. In fact, the lack of grief and mourning where it would be expected may lead to psychopathologic outcomes.

According to Dizmang grief occurs normally after a significant loss.[21] He says,

> Shock, disbelief, puzzlement, and a profound feeling of anguish, accompanied eventually by intermittent surges of anger, characterize this state. Mourning is the process by which, after the initial grief, the cathected object gradually is relinquished . . . and the bereaved individual eventually can reestablish new object ties.

In a similar vein Bowlby says that grief is the "sequence of subjective states that follow loss and accompany mourning" and says that mourning is "the psychological processes that are set in train [motion] by the loss of a loved object and which commonly leads to the relinquishment of the object."[22]

Symptomatology of Normal Grief. Lindemann combines grief and mourning and discusses the symptomatology of normal grief.[23] He says,

> Common to all is the following syndrome: sensations of somatic distress occurring in waves lasting from twenty minutes to an hour at a time, a feeling of tightness in the throat, choking with shortness of breath, need for sighing, an empty feeling in the abdomen, lack of muscular power and an intense subjective distress described as tension or mental pain . . . these waves of discomfort can be precip-

itated by visits, by mentioning the deceased and by receiving sympathy.*

In addition, the bereaved tends to be intensely preoccupied with the deceased, and thus seems to be emotionally distant. This distance is often expressed in feelings of anger and irritability, and a wish not to be bothered by others. The bereaved also is preoccupied with guilt feelings as he searches the time before the death for evidence of his letting the deceased down. He may exaggerate minor omissions or accuse himself of other neglects.

Although lacking the capacity to continue any organized pattern of activity for a length of time, the bereaved is restless, moves about aimlessly, and seems unable to sit still. He also talks frequently about the deceased.

BEHAVIORAL SEQUENCE OF GRIEF. The loss of a loved one leads to a behavioral sequence that is to some degree predictable. In humans, this sequence is accompanied by feelings of anxiety and anger, then pain and despair, and usually ends with hope.

Bowlby has described the phases of behavior in grief, as follows:[24]

PHASE 1: PROTEST

> The bereaved is in disequilibrium and experiences shock and disbelief. During this phase there may be a tendency to continue to act as though the loved one was still present, and there are strenuous efforts to recover the deceased. These efforts at recovery can be seen in the hopes and fantasies, dreams and actions of the survivor. Weeping and anger are the prominent features of this phase, although accusations and ingratitudes may also be present as the bereaved tries to recover the lost object and is brought back to reality by those trying to comfort him.

PHASE 2. DISORGANIZATION OF ADAPTIVE PROCESSES

> As the bereaved realizes that the lost partner is gone and his efforts at reunion are futile, he moves into phase 2. Here each memory of the deceased and the awareness that he no longer exists is met with painful disappointment and despair, and lacking an object toward which to organize, behavior becomes disorganized. At this time he becomes restless, irritable, unable to sit still, and is unable to carry out organized activities as mentioned before.
>
> Depression may also be present during this stage because of the lack of interchange between the bereaved and the external world resulting from the grief process. This depression results in disorganization of the bereaved, is painful, and carries with it the possibility that satisfactory reorganization will never be achieved. However, disorganization is necessary if the bereaved is to readapt.

PHASE 3. REORGANIZATION

> This phase involves the reorganization of the system to the new reality and detachment from the old. However, there may still be some socially acceptable (and thus what would be considered normal) thoughts of the lost object. In general, such thoughts include the belief in his existence in another world, or maintaining values and pursuing goals that have been associated with the deceased and which remain linked with him, but can be pursued realistically in reference to his memory.

The duration of this process seems to depend upon the success with which a person does the "grief work," that is, achieves emancipation from the bondage of the deceased, readjusts to the environment in which the deceased is missing, and forms new relationships. Progress can be judged in terms of whether there is a gradual return to the level of functioning prior to the loss and the establishment of or interest in new relationships. Aguilera says that when the bereaved is able completely and realistically to remember the pleasures and disappointments of the lost object, mourning has been successfully completed.[25] Even at the latest stages of this process, reminders of the deceased such as pictures, songs, or old haunts may bring forth short periods of grief.

The time span for normal grief is usually 6 months to 1 year. However, it has been found that therapy reduces this period to 4 to 6 weeks in uncomplicated grief reactions.

* The American Journal of Psychiatry. Vol. 101. September, 1944. Copyright 1944, The American Psychiatric Association.

Morbid Grief Reactions. When one is unable to overtly express normal urges to recover the lost object and represses such reactions, pathologic mourning will follow. With assistance, most of these morbid reactions can be transformed into normal reactions leaving the individual at an equal or higher level of coping. Most frequent among such morbid reactions is the **delayed reaction** or postponement of grief that occurs when the bereaved is required to continue important tasks or to support others experiencing the loss. In such situations, the bereaved may show little or no immediate reaction to the loss and may delay it indefinitely. These delayed reactions often appear around important dates such as the anniversary of the death, the wedding or when the bereaved reaches the age of the deceased; they may also follow another loss. At such times, the individual will go through the grief process. An adequate assessment is necessary to distinguish the delayed grief reaction from situations in which the survivor would not be expected to grieve. For example, absence of grief would not be maladaptive if the survivor had moved away from the intense relationship prior to death, if he was separated, had established new relationships, or if the relationship was predominantly negative.

A second kind of morbid reaction is the **distorted reaction.** Such reactions involve alterations in the client's conduct following a period after the loss. The individual may become overactive and incorporate aspects of the deceased person's activities into his or her behavior or take on symptoms from the last illness of the deceased. Illnesses may also develop having psychosomatic components such as ulcerative colitis, rheumatoid arthritis, and asthma. These individuals may also become irritable toward, avoid, or in other ways alter their behavior toward friends and relatives. They may also become hostile toward specific individuals such as the doctor who they may accuse of neglecting his or her duties. These behaviors may be accompanied by tension, agitation, insomnia, feelings of worthlessness, and a need for punishment, which are characteristically seen in agitated depression.

Pregnancy. Pregnancy may create a situational crisis in families because of the changes and disruptions introduced into the family system. During pregnancy the woman has increased dependency needs, which places new demands and responsibilities on others in the family system. In addition, her tastes and desires change and she may wish to forgo sexual and other activities. She must also develop the skills and knowledge needed to care for a newborn and this responsibility may create anxiety. Both parents may worry about whether the child will be normal and healthy, whether they can care for it adequately, and whether they can even afford the child.

An unwanted pregnancy may also create a crisis for the woman and her family. She must make a decision about abortion, about putting the child up for adoption or even keeping the child. In addition to conflicting feelings that evolve around what to do about the developing fetus, she may not be in agreement with the child's father or her parents if she is unmarried and living at home.

Unemployment. Loss of a job and inability to locate work may create a crisis for the worker and his or her family. The loss of a job is a blow to the ego in our society because we are considered successful when we can provide for ourselves and our dependents. Loss of a job may lead to feelings of grief, loss, despair, and depression, which may interfere with locating another job. In addition, other dependent members of the family may be affected because of the decreased or lost income.

Divorce. Divorce is a common occurrence in the American culture and can lead to crisis. It has been estimated that about 50% of all marriages end in divorce. This indicates that many are not adequately prepared for marriage. Rappaport says that there are three sub-phases of marriage when stress is most common.[25] These include the engagement, the honeymoon, and early marriage. During the engagement phase the individuals must review their readiness for marriage and must develop satisfactory interpersonal relationships with each other. During the honeymoon, the couple develops a basic sense of harmony, and during the early marriage phase they accommodate and change to become a single system in such areas as authority, decision making, and patterns of sexual relationships.

The majority of divorces in childless couples occur during the early years of marriage; the peak is reached during the second year of marriage. Factors identified with divorce include early marriage, short courtship and engagement, dissimilar backgrounds, unhappy parental marriages, and mixed social, racial, or religious marriages. In addition, there may be communication and sexual problems, economic difficulties, and a lack of emotional love, which influence the decision to divorce.

Divorce is always difficult for a couple regardless of the length of the marriage. This change in the family structure requires adjustment to living alone or with friends and changing one's self-perception and role from a married to a single person. There may be strong feelings about the partner that must be dealt with. In addition, there may be court battles over custody and child support, if children are involved.

MATURATIONAL CRISIS

Stress is experienced by all human systems during the transition period of moving from one stage of physical, social, psychological, and intellectual growth to another (negentropy). These transition periods, which usually extend over an interval of time, are potential crisis situations. Often individuals are required to take on new roles as a result of the growth experienced and crisis may result from an inability to take on these new roles. Murray and Zentner identify three reasons why human systems may be unable to take over new roles and so prevent a maturational crisis.[27]

1. An adequate role model may be absent and the individual is thus unable to model the role behavior and learn the skills needed in the role.
2. The system may lack the intrapersonal resources to make the role change. For example, communication skills or the ability to see alternatives to the present life style may be lacking.
3. The system may be locked into a role by others in the environment and is thus unable to take over new role behaviors.

Because a family or group must change as a system and a change in a part affects the whole, all role behaviors are affected by the developmental changes in any one part. Feedback is discussed in Chapters 1 through 4 as the process whereby an individual in a family or group may take over new roles that fit with the other roles. Community health nurses may help families confront the growth needs of members and teach techniques for moving the family or group system to new levels.

The phases of growth for individuals are mentioned in Chapter 2 as negentropic processes and are reviewed here briefly. Transition periods fall between one phase and the next, at which time the human system attempts to reduce the conflict and tension experienced by learning the new roles and behaviors expected.

Erik Erikson has identified eight psychosocial stages or phases of the life cycle.[28] These include trust versus mistrust, autonomy versus shame, initiative versus guilt, industry versus inferiority, identity versus diffusion, intimacy versus isolation, generativity versus stagnation, and integrity versus despair. Piaget has identified four stages of intellectual development and they are sensorimotor, preoperational thought, concrete operations, and formal operations. Readers interested in more detail on these and other developmental phases are referred to Sutterley.[30]

Although the phases of growth discussed by Erikson, Piaget, and others occur at different ages and the transition periods for one or another aspect of growth may vary, they can be combined into a developmental model of stress producing transition periods that will be appropriate to individual human systems. The developmental phases to be discussed here include infancy, school years, young adulthood, middle age and old age.

Infancy. One of the first developmental tasks of the human system is learning to trust the maternal figure and developing confidence in the sameness and continuity of the environment. Since the infant is almost totally helpless and dependent, trust and dependability are learned when the mother figure is dependable. Thus, a mother figure must be available to satisfy the infant's needs and to provide love, warmth, and security. When a consistent mother figure is absent or undependable, the infant may have a maturational crisis and not learn to trust. The infant may feel insecure and cry, appear depressed and withdrawn. In severe cases, the infant may die. Infants who do not develop trust often have retarded sensorimotor and intellectual development and do not progress adequately through the other stages of psychosocial development. As adults they are often chronically mistrustful, dependent, depressed, withdrawn and incapable of developing deep interpersonal relationships.

Intellectual behavior of the infant is described by Piaget as sensorimotor.[31] The infant strengthens the reflex patterns of birth through repeated use. Such reflex patterns include grasping, sucking, auditory, and visual pursuits. By the end of the first year of life these actions become internalized as thought patterns and by the second year of life new patterns such as eating, washing oneself and walking have been learned.

Autonomy is developed during the second year of life in which infants move from a dependent stage to independent actions. Infants explore and learn and begin to differentiate themselves from others. Their muscular system is also developed to the point where they can hold on or let go and conflict or power struggles may arise between children and parents in such areas as elimination or exploration. In addition, the origins of concrete literal thinking are developed over the next several years. Self-esteem and self-control result from the child's reaching out and exploring. If children are not allowed to reach out and grow a crisis develops and they may lack the sense of independence to function effectively as an adult.

During the remainder of the preschool period children have the task of developing initiative. Children ask many questions and in the process of exploring discover what kind of persons they are and are governed by their conscience. Shame may result either from being exposed or from fear of exposure and guilt may result from thoughts or deeds. At the end of this period children have developed a social conscience with gender roles and can fantasize about what they will become. If they are thwarted in their development they may be confused about their psychosocial role, experience guilt in interpersonal relations, and lose their initiative regarding the exploration of new skills.

School Years. During the school years individuals develop a sense of industry and feel adequate if they are able to make things and do things well. They want to be shown how to do things and win recognition by accomplishing things. Cognitively, children begin to solve concrete problems. Peer groups are important during these years. If children do not develop a sense of industry, they may feel inadequate and may experience a maturational crisis.

As school-age children enter adolescence they must develop an identity in the sexual, occupational, and other adult areas. This has been labeled one of the most stressful periods of life and is a period when crisis is most common. The peer group is very important to the adolescent who tests out and develops an identity with the group. The adolescent also must work through the need for independence from parents. At times, when adolescents face new experiences, they need the support of and dependence on parents, and at other times, they will strike out on their own. This behavior may be confusing to parents who may hamper the adolescent's development. If the adolescent is unable to establish a satisfactory sexual identity, occupational identity, and independence from parents a maturational crisis may develop.

Young Adult. During young adulthood the individual must choose and settle into occupational roles. Some individuals get jobs, marry, and begin raising a family. Others go to college, professional, or technical schools in preparation for occupational roles. The young adult must also develop sexual and nonsexual intimate relationships with others. Maturational crisis may result from the inability to choose and settle into occupational roles or from the inability to develop intimate relationships. Failure to develop intimate relationships may lead to self-isolation or "highly stereotyped and formal interpersonal relationships, characterized by a lack of spontaneity, warmth, and an honest exchange of emotional involvement."[32] Cognitive development at this age involves deductive and inductive logic and the beginning of creativity.

Middle Age. Crisis may also occur during middle age because of physical, economic, and psychological stresses. Body changes such as sagging skin, irregular menses, and baldness are all signs that death is imminent and that the body is not functioning as it once did. Psychosocial development involves generativity versus self-absorption, or stagnation. The concern here is with what individuals have generated or helped to generate and their feelings about their successes or failures. When individuals turn inward, become self-absorbed and indulge themselves rather than attempt to make society better by their efforts, they do not successfully meet this developmental stage and a crisis may follow. This may be a result of a failure to accomplish at work, in producing children to be proud of having, or a failure in a marriage.

Old Age. There are many potential crisis situations revolving around old age. Individuals must work through the rejection experienced at retirement and fill what was previously work time with other activities. This age group is also subject to many chronic illnesses for which there may be no cure and for which the cost of care may be high. This may be at a time when the economic base of the family is low because of retirement. There may also be fears of dependency resulting from illness or fears of being moved from a usual home base to a nursing home. Death of friends and relatives may also lead to loneliness and potential crisis situations. There is also the recognition that death is close at hand and feelings about death must be dealt with.

The psychosocial development of old age involves integrity or despair. Those who have adapted successfully to the successes and failures of life are integrated and can reflect upon and enjoy what has been. Despair results when there are misgivings about how life was lived and in realizing that time is too short to accomplish what has not yet been done. Fear of death may result from this despair and create an additional crisis.

SHEEHY MODEL OF MATURATIONAL CRISIS

Sheehy has also developed a model of predictable crises that deals more with adults than those developed by Erikson and Piaget.[33]

Pulling Up Roots. Before age 18, children frequently think they must get away from their parents but seldom take action in that direction. However, after age 18, they act upon this thought by going to college, taking a job, going into the military service, and so forth. They are intent upon developing their own views of the world and look outside the family for views they can call their own. The individual joins with others in clubs and makes alliances, but underneath feels like a child. These feelings are covered up by acts of defiance and pretended confidence. Club and peer alliances continue as long as the values are not basically contrary to family values. When there is a conflict, the individual rebounds back to the family.

The tasks of this group are to participate in a peer-group role, a sex role, plan occupational roles, and develop a view of the world. Accomplishment of these tasks allows the individual to move physically and psychologically from the family and to find out who they are and what is truth for them. If individuals fail to develop an identity during this period they may have an identity crisis or it may be delayed until later in life when it will be more difficult to deal with.

Trying Twenties. Sheehy labels the next stage of passage as the trying twenties. During this stage individuals must prepare for an occupation and develop the capacity for intimacy without losing their self-concept or identity, which is still loosely defined. Individuals may search for models to meet these tasks during this stage.

This stage is characterized by doing what we "should" do and the shoulds are defined by family and peers. Peers often have influence and may be a factor in determining whether an individual gets married and has a family or chooses an alternate life style. Choices during this stage are controlled by an inner conviction that choices made are irrevocable. Although this is not realistic, these choices do influence a later life pattern, which may range from being locked into a commitment made for life, to an unwillingness to make firm commitments. These patterns will follow the individual throughout life.

Catch 30. As individuals approach 30 they feel restricted by the career and personal choices of the 20s and alter their shoulds by making new choices and altering or deepening committments. Moving from the previous "shoulds", which were useful in the last stage but are now restrictive, creates turmoil and sometimes crisis for the individual. A common response is to undo most of what they have spent the last period accomplishing. If single they may marry and if married they may divorce.

Or, they may start in a different career direction feeling discontent with their occupational choice.

Thereafter, throughout the early thirties, individuals settle down, buy homes, and work diligently to become a success. Life becomes more rational and orderly, but satisfaction with marriage may go downhill compared with the feelings experienced during the twenties.

The Deadlock Decade. During the midthirties individuals reach the halfway mark of life and begin to see that their life and successes end despite their being in the prime of life. They begin to lose the physical ability that they have taken for granted and see that they have no absolute answers. A crisis may occur in which they must reexamine their purposes and determine how they can best use their resources in the future. Suppressed desires and feelings are acknowledged during this stage.

There is a reintegration of the personality during this stage. Individuals discover that they are alone and must assume resonsibility for themsleves. They also discover masculine and feminine aspects of the ego that have previously been suppressed. A part of the self also dies during this reintegration, and grieving is often a part of the process. Reintegration provides the individual with a sense of self-identity not experienced by the previous identity, which was put together with parts composed of parents, mates, and peers.

Realizing that time is moving on and that it is the downward side of the hill, individuals may accelerate their push for success during the midthirties. However, by forty they may move away from this drive for success and become more tender and emotional owing to thoughts about their health and future.

Renewal or Resignation. An equilibrium that is more or less satisfying to the individual is established by the mid-forties. Individuals who have not resolved previous crises, however, become stale and resigned. The career is now just a job, children and mates move away or grow distant, and the individual feels empty and abandoned. Such individuals may experience earlier unresolved crises around age 50 and be pushed into seeking revitalization.

Individuals who confront themselves in the previous stage will experience good years as a result of the renewed purposes of life. After 50, the individual has a new warmth and mellowness. Both friends and privacy become more important.

FAMILY CRISIS

Many of the crises discussed above for individuals also affect the family. For example, a maturational change in a family member, which produces stress and possibly crisis requires changes in the role behaviors of all family members. (See Chap. 3.) In addition, situational crisis such as divorce, death, illness, or unemployment of a family member also affects the roles of other family members.

Hill looks at families under stress and develops the following classification systems for crisis.[34] The first system involves the source of trouble, which may be extra-family or intra-family. Intra-family events that may lead to crisis include illegitimacy, nonsupport, mental illness, suicide, infidelity, and alcoholism. The intra-family events are usually more stressful and disorganizing to the family, because they reflect on the family's internal adequacy. Extra-family stressors that may lead to crisis include war bombings, political or religious persecution, tornadoes, hurricanes, floods, war separation, forced migration, premature births, and sudden decreases in income due to a depression. These are often defined as stressful but may solidify rather than disorganize families, because they are external to the family and other families may be experiencing the same catastrophe.

A second classification system involves combinations of loss of family members (dismemberment), or an unprepared-for addition of another member (accession), and loss of morale and family unity (demoralization). Dismemberment in a family would include such things as the death of a member, the hospitalization of a spouse or war separation, whereas, accession would include an unwanted pregnancy, adoptions, war reunions, or addition of a step parent. Demoralization would include nonsupport, infidelity, alcoholism, delinquency, and drug addiction. In addition, demoralization plus dismemberment or accession would include illegimacy, runaways, desertion, divorce, suicide, institutionalization for mental illness, or imprisonment.

Hill says that stressors leading to crisis may also involve status shifts. These stressors may include sudden loss of income and savings, prolonged unemployment, sudden wealth and fame, war bombing and deprivations, disasters, tornadoes, floods and explosions.

Crisis may also be precipitated as a family moves from one stage of development to another. As a family moves from a couple to parents with small children, to a family with school-age children, adjustments must be made in roles and autonomy of members. Changing needs and goals increase the tension on members until the new roles are learned. Some families adjust better to these developmental changes than others.

FACTORS INFLUENCING A CRISIS

Factors that influence a crisis in a family are basically the same as those for an individual. An individual affected by a stressor may or may not experience a crisis depending upon their perception of the problem, their coping skills, and the situational support. Hill says that the factors making for crisis-proneness in families include the event that is interacting with the family's crisis-meeting resources and the members' definition of the event producing crisis, but the event is less important than these other two factors. The family crisis-meeting resources include both the family's support structure and coping skills, whereas, the members' definition of the event includes their perception of the problem. Thus, one model, which incorporates the perception, coping abilities, and support can be used for both individual and family crisis assessment and planning. This model is presented in the section on Nursing Process and Crisis later in the chapter.

Family Adjustment to Crisis. Hill says that the course of adjustment to crises varies from family to family but the overall form of the adjustment is like that of a roller coaster.[36] Initially, family members are collectively numbed by the stressor and there is a failure of their coping skills. However, they may hide this from friends and others outside the family. Later, as they assimilate the facts there is a downward slump in family organization where roles are performed less effectively, and resentment and conflict may be expressed or smothered and converted into tension, which affects the family relationships. At a certain point relationships improve in the family and they are again able to perform appropriate roles. The components of this adjustment are crisis, which leads to disorganization, followed by recovery and later by reorganization. Hill pictures this adjustment as the downward aspect of the roller coaster ride as disorganization follows the crisis. The upward trend begins with recovery and then levels out when the family has reorganized.

Factors in Family Crisis Adjustment. There are factors that influence the family's adjustment to a crisis. Many of the factors that are conducive to a good adjustment following a crisis are the same as those that help a family adapt to any change in one of its members or the family as a whole. (These were identified in Chap. 3.) Hill says that the important factors in helping families adjust to a crisis include family adaptability and integration, affectional relationships, compatible husband and wife and parent-child relationships, democratic decision-making processes, social participation of wife and previous experiences with crisis.[37]

ORGANIZATIONAL CRISIS

In a process similar to an individual or family crisis, an organization may experience a crisis when its coping responses are inadequate to resolve a problem that poses a threat to the system. Organizational crisis may result from internal or external events such as the loss of financial assistance, the failure to achieve important organizational objectives, the death of a key person, or the discovery of major inadequacies in the system. Any of these events may be experienced by the organizational group as a threat to its survival.

In Chapter 1, three aspects of feedback in systems were identified. These included steady state, entropy, and negentropy. Thus, an organization as a system may maintain the status quo, may move backwards, or may move ahead and grow. Ideally, an organization does not move backwards toward destruction. Growth or negentropy is necessary for the organization to continue to meet the needs of society and thus to continue to exist. However, periods of maintaining the status quo, similar to those seen in an individual, may also be necessary. Thus, the normal system is marked by periods of growth and periods of maintenance. In the initial phase of an organizational crisis the maintenance forces predominate and there is a strong resistance to change. In a later phase of a crisis, the growth-forces predominate and provide for the necessary adaptation to the crisis.

STAGES IN AN ORGANIZATIONAL CRISIS

There are four stages in an organizational crisis that are somewhat similar to an individual crisis. These are now identified.

Shock. Fink says that during the initial stage of an organizational crisis individuals become concerned about themselves, their job security, and so forth.[38] As a result, there is a fragmentation of interpersonal relationships and energy goes into worrying rather than relating and carrying out roles effectively. Decision making, communications, and activities related to planning and goal setting are all affected.

Defensive Retreat. A control system is imposed upon the organization during this stage to guarantee the survival of the organization. As a result, the status quo is maintained. In the group versus out-groups, roles are assumed in interpersonal relationships where the focus is upon unconditional loyalties, rather than realistic appraisals of the situation. There is also an effort to find a scapegoat in the out-group. Communications become ritualistic and controlled because there is a fear of losing control and reexperiencing the chaotic state of the shock phase.

The fear of loss of control also leads to highly centralized leadership and decision making and the handling of problems is done in a way that disposes of them rather than solves them. Planning and goal setting focuses on getting the job done today rather than on a long-range focus on the next month or the next year. Thus, decisions made may handle an immediate goal, but run counter to any long-range goals. The structure and functioning of the organization becomes highly traditional during this phase and there is a move toward autocracy and patterns that have been effective in the past. During this phase the organizational patterns allow for survival, but not for solving the problem encountered.

Acknowledgment. The acts of expediency of the previous stage of organizational crisis fail to meet the goals of organizational growth and cannot be continued indefinitely. Thus, the group must come to grips with the problem. Individuals begin self-examination and interpersonal confrontation, which may lead to support and forward movement or accusation and blame with backward movement temporarily using defensive retreat. The process at this time is similar to the process in a family when change is indicated. (This is discussed under Feedback in Chap. 3.) Eventually, individuals engage in interpersonal relationships that focus on present issues rather than past failings and begin to see the out-group as an essential resource carrying equal responsibility for the crisis, rather than as a threat. New ways of communicating are established, leadership and decision making become open and more democratic, and problems are explored. As a result, solutions are more related to the presenting problem. In addition, planning and goal setting become future rather than present oriented.

Adaptation and Change. During this phase the organization again begins to grow (negentropy). Dysfunctional behavior gives way to interdependent functioning, coordinated intergroup relations, accurate communications, and appropriate leadership and decision-making processes. At this stage, the organization is adequately coping with the problem and new solutions and alternatives are explored and identified for implementation.

THE NURSING PROCESS AND CRISIS

Community health nurses have many opportunities to assist individuals, families, or organizations to prevent or to resolve crises. As a result of long-range contact with individuals, families, and organizations in the home, clinic, school, industry, and other settings, they may identify and work with human systems who are in potential crisis-producing situations. In addition, individual human systems may seek out the community health nurse for assistance in such situations. In many situations community health nurses should identify and help the human system resolve the potential or actual problem. However, in some situations the nurse may identify the problem, but choose to refer the individual to other community resources.

ASSESSMENT

Knowledge of stressful situations for human systems should alert community health nurses to the times in the life span when crises may occur. These times include the situational and maturational crisis situations discussed earlier. At such periods nurses should do an adequate assessment to determine how well the system is coping with the stressor and how they can be of assistance to the particular individual or group.

Aguilera has presented a model that should be useful to community health nurses in determining whether or not a stressful situation will or has produced a crisis.[39] The author identifies the following balancing factors that can effect a return to equilibrium for the individual, family, or group following an encounter with a stressful situation. These are (1) the perception of the event, (2) the available situational support, and (3) the coping mechanisms of the human system. When any one or more of these factors are faulty, a crisis may be precipitated.

Perception of the Event. When individuals are able to perceive the event realistically, they are able to recognize the relationship between the event and the feelings about it and solve problems to reduce the tension felt. A successful resolution of the problem is likely. On the other hand, a distorted perception of the event may lead to a failure to recognize the relationship between the event and the feelings experienced. Thus, problem solving will be ineffective and tension will increase.

With such individuals, the nurse must help them identify the crisis-precipitating event and their perception of the event. Questions and observational skills must be used in this process. Observations may be made about the level of anxiety, expressive movements, emotional tone, and verbal responses. Questions revolve around the following: What has gone on in the person's life to bring about the change? How does he perceive the situation? What does it mean to the person? How does it affect his future? From these or similar questions, an assessment can be made regarding the precipitating event and the person's assessment of it.

Situational Support. A second balancing factor is the support available. "Situational support means those persons who are available in the environment who can be depended upon to help solve the problem."[40] If these are lacking, the individual may be vulnerable to crisis.

Hogue defines a support system as a "defined set of persons consisting of a focal or anchor person, all the family, all the friends and all the helping persons who stand ready to serve the anchor person, and the linkages or relationships among these people."[41] Thus, the community health nurse must help persons in crisis identify their usual source of help by asking questions such as, "Who do you usually talk with when you have something on your mind?" "Who are your closest friends?" "Do you talk over concerns with members of your family?" or "Who do you trust?" In some instances, when situational support is lacking, the nurse may serve in this capacity or may refer the client to other helping agencies.

Coping Mechanisms. In the process of living the human system learns patterned responses that are used to reduce stress and tension. These can be overt or covert and consciously or unconsciously activated. Because these patterned responses often become habitual as a result of previous successes in reducing stress, the individual may automatically reduce stress and lose awareness of how and why he or she reacts to stress in a given situation. Thus, when a new unfamiliar situation occurs, in which the patterned responses are inappropriate, feelings of discomfort and tension are experienced. The tension and discomfort may lead to a narrowing of perception to the point where the person becomes so involved in his feelings that he is unable to identify or solve the problem.

Available coping skills include such things as withdrawing and thinking through the problem, talking it over with a friend or family member, crying it out to get rid of the anger and hostility, complaining, using projection or any of the other defense mechanisms. If the person is aware of the problem and can use his coping skills, a crisis may not follow a stressor. However, if the individual is so engrossed in the feelings that perspective on the problem and problem-solving skills are lost, a crisis may follow.

The nurse must elicit information from the person that assists in activating the coping mechanisms. The client may be questioned about previous similar stressors and the method of dealing with them or about the usual method for dealing with tension and anxiety. If usual methods have been unsuccessful, the nurse may ask the client why he thinks this has been so and what he thinks might work? Often when the problem is identified clearly by the nurse and the client, an appropriate coping mechanism can also be identified.

Organization. Assessing a crisis within an organization, a nurse must use a similar process of helping the group look at their perception of the problem, their coping skills, and any support systems. However, some aspects of the assessment may be more difficult. The characteristics of the defensive-retreat stage of crisis in an organization are similar to a highly traditional bureaucracy and a distinction must be made between the defensive-retreat stage of a crisis and an organization in which this is the usual pattern. Data about the background of the organization regarding decision making, leadership style, communication, and interpersonal relationships are useful in making the distinction.

During this phase the nurse must support the individuals in the system regarding their need to protect themselves, but must also be honest in terms of the organizations ineffective management of long-term survival and growth. Failure to point out the reality of the situation may prolong the stage of defensive retreat. During this phase, the nurse may encourage members to collect data on themselves and help them interpret the data. This may influence the members of the organization to examine the situation realistically. Support and confrontation are both important.

During the acknowledgement stage of organizational crisis, the nurse may more realistically support both the members and their actions. The nurse can be most therapeutic in supporting during this stage, and confrontation is no longer necessary.

Instrument. Holmes and Masuda studied people and found 43 life stresses that create the need for change in ongoing life adjustments.[42] The leading stressors for Americans are death of a spouse followed by divorce, marital separation, and marriage. Other stressors in the order of severity include death of a close family member, detention in jail, major personal injury or illness, retirement, being fired, marital reconciliation, sexual difficulties, a major change in the health of a family member, and the addition of a new family member. These and other life stresses are identified by the authors in the Schedule of Recent Experiences, which is a self-administered questionnaire. In this instrument items are checked by an individual for a year and assigned values consistent with the importance of the event to large numbers of people, and then they are totaled to give an overall value for the year. This value is known as the total Life Change Units (LCU). The instrument has been used with many groups and a LCU of 150 in 1 year has been identified as likely to precipitate a crisis.

PLANNING

Plans should be made with the individual to restore equilibrium, rather than to make changes in the personality structure. Thus, the interventions should be based upon the current rather than past situation of the person. These plans should follow from the identification of the event and the factors influencing the disequilibrium. A determination should also be made about the person's ability to carry out the activities of daily living.

After the strengths of the individual are identified regarding coping skills, resources, and perceptions, the nurse should consider alternative solutions with clients and assist them in selecting an appropriate one. Tentative solutions may be suggested by the nurse based upon the assessment of the situation and the theoretical base of knowledge. According to Aguilera, planned interventions may include helping the person understand the crisis and ventilate feelings, explore feelings, find new and more effective coping mechanisms, or in identifying support systems.[43]

INTERVENTION AND EVALUATION

After plans are made, the individual tries out the new behavior. If the plans have been appropriate, the crisis will subside and the person should be at a level of functioning that is equal to or higher than the pre-crisis level. If plans have been inappropriate, new plans must be made and tested. Once the appropriate behavior has been identified and used successfully by the individual, it may become a part of his patterned behavioral responses to future situations.

Caplan says that interventions may be on an interpersonal or community-wide basis.[44] The previously discussed interventions fit his interpersonal category and are most appropriate for community health nurses. However, if community health nurses identify large numbers of people being affected by similar situations, they should report this change to the supervisor who will report it to other officials. In this process, it is possible that environmental or other changes can be initiated on a community basis to reduce the risk. For example, crisis resulting from unemployment may be countered by increased job opportunities using local, state, or federal funding, or, crises resulting from divorce may be countered by the development of community agencies for premarital and marital counseling. Such efforts may prevent crises for others and are thus primary-prevention activities.

Nurses in the community may also prevent crises in their interpersonal approaches to families and individuals. Anticipatory guidance is an important aspect of health promotion and may be used to prepare humans beforehand for developmental changes. For example, if mothers expect changes in their children's growth and development, they are better able to cope with these changes and adjust their behavior accordingly. Anticipatory guidance may also reduce the stress of situational crises such as marriage, retirement, divorce, death, and illness. Fromer has identified the following group activities which may prevent crises: premarital counseling, prenatal classes, preretirement counseling, counseling of the terminally ill and their families, and pre-operative teaching.

Self-Help in Crisis. Although not usually associated with crisis, dreams are an excellent way of using the unconscious mind to help solve problems. If the individual or outside resources can reduce the tension and anxiety to manageable levels and identify the precipitating stressor, dreams may help the individual identify alternate solutions to the problem and ways of coping.

The process of dream recollection and interpretation is an ongoing process. Initially the individual must make a concerted effort to recall dreams and to write down key points if he awakens during the night or the whole dream upon awakening in the morning. This should be done prior to leaving the bed because alertness of the conscious mind causes dreams to fade. Thus, a pad and pencil should be kept at the bedside.

Dream interpretation is usually based upon individual symbols rather than universal symbols, although universal symbols may provide insight for the individual. Most books on dreams provide the universal symbols; it is then up to the individual to apply individualized meaning to the symbols. For example, for a nurse, a dream about a hospital could mean work or an illness. The other aspects of the dream should differentiate between the two possibilities. For a carpenter, a dream about a hospital would probably indicate an illness rather than a work situation.

Dreams are best understood in series. Often several different dreams in one night carry the same basic message, when interpreted. In addition, if dreams are not acted upon, the basic message may be repeated for days, months, or years.

Nurses who are knowledgeable about dream symbology could help clients interpret dreams in crisis situations by offering interpretation of universal symbols identified in the dreams. Often, dreams are very clear when the individual is aware of the problem, as in the instance of crisis.

SUICIDE

An important aspect of any crisis assessment is a suicidal assessment. Suicide may be the only alternative method of coping considered by the individual when overpowered by a crisis.

GROUPS AFFECTED

Suicide rates are lower for Blacks and Japanese in the United States than for Caucasians, but American Indian and Chinese suicide rates are slightly higher. However, there are many problems with these rates because they may vary by age, sex, area of the country, and honesty in reporting. For example, is an automobile accident an accident or is it a suicide? In the United States in 1976, there were 13.2 suicides per 100,000 population per year for Whites and 7.0 per 100,000 for non-Whites.[46] However, foreign-born White males had two times as many suicides as American born, and also suicides for Whites ranged from 6.2 per 100,000 Whites in New York to 26.9 per 100,000 Whites in El Paso, Texas. Thus, generalities should be avoided.

There is also great variation in suicides among occupational groups. However, there is a tendency toward higher suicide rates in the highest and lowest prestige occupations. Professionals such as dentists, teachers, lawyers and certain physician groups have suicide rates higher than the general population. On the other hand, the consistently unemployed also have higher rates of suicide than the general population.

Health may also be a factor in suicide. Among the mentally ill, suicide is eight to twelve times higher among depressed clients, manic-depressive clients, and schizophrenic clients than among the general population. Suicide is also higher among individuals having physical disorders, especially among the older age group. There is also a strong relationship between alcohol and drug dependency and higher suicide rates.

SUICIDE ASSESSMENT

Because of the suicide potential in crisis and the problems with interpreting rates, everyone experiencing a crisis should be assessed One area of assessment should involve suicidal ideas and behavior. Is there a history of suicidal behavior or a recent personality change with an attempt at suicide? Is depression, agitation, or psychosis present? Are there disturbances in sleep, loss of appetite, weight loss, social withdrawal, or signs of hopelessness and helplessness? Is there extreme tension, anxiety, guilt, shame, or loss of contact or disorientation? Are suicidal ideas communicated to others? Are these ideas communicated directly in the form of such statements as, "I wish I was dead" or "I can't go on any longer," or are they indirect in the form of a preoccupation with the death of someone else, or are they expressed in behaviors such as suddenly making a will or giving away prized possessions? These and other questions and observations should elicit answers about suicidal ideas and behavior.

Other areas associated with suicide and presented earlier might also be evaluated. Does the person have an isolated life-style with limited support from others? Is psychiatric or physical illness present? Has there been a withdrawal from meaningful relationships or a recent significant loss?

The community health nurse should also assess the lethality of the suicide potential. Freeman and co-workers consider this the most significant criteria of a suicidal potential.[47] The three elements of the lethality include (1) the lethality of the proposed method, (2) the availability of the means, and (3) the timing and planning of the details. If the individual plans to commit suicide by shooting, hanging, or drowning the lethality is higher than if the plan is to use pills or to slash the wrists. If the person plans to commit suicide by shooting, and a gun is available, the lethality is even higher. And if the time and details are planned, the potential is very high. Thus, the community health nurse should explore these three areas with the client. The intent should also be investigated. If an individual knows the effect of aspirin and plans to take them before a spouse arrives home, there is the likelihood that the attempt is being used to manipulate rather than to commit suicide. However, if individuals do not know the action and effects of aspirin and plan to take a handful all at once when there is no likelihood of someone discovering them, the lethality is higher. Overall questions that might be asked about potential suicide include questions about how life is going, how the individual is feeling, the person's mental outlook, any wish to be out of it or dead, how close they are to suicide now, how they would do it, and what is their plan?

INTERVENTIONS

Interventions should be based upon the seriousness of the suicide potential. If individuals are at high risk they should be hospitalized for self-protection until they are able to cope with the situation. If there is no immediate danger to the individual's life, he or she should be assisted to cope with the situation, to develop realistic perceptions, and to identify support persons in the same manner as in any crisis.

REFERENCES

1. Taber's Cyclopedic Medical Dictionary, p. C126. Philadelphia, F A Davis, 1977
2. Murray R, Zentner J: Nursing Concepts for Health Promotion, p 207. Englewood Cliffs, Prentice-Hall, 1975
3. Caplan G: Support Systems and Community Mental Health, p 201. New York, Behavioral Publications, 1974
4. Caplan G, Ibid, p 202
5. Caplan G, Ibid, p 203
6. Caplan G: Principles of Preventive Psychiatry, p 38. New York, Basic Books, 1964
7. Aguilera D, et al: Crisis Intervention Theory and Methodology. St Louis, C V Mosby, 1974
8. Aguilera D, Ibid, p 3
9. Lindemann E: Symptomatology and management of acute grief. Am J Psychiatry 101: 141–148, Sept 1944
10. Caplan G: Support Systems and Community Mental Health. pp 208–209
11. Janis L: Psychological Stress: Psychoanalytical and Behavioral Studies of Surgical Patients. New York, John Wiley & Sons, 1958
12. Murray R, Zentner J, Ibid, p 209
13. Mason E: A method of predicting crisis outcome for mothers of premature babies. Public Health Reports Vol. 78, No. 12: 1031–35, Dec 1963
14. Kaplan D M, Mason E: Maternal reactions to premature birth viewed as an acute emotional disorder. In Parad H J (ed): Crisis Intervention, pp 118–128. New York, Family Service Association of America, 1965
15. Mason E, Ibid
16. Parsons T: Definitions of Health and Illness in Light of American Values and Social Structure. In Jaco E C (ed): Patients, Physicians and Illness, pp 107–127. New York, Free Press, 1972
17. Hall J, Weaver B: Nursing of Families in Crisis. Philadelphia, J B Lippincott, 1974
18. Janis I, op cit
19. Crate M: Nursing Functions in Adaptation to Chronic Illness. Am J Nurs Vol. 65, No. 10: pp 72–76, Oct 1965
20. Crate M, Ibid, p 72
21. Dizmang L: Loss, bereavement and depression in childhood aspects of depression. In Shneidman E (ed): International Psychiatric Clinic, Vol. 6, No. 2, 1969
22. Bowlby J: Process of mourning. Int J Psychoanal 42: 317–340, 1961
23. Lindemann E, op cit
24. Bowlby J, op cit
25. Aguilera D, op cit
26. Rappaport R: Normal crisis, family structure, and mental health. Family Process 2 68–80, 1963
27. Murray R, Zentner J, op cit
28. Erikson E: Identity and the Life Cycle. Psychological Issues, Vol. 1, No. 1, Monograph 1. New York, International Universities, 1959
29. Piaget J: The Child's Conception of the World. Totowa, Littlefield Adams, 1963
30. Sutterley D, Donnelly G: Perspectives in Human Development. Philadelphia, J B Lippincott, 1973
31. Piaget J, op cit
32. Aguilera D, et al, op cit, p 120
33. Sheehy G: Passages: Predictable Crises of Adult Life. New York, Bantam, 1977
34. Hill R: Generic Features of Families Under Stress. In Parad H (ed): Crisis Intervention, pp 32–52. New York, Family Service Association of America, 1965
35. Hill R, Ibid
36. Hill R, Ibid
37. Hill R, Ibid
38. Fink S, et al: Organizational crisis and change. Article pending publication in J Appl Behav Sci
39. Aguilera D, et al, op cit, p 60
40. Aguilera D, Ibid, p 64
41. Hogue C: Support systems for health promotion. In Hall J, Weaver B (eds): A Systems Approach to Community Health, pp 65–80. Philadelphia, J B Lippincott, 1977
42. Holmes T, Rahe R H: The social readjustment rating scale. J Psychosom Res 11: pp 213–218, 1967
43. Aguilera D, op cit, p 51
44. Caplan G, op cit
45. Fromer M: Community Health Care and the Nursing Process, p 347. St Louis, C V Mosby, 1979
46. U. S. Department of Health, Education, and Welfare. Facts of Life and Death, p 46. Washington, D C, National Center for Health Statistics, 1978
47. Freeman D, et al: Assessing intent to die in self-injury behavior. In Neuringer C (ed): Psychological Assessment of Suicidal Risk, pp 18–42. Springfield Charles C. Thomas, 1974

PART IV

APPLICATION OF THEORIES, CONCEPTS, AND PROCESSES

11

High-Risk Considerations Throughout the Life Span

Sheila Spelman

With the notable exceptions of sexually transmitted diseases, which have reached epidemic proportions in this country, communicable diseases are no longer the major threat to life that they have been throughout world history. Scientific achievements in the areas of immunization, water and food purification and preservation, pharmacology, and sanitation have minimized the impact of communicable diseases on human longevity. Coronary heart disease, malignant neoplasms, cerebrovascular disorders, and accidents are the major causes of death in the United States (Table 11–1). These conditions are not the result of any single etiologic agent but are influenced by many factors: the individual's innate biologic potential (internal environment) and his relationship with the physical, social, and psychological external environment. The ability to maintain a state of equilibrium between these internal and external environmental forces results in an optimal level of functioning and well-being; imbalance between the two results in physical, emotional, and/or social pathology.[1] As noted by Suchman, "Man is an inherent part of his environment; he both shapes and is shaped by it."[2]

Carter states that "The development of an individual from conception to the grave depends on two sets of interacting influences—genetic factors and environmental experiences."[3]

He further contends that while all diseases contain varying degrees of genetic influences, diseases in general can be categorized as follows:

1. Those due entirely to genetics such as phenylketonuria, galactosemia, and sickle cell disease.
2. Those in which genetic components and environmental forces share causation such as congenital hip dislocation, schizophrenia, and hypertension.
3. Those in which environmental factors are the predominant causative factors such as communicable diseases, accidents, and many forms of cancer.[4]

The Center for Disease Control of the Department of Health and Human Services has also analyzed the impact of internal and external environmental influences on mortality rates. They categorized the primary contributing factors to health status into the following four areas: (1) life style, which includes personal habits and behaviors related to diet, exercise, substance abuse and safety practices, (2) hereditary or biologic factors, (3) natural and man-made environmental influences,

TABLE 11–1. Ten Leading Causes of Death U.S.A. 1977

CAUSE	NO. OF DEATHS	RATE PER 100,000	% OF TOTAL*
Heart disease	717,320	331.6	37.8
Malignant neoplasms	387,430	179.1	20.4
Cerebrovascular disease	182,840	84.5	9.6
Accidents	105,020	48.5	5.5
Influenza and pneumonia	49,960	23.1	2.6
Diabetes	33,570	15.5	1.8
Cirrhosis of liver	31,260	14.5	1.6
Arteriosclerosis	29,040	13.4	1.5
Suicide	28,390	13.1	1.5
Mortality in early infancy	23,310	10.8	1.2

* % column does not add up to 100% because all causes of death are not listed
From Monthly Vital Statistics Report, Annual Summary for the U.S., 1977

and (4) limitations or constraints inherent in the health care system.[5] Their findings are noted in Figure 11–1 and strongly suggest that changes in individual and societal health states are more a function of human behavior and environmental influences than medical technology. Eckholm observes that ". . . increasingly, the forces that shape health patterns are set in motion by human activities and decisions. Indeed, in creating its way of life, each society creates its way of death."[6]

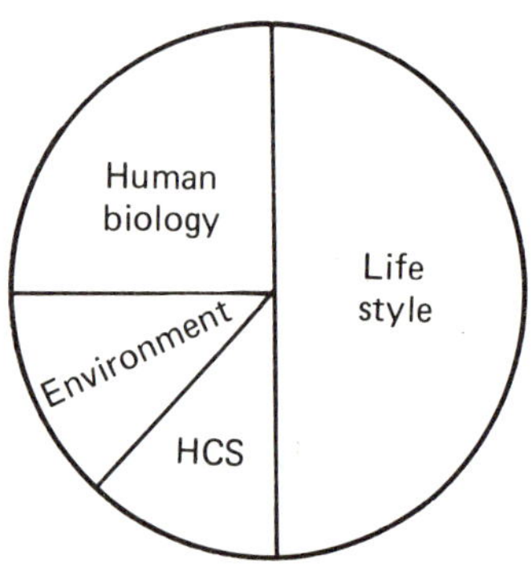

Figure 11–1
Proportional allocation of the contributing factors of mortality to the four elements of the health field (ten leading causes of death among the total population 1+ years of age [U.S.A., 1975]). HCS = Health care system.

What are the implications for nursing? At each stage of individual and family development certain tasks must be performed and objectives met to assure optimum growth and well-being. In this section we explore several internally and externally induced factors that can produce increased risk for individual and family systems as they seek to attain and maintain a state of equilibrium, and we offer suggestions for joint nurse-patient interventions.

GENETICS

An estimated 7% of all births result in an infant with some degree of physical anomaly or mental retardation.[7] In addition, approximately 20 million Americans are afflicted with the often devastating physical, emotional, social, and economic effects of genetic diseases. Despite the overwhelming proportions of the problem, it is only within recent years that components of the health professions, including nursing, have directed attention toward the primary, secondary, and tertiary preventive measures associated with genetic defects. The National Research Council has noted that "The exuberant growth of knowledge of human genetics has been both a cause and a result of some changes in medicine . . . a cause because it has supplied the conceptual approach to the clarification of many newly described diseases, and an effect because the changing patterns of disease have made hereditary problems more visible and their education more urgent."[8]

While there is some disagreement among authorities as to the appropriate classification of genetic disorders, for our purposes the following simplified classification suggested by The March of Dimes and Hendin and Marks are used:[9,10]

1. Single-factor genetic disorders that follow mendelian patterns of inheritance.
2. Multifactorial disorders resulting from combinations of interaction between genetic material and the environment.
3. Aberrations of the structure, number, or arrangement of chromosomes.

It was only within the past three decades that science had determined that all normal human cells contain 23 pairs of chromosomes (a total of 46), which carry the basic genetic materials in DNA (deoxyribonucleic acid). One chromosome of each pair is "donated" by the father and one of each pair by the mother. Twenty-two of these pairs, called autosomes, are responsible for our characteristics that are inherited according to the mendelian principle of dominant and recessive genes—eye color, hair color, skin color, and so forth. The remaining pair, or sex chromosomes, determine if we are male or female. Normal females have two X chromosomes and normal males have one X chromosome and one Y chromosome. Females do not possess a Y chromosome, therefore, the old adage that fathers determine the sex of the child is accurate. Table 11–2 identifies some of the almost 2000 single-factor genetic disorders known with their probability of occurrence.

The precise method of genetic transmission in

TABLE 11–2. Examples of Genetic Disorders and Their Probability of Occurrence

AUTOSOMAL DOMINANT	AUTOSOMAL RECESSIVE	X-LINKED
Achondroplasia Congenital Cataracts Chronic simple glaucoma (some forms) Huntington's chorea Hypercholesterolemia Polydactylism	Albinism Cretinism Cystic fibrosis Friedreich's ataxia Galactosemia Maple syrup disease Phenylketonuria Sickle cell disease Tay-Sachs disease Thalassemia	Agammaglobulinemia Color blindness Hemophilia Lesch-Nyhan syndrome Muscular dystrophy (Becker, Duchenne's) Spinal ataxia
With one affected parent: 1. 50% chance of disease 2. 50% chance no affect	With both parents carriers: 1. 25% chance of disease 2. 25% chance of no affect 3. 50% chance of being a carrier	*Male child* with carrier mother: 1. 50% chance of disease 2. 50% chance no affect
With both affected parents: 1. 75% chance of disease 2.* 25% chance of no affect	With one parent unaffected: 1. 50% chance of being a carrier 2. 50% chance of no affect	*Female child* with carrier mother: 1. 50% chance of being a carrier 2. 50% chance no affect

* Probability rates apply to each pregnancy

multifactorial genetic disturbances is not clearly defined and the extent of the number of diseases involved is unknown. Spina bifida and anencephaly, both neural tube defects, occur in approximately 1 in every 500 births; cleft lip and palate occur in about 1 in 1000 births, and pyloric stenosis in about 1 in every 300 births. With any of these disorders, there is a 2% to 8% chance of recurrence in future pregnancies.[11]

The chromosome disorders are generally not transmitted from generation to generation, but are considered genetic in origin. The development of these diseases is very complex and are not dealt with here in great detail. Changes in the structure, arrangement, and number of chromosomes are thought to occur during the separation and formation phases of the reproductive cells at the time of conception. It is now believed that about 50% of all spontaneous abortions are caused by chromosomal abnormalities of sufficient severity to prevent the further development of the embryo.[12] Trisomy 21 (Down's syndrome) is one of the more common chromosomal disorders and its incidence has been shown to be related to maternal age.

As yet unmentioned are those congenital defects not related to genetic factors, but resulting exclusively from teratogenetic environmental influences, such as rubella, radiation, heavy alcohol consumption, drugs, pesticides, and fertilizers. The probability for recurrence is determined by continued or repeated maternal and fetal exposure.

GENETIC SCREENING AND COUNSELING

Community health nurses are well acquainted with certain aspects of health care related to genetic disorders. Virtually all states now require PKU testing, and sickle-cell screening is common in clinic, school, and community settings. State programs for services to medically indigent, handicapped, or crippled children have involved community health nurses in providing direct physical and rehabilitative care to these children in their homes and schools, counseling and support to parents, and guidance to families in assisting the child toward optimal physical, emotional, and social development.

Figure 11–2 provides a framework for visualizing the process and desired outcomes of screening programs initiated after the birth of a child. Holtzman views the process as interdisciplinary but also under the administrative control of a central agency, such as, a state health department or regional branch of a state health department, in order to assure coordinated programs and patient services. He further states that screening programs to detect any disorder should only be developed based on the following considerations:

> (1) Frequency and severity of the conditions; (2) availability of a therapy of proven efficiency; (3) extent to which detection by screening improves the outcome; (4) validity, reliability, and safety of the screening test; (5) adequacy of resources to assure effective screening and follow-up; (6) costs, and (7) acceptance of the screening program by the community, including both consumers and practicing physicians.[13]

Holtzman emphasizes that the existence of a screening test alone, without consideration of the other ethical, legal, and cost-benefit criteria cannot justify the implementation of such a program.

The traditional role of the community health nurse can be readily identified in the Holtzman model—casefinding and follow-up in the management of the disease process. These activities involve aspects of secondary and tertiary prevention and are reflective of the screening process associated with PKU identification and treatment. Consider the following case study:

> Mrs. Green, age 24, presented herself at the health department clinic requesting family planning services. Mrs. Green, along with other patients, was shown a film on the various methods of birth control, which was followed by a nurse-led question-and-answer period. Following the group session, Mrs. Green met with the nurse for a review of her current, past, and family medical history. During the interview Mrs. Green revealed that although she had been married for almost a year, it was only recently that her husband informed her that he did not want children. Her husband had a brother "in a mental institution" and he was afraid of fathering a child who would be similarly affected. The young wife admitted she had been terribly hurt by this unexpected

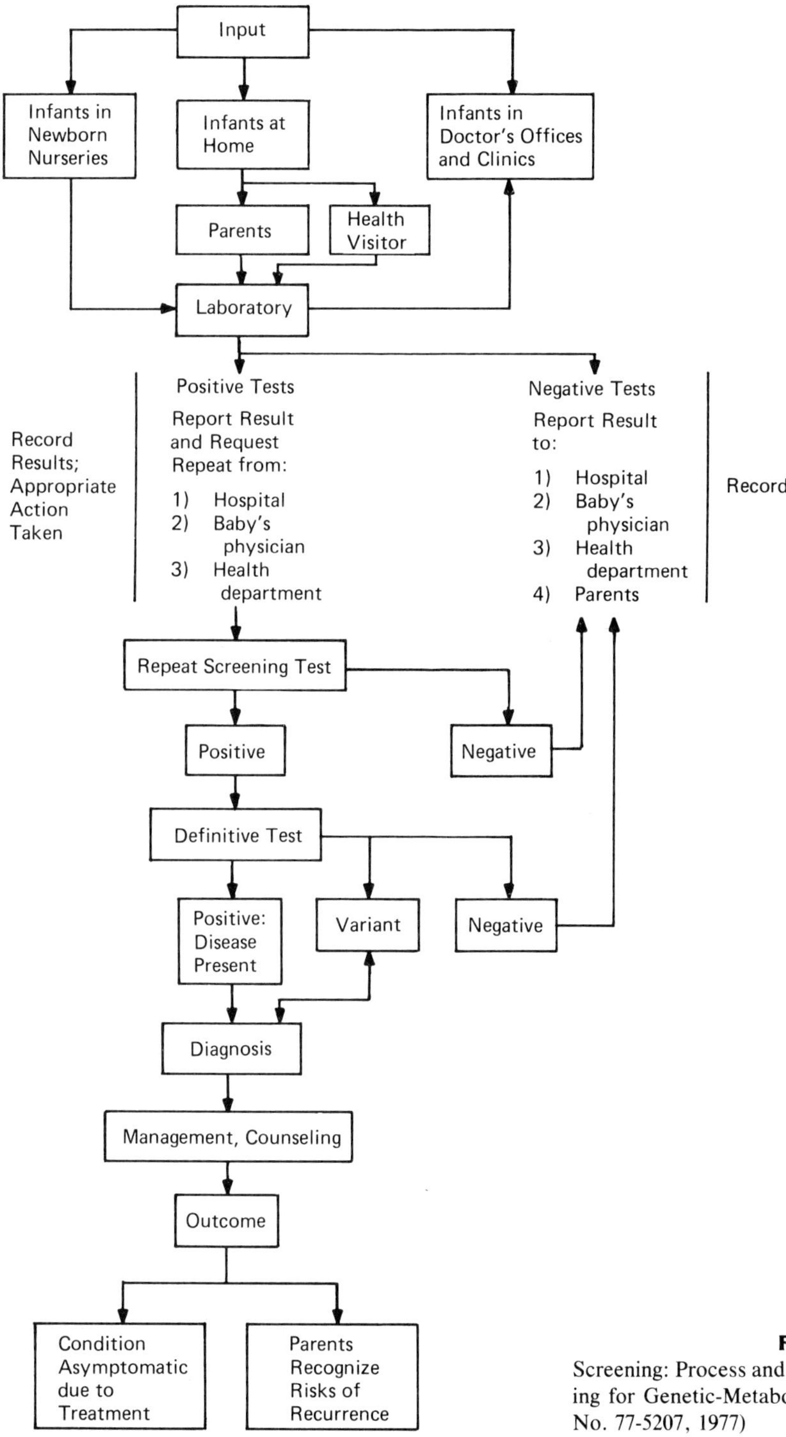

Figure 11–2
Screening: Process and outcome. (Holtzman NA: Screening for Genetic-Metabolic Diseases. DHEW Publication No. 77-5207, 1977)

disclosure since she had looked forward to motherhood. The ordeal had placed a tremendous strain on the marriage. Upon further questioning, the nurse was able to ascertain that the brother was severely retarded and that he had been born when his mother was well into her forties. Neither Mr. nor Mrs. Green was aware of the genetic counseling program available through a nearby medical center, but Mrs. Green demonstrated interest in receiving more information about it. Mrs. Green left the clinic with her birth control method of choice and a referral to the Genetic Counseling Center.

This case study illustrates genetic counseling and screening programs directed toward primary prevention. The focus is shifted from the early identification and treatment of children at risk, to the identification of at-risk parents capable of producing a genetically disabled child.

Riccardi, in his description of the Colorado-Wyoming Regional Genetic Counseling Center, advocates "the genetic approach to human disease" as an integral part of primary health care directed toward the reduction in numbers of infants born with congenital and genetic disorders and maximizing support to families and individuals when birth defects occur.[14] The prevention aspects of the program include (1) identification of at-risk families prior to conception and (2) early prenatal diagnosis in high-risk pregnancies. Screening in the former category is directed toward carrier detection. The National Foundation—the March of Dimes—reports that nearly 60 carrier states such as sickle cell anemia, thalassemia, and Tay-Sachs disease can now be identified through parental blood-and-cell analysis.[15] Certain chromosomal rearrangements in normal adults, such as translocation, are also available through cytogenic studies. Counseling is directed toward alerting prospective parents to the probability of genetic disorders occurring or recurring in their offspring in order that they, the family, can make informed decisions regarding childbearing.

Prenatal diagnosis of many genetic disorders may be accomplished through amniocentesis, fetoscopy, fetal x-ray films, or fetal ultrasound examinations.[16] All chromosome disorders, some 60 single-factor disorders, and some multifactorial disorders, such as anencephaly can be diagnosed early in the pregnancy. Should the results of the studies reveal a defective embryo, the parents can then decide whether termination or continuance of the pregnancy is appropriate for them. Whichever decision is reached, extensive emotional support is indicated to assist the couple in coping with the feelings that might result of guilt, shame, or failure. If the pregnancy is brought to term, the couple will also require guidance in planning to rear a handicapped child.

IMPLICATIONS FOR NURSING

As previously noted, community health nurses have been concerned with the treatment aspects of genetic disorders, but insufficient attention has been given to the preventive approach. Appropriate areas for community-health nursing involvement should include (1) The early identification of individuals and families at risk for producing a genetically handicapped child. These include women 35 years of age or older and men over 55; persons with a known genetic problem such as PKU, or sickle cell disease or trait; siblings of those with genetic handicaps; women with a history of several spontaneous abortions; families with at least one child with a diagnosed genetic defect; normal adults with known chromosomal aberrations; and persons belonging to certain racial or ethnic subgroups, such as Blacks (sickle-cell disease), Jewish people from Eastern Europe (Tay-Sachs disease), White persons of European descent (cystic fibrosis), and those of Mediterranean descent, particularly those of Italian or Greek heritage (thalassemia); (2) referral of high-risk individuals and families to genetic screening and counseling programs. This includes assisting families in gathering personal and family health histories, which may be needed to aid genetic counselors in defining the problem; (3) providing information and referral services to family planning programs for couples interested in this alternative; (4) acceptance and support of families once they have reached a decision, regardless of what that decision might be; (5) participation in community and school educational programs directed toward public awareness and acceptance of genetic screening and counseling services. The National Research Council recommended that "It is essential to begin the study of human biology, including genetics and probability, in primary school, continuing with a more health-related curriculum in secondary school. . . ."[17]

ENVIRONMENTAL INFLUENCES

Auger notes that the "physical characteristics a child is born with influence the environmental response to the child and his response to his environmental perceptions."[18] The responses toward healthy well-developed infants are more likely to be positive, accepting, and serve to reinforce a sense of high self-esteem and promote optimal emotional growth and social development. It must be remembered, however, that visible inherited traits are not limited to physical structure. Societies place values on other physical characteristics, such as sex, eye color, hair color, and skin color.[19] Even in this enlightened age of equal rights for women, our culture still values the arrival of baby boys over that of girls.

It is also a tragic reality that for several centuries the American society valued one skin color over all others. Persons of color, especially Native Americans and Blacks, were perceived as being genetically inferior. Despite its irrationality, the color of one's skin dictated placement in the social hierarchy and became a "primary determinant of whether an individual's chances for full human development were to be actualized."[20] The social climate is gradually changing and opportunities for all minorities will hopefully equal those of the majority. However, the physical and emotional environmental stresses induced by social segregation continue to be reflected in health-status data. Mortality rates for non-white populations suggest social stress factors operating in deaths caused by cerebrovascular accidents, homicide, motor vehicle and all other accidents, and cirrhosis of the liver to a greater extent than in the White population. Despite a general decline in the incidence among the population as a whole, the rate of tuberculosis in minorities is four times that of the White population; the death rate for non-White infants and children under 5 years is twice that of Whites and an overall death rate is 1.4 times that of Whites.[21] The actual or perceived social isolation and segregation of persons of color or varied ethnic backgrounds creates a self-perpetuating cycle of inadequate education, low income from decreased employment opportunities, malnutrition, increased incidence of physical and emotional disease, and low levels of self-esteem.[22]

By virtue of our living in a technologic, industrialized society, our bodies are continuously subject to invasion by hazardous materials through the food we eat, the air we breathe, and absorbtion through the skin. This attack is more likely to come from toxic substances of our own making than from infectious agents.

CHEMICAL HAZARDS

Cancer is a leading cause of death in this country. It is estimated that 60% to 90% of human malignancies are related to environmental influences.[23,24] Approximately 10% of the 10,000 chemicals in the environment are known to be carcinogenic.[25] Workers exposed to these chemicals daily in the performance of their jobs are at particular risk. Unfortunately, the effects of exposure may not be evident for 20 to 30 years. There also appears to be a strong relationship between the carcinogenic and mutagenic effects of certain chemicals. For example, personnel working in operating rooms have increased rates of cancer and females experience more spontaneous abortions than would be anticipated. Chemicals in anesthetics are thought to be the predisposing factors.

Individuals living with persons who are exposed to carcinogens, or who live in proximity to industries using or manufacturing such chemicals are also at risk. Studies have shown that families of asbestos workers have higher incidences of mesothelioma than the general population, while wives of polyvinylchloride plant workers have more stillbirths and miscarriages than the general public. The Love Canal tragedy in Niagara Falls has resulted in birth defects, cancers, stillbirths, and miscarriages in residents living in the vicinity of the canal, which was a chemical waste dump.

Skin cancer is on the rise and has generally been associated with outdoor occupations. However, some of the increase is thought to be related to the more frequent use of synthetic fibers in clothing. Synthetic fibers are only 40% to 60% as efficient as cotton in blocking ultraviolet rays from the sun. Changing standards of dress plus the perceived status of a deep tan are also contributing factors.

Our homes are a common source of chemical contact. Lead poisoning, a particularly dangerous condition to young children, can result in renal disorders, blindness, anemia, and central nervous system disorders leading to retardation, epilepsy, or death. The most frequently identified source of lead is the lead-based paint in wall-paint chippings, which are ingested by children. While older, run-down housing has generally been acknowledged as the primary source of lead poisoning, other sources of lead in the child's environment include paint on toys or furniture. Comic books, magazines, and newspapers using red, orange, or yellow inks and dirt (soil) are other potential sources of exposure.

Treatment is lengthy and painful and involves removing the child from the leaded environment or removing the lead source from the environment.

Foodstuffs have also been identified as sources of chemical or other nonmicrobial pollutants. Substances absorbed by plants can be consumed by humans either directly or through animals, fowl, or fish who have fed on the plants or other toxic materials. Food additives ranging from preservatives to coloring have also been implicated as sources of health hazards.

AIR POLLUTION

Approximately 80% of this country's population resides in urban areas with air that is polluted by particulate matter, toxic gases, or both. Particulate matter includes dust, pollens, industrial dirt and ash, carbon, tar and metallic oxides.[26] The greatest source of air pollution is the automobile. Industrial contributors include oil refineries and smelters, steel mills, paper mills, and industries using coal for energy sources. Burton and Smith poignantly write, that "unless gas masks are to become an acceptable part of our dress, we must recognize the dangers and adopt adequate measures to reduce air pollution in our country effectively."[27] Cancer of the lung, asthma, emphysema, and chronic bronchitis are all related to air contaminants. Severe occurrences of prolonged, intense pollution have led to deaths.

WATER POLLUTION

Water may be polluted by infectious agents, sewage, soil from land erosion, human and animal wastes, and chemicals such as insecticides, pesticides, and detergents.[28] All are potential sources of disease to all forms of life. Large amounts of the pesticide Kepone entered the James River in Virginia and virtually destroyed the fishing and crabbing industry of the area. Of even greater tragedy was the effects on the workers exposed to the pesticide at the plant in Hopewell, Virginia. The victims have developed tremors, nervous disorders, reproductive failures, and are at increased risk for developing cancer.

ACCIDENTS

Accidents, motor vehicle and other types, are the leading cause of death for persons aged 1 through 34 years.[29] Accidents, poisonings, and violence account for 14% of the hospitalizations for children under 15 years of age. Motor vehicle accidents are the leading cause of death in persons 25 to 34 years of age. Accidental injuries are also a major cause of permanent disability. Falls are the leading cause of accidental death in homes, followed by fires.[30] Occupationally related deaths are declining, while other types increase in number.

Virtually all accidental deaths are preventable; yet, despite the horrifying statistics, people persist in placing themselves and others in jeopardy. Seat belts are not worn; motorcyclists abandon their helmets; swimming takes place in unsupervised or unauthorized areas; children are left unattended, and drinkers of alcohol continue to drive. Educational efforts have demonstrated limited positive behaviorial changes; self-destruction and mutilation persist. A number of researchers support the theory that this type of violent or careless behavior is symptomatic of the "diseases of adaptation," as are illnesses, such as hypertension, which are associated with persistent exposure to stressful stimuli.

NOISE POLLUTION

Noise is more than unpleasant sound; permanent hearing loss resulting from job-related exposure to loud noises has for some time been recognized as an occupational health hazard. The Occupational Safety and Health Administration (OSHA) has established safety standards for noise exposure and protection in the job environment to minimize the hazards. However, the detrimental effects of noise are not limited to industrial sources: Noise is everywhere. It is estimated that 20 million Americans are exposed daily to noise in their neighborhoods, schools, or home environments at levels severe enough to cause permanent, irreversible hearing loss.[31]

Prolonged exposure to excessive noise is now thought to damage our health and well-being in other, more subtle ways. Noise is a stressful stimulus and the body reacts accordingly with changes in adrenal enzyme levels and in the cardiovascular system. Research suggests strongly that these changes are associated with hypertension, ulcers, low-birth-weight infants, and possibly certain congenital defects. As a result of noise exposure interfering with auditory perceptions, children may exhibit delays in language development and reading ability. Inattentiveness, exhaustion, forgetfulness, and decreased perceptual abilities are other results of noise exposure, which interfere with our ability to perform at optimal levels of functioning and increase the probability of accidents.

LIFE-STYLES

Much has been written on the American life-style and its negative impact on the health and well-being of the citizenry. We are generally considered a sedentary, overfed, self-indulgent people. Recent data suggests that perhaps we are taking a second look at ourselves. Although still the leading cause of death, coronary disease is showing a slow but steady decline. Credit for this change is being attributed to shifts in dietary and smoking patterns and adoption of regular exercise programs. Weight-control groups, exercise and athletic clubs, and "health" food stores are becoming as commonplace as fast-food chains. "No Smoking" signs and sections are visible in most public places and many private homes. Jogging, running, and even walking have become our new status symbols.

These are all positive changes; however, problems still exist. Alcoholism and other forms of substance abuse remain deterrents to optimal wellness. The scourge of smallpox has been replaced by fetal alcohol syndrome. Despite a decrease in the number of adult males who smoke, women (especially teenage females) continue to smoke and ignore the risks to health. Pulmonary cancer in females is rapidly approaching the incidence rates in males. It has also been demonstrated that women who smoke during pregnancy give birth to lower-weight infants.

Sexual behavior must also be considered in the context of life-styles. Sexual activity, especially by girls, is starting at earlier ages. Adolescents are particularly susceptible to the often explicit sexual overtones of advertisements, recordings, movies, and magazines. Cohabitation and giving birth out-of-wedlock are no longer the social stigmas as in past generations. Unfortunately society's zeal in promoting sexuality and "sexual liberation" for women has focused on sexual acts rather than the mutual responsibilities of sexual partners to each other. Pregnancies in women 15 to 19 years of age are increasing. These infants are more likely to be born too small or too soon and have greater numbers of physical and mental handicaps. Teenage mothers and fathers are often unable to continue their schooling owing to the demands of parenthood. Employment opportunities for them are limited. They fall victim to the health risks of the under-employed and undereducated.

IMPLICATIONS FOR NURSING

Consider the following case study:

> The Osborne family live in a middle-sized urban community. Mr. Osborne, age 40, was recently promoted to a supervisory position at the plant where he is employed. The plant manufactures herbicides and pesticides. Mrs. Osborne, age 38, works part-time as a receptionist at the nearby nuclear energy plant. The eldest Osborne son, age 18, is a lifeguard during the summer months, while the yougest son, age 16, plays the lead guitar in a rock and roll band at school dances and parties. The Osbornes also have a 6-year-old daughter who attends the elementary school near the airport.

Mr. Osborne's promotion has made it financially possible for the family to purchase a larger home. The house is in an older section of town and will require considerable renovations of the plumbing and heating systems plus plastering and painting.

The Osborne's assess their own health status as being excellent. Mr. Osborne takes pride in the fact that he has only missed 2 days of work in the past 10 years. He attributes his minor cough to smoking a pack of cigarettes a day. Except for two miscarriages, Mrs. Osborne's health history is also unremarkable. Her mother died recently of breast cancer. Both Mr. and Mrs. Osborne are about 15 pounds overweight.

The children have had no serious illnesses although the daughter has been inattentive and listless lately. The parents attribute this change in behavior to their recent move.

The eldest son is the only family member to participate in a regular exercise program. He is a member of a swimming club. He also plans to purchase a motorcycle with his summer earnings.

Mrs. Osborne generally prepares the family meals. Her husband is a "meat and potatoes" man and despite escalating food costs, she has managed to meet his needs.

The Osborne family is not unique. They are functioning as a family unit to achieve family goals. Are they aware however of the potential risks they face from environmental and genetic influences as well as their adopted life-style? The role of the community health nurse is to promote awareness of consumers' personal environments so that they, the consumers, may make informed decisions about their present and future health statuses. The nursing assessment of individuals and families must include a database that clearly identifies areas of potential and actual risk, so that both nurse and consumer can plan and implement realistic strategies to achieve desired health goals. The control of individual health is the primary responsibility of the individual, although the individual may need assistance in defining options. Does Mrs. Osborne know of the need to perform breast self-examinations? Does she know how to examine herself? Is Mr. Osborne aware of the hazards of smoking? Are the parents aware of the relationship between diet, exercise, smoking and coronary heart disease?

It must also be recognized that in some situations the individual is limited in controlling the physical and economic environment. The Osborne's can handle the changes required to turn their new house into a safe home. But is it practical, feasible, or advisable for Mr. Osborne to resign from his job? How many homes, schools, hospitals, and industries are dependent upon the electricity generated by the nuclear energy plant? Are the noise levels in the school by the airport at or near dangerous levels?

What are specific actions that nurses might consider in providing assistance to the Osborne family? Is the occupational health nurse at Mr. Osborne's plant aware of the chemicals being handled by employees that may cause health problems? Are there controls established by management or government for the processing and handling of these chemicals? Are controls being adhered to? Are employees informed of potential risks? Is there a screening program to detect early symptoms of illness?

Has the school nurse requested a noise-level appraisal from the appropriate agency in the community? Does the curriculum include topics addressing nutrition, accident prevention, and family life?

Has the generalized community health nurse discussed breast self-examination with Mrs. Osborne? Has there been coordination between the generalist and the school nurse in the evaluation of the daughter's symptoms? Has the relationship between diet, exercise, smoking and illness been discussed with the family? Have they been informed of the appropriate resources in the community available to provide guidance in changing lifestyles?

These interventions are not all-inclusive but designed to illustrate the pivotal role community health nurses play in assisting individuals and families in fulfilling their health potential.

CULTURE

In 1676, Spinoza wrote, "Whenever I have studied human affairs, I have carefully labored not to mock, lament, nor condemn, but only to understand."

From the moment of our birth to our final destination on earth, our behavior is molded by the influences of the culture of our society. As noted succinctly by Krech, Crutchfield, et al, "Culture is as people do."[32]

Culture is a way of life. It encompasses the ideals of a given group—their folklore, science, religion and philosophy; the ethos of a people—their norms, which govern morality, interpersonal relationships, art forms, family and social institutions, and verbal and nonverbal behavior; and the material values such as dress codes, food habits, shelter, tools and occupations. Culture is learned behavior that is passed on from generation to generation through members of a given society and represents ". . . the traditional ways of solving the problems of its members."[33] Culture is not stagnant, but rather it is dynamic, adaptive, and within limits, permits individual freedom and self-expression, thus allowing social change to occur.

American culture reflects such beliefs as free elementary and secondary school education for all; that "all men are created equal" (in philosophy if not in practice); and the innocence of those accused until proven guilty. Baseball is our national game and we are noted throughout the world for our hot dogs and hamburgers.

However, within our total cultural climate, differences in values do exist. We are a nation of diverse ethnic backgrounds, geographical variations, social class and occupational differences. The term **subculture** is used in reference to those segments of a society, which although they share many of the same beliefs, values, and norms of the dominant culture, also exhibit distinctive traits. Grits and greens are characteristic of southern food preferences; scrapple is unique to the Pennsylvania-Dutch communities; matzoh balls are Jewish; and fried bread is associated with the Navahoes. The cultural patterns of a society also provide explanations for life—events such as birth, death, puberty, childrearing, illness and disease—and prescribe the norms or acceptable behaviors of response to these situations.[34]

All persons, regardless of their cultural conditionings, like to think well of themselves and of those values and beliefs that give substance, stability, and meaning to their lives. When value systems are perceived as being threatened, barriers to communication arise. Consider the following example.

A program for improving the health care for migrant workers was established within a rural county health department. Priority was given to updating the immunization levels of the preschoolers. Arrangements were made for teams of public health nurses to visit the migrant farms, instruct parents in the desirability of adequate immunizations, and to administer the needed vaccines. The majority of the migrant families were of Spanish-American descent. Upon arrival at the farms, the nurses found that many of the children were, indeed, at risk. The mothers appeared receptive to the nurses' explanations about the benefits of immunizations; however, few mothers consented to sign the permission forms needed for the nurses to administer the vaccines. The nurses finally left feeling frustrated that their goal had not been achieved.

The nurses, influenced by the values of the scientific health-care system, anticipated patient compliance. Failing to obtain this desired outcome, the nurses interpreted the parents' behaviors as rejection of their belief that immunizations were essential to optimal health. The mothers on the other hand were not objecting to the content of the nurses' messages, but to the method of implementation. In their patriarchal subculture it is the father who is responsible for major decision making.[35] It is highly probable that these nurses now view Spanish-Americans as "unmotivated", and "non-compliant," while the nurses are perceived as "insensitive" and "uncaring".

Mechanic states that "The cultural approach to health involves study of the relationships between cultural content and cultural lifestyles on the one hand and definitions of health and responses to illness on the other."[36] It is not our intent to provide community health nurses with a detailed content analysis of all the cultural or subcultural groups they might interact with during a professional lifetime, but rather, to identify some cultural components in general that guide people in their decision-making processes relating to health and illness. Progress toward achieving health goals must be pursued in ways that are culturally acceptable and congruent with the values of the client system. Nurses must develop a sensitivity to the fact that difference need not imply deviance.

PERCEPTIONS OF HEALTH AND ILLNESS

The perceptions persons hold toward their physical and emotional state of well-being are influenced by, and, in turn, influence the cultural canons of the societal climate. Wellness or health may be perceived as the lack of physical or emotional discomfort, or the ability to continue to perform those role-specific activities sanctioned by the subcultural group.

Parsons defines health as, ". . . the state of optimum capacity of an individual for the effective performance of the roles and tasks for which he has been socialized. It is thus defined with reference to the individual's participation in the social system."[37] Hypertension is generally asymptomatic; therefore, being pain free the individual is able to carry on the tasks of a family breadwinner, parent, or otherwise fulfill the obligations associated with his or her culturally defined role. The scientific concept of hypertension as a chronic disease that if left untreated can result in death or disability is not congruent with the patient's beliefs, which have been internalized as a result of the normal learning process of socialization. Neither the patient nor his or her group of cultural orientation would view noncompliance with a treatment regimen as deviant behavior.

Illness as defined by Parsons is, ". . . some imputed generalized disturbance of the capacity of the individual for normally expected task or role performance which is not specific to his commitments to any particular task, role, collectivity, norm or value."[38] He adds further that cultural canons not only identify states of health and illness, but also specify the appropriate behaviors involved in sickness and in being well. Implicit in the valuation of health is the individual's obligation to take preventive measures when illness threatens. Illness is an undesirable state and expectations of the individual assuming the sick role include the following:[39]

- The person cannot overcome his illness by desire or will power, therefore, cannot be held responsible for the condition.
- Depending upon the nature of the disorder, sick persons are exempted from carrying out their usual social roles and tasks.
- The person is expected to desire to get well.
- The individual must seek technically competent help, and is obliged to cooperate with the caregivers in getting well.

The cultural or subcultural groups, therefore, define the conditions under which the sick role may legitimately be assumed, establish behaviorial expectations for that role, and, because cultural concepts are dynamic in nature, alter the role and behaviorial expectations based on changing group needs or current knowledge. Alcoholism, for instance, was long viewed as a self-inflicted behaviorial disorder that could be overcome by self-discipline alone; this perception was not limited to the lay members of society. Studies reveal that physicians frequently omit documenting the diagnosis of alcoholism on patient records, especially if the patient fails to fit the "skid-row" stereotype.[40] Society's denial of the "sick role" to the alcoholic was therefore reinforced by the actions of those judged technically competent to distinguish between stages of illness and health. While considerable controversy remains as to the illness concept of alcoholism and appropriate methods of treatment, societal attitudes over the past decade appear to be reflecting a gradual acceptance of alcoholism as an illness, with the alcoholic viewed as a suffering individual rather than one who is weak-willed and self-indulgent.

FOLK MEDICINE

Folk practices addressing disease prevention, health maintenance, and acceptable methods and sources of treatments are tenets of all cultures.[41] These beliefs are often interrelated with spiritual or religious values and are not always congruent with the community health nurse's scientific knowledge of disease causation and therapeutic interventions. Folk medicine practices may include attributing illnesses to "evil spirits," witchcraft, envy, or other "bad thoughts," emotionally traumatic experiences, the "will of god," or an "imbalance with nature," as examples. Depending upon the perceived source of the disorder, assistance may be sought from family, or a variety of folk practitioners; shamans, herbalists, medicine men, midwives, acupuncturists, or other individuals the subculture recognizes as being expert in diagnosis, treatment, or prevention. This is not to imply that assistance is never sought from what we consider traditional sources of care—physicians, clinics, and so forth. Certain symptoms may be classified as indicative of a "White man's" or "Angelo" disease, while other symptoms may be perceived as being unique to members of that group. According to their beliefs, "White man's" symptoms require "White man's" treatments. The severity of the symptom or disorder might also influence the source of preferred care. Minor physical complaints, or emotional disturbances might be viewed within the expertise of the indigenous health practitioner, while life-threatening events such as hemorrhage might be referred to a physician or a hospital. Consider the following case study:

> Mrs. Luna, a 35-year-old Native American residing on a reservation in the Southwestern part of this country, was pregnant with her fifth child. She was diagnosed as diabetic a year prior to this pregnancy and, until recently, had been fairly well controlled with diet and insulin. Mrs. Luna was now 34 weeks pregnant. Her diabetic condition was unstable, her blood pressure was markedly elevated, and weight gain totaled 55 pounds (25 kg). Mrs. Luna presented other laboratory and neurologic evidence of severe pre-eclampsia. The doctors at the Indian Health Service Clinic advised immediate hospitalization for mother and fetal monitoring, stabilization of the diabetes, rest and diet, and a probable cesarean birth. Mrs. Luna stated that she would discuss these recommendations with her family and return in the morning. When she did not return, a referral for a home evaluation was submitted to the community health nurse.
>
> The nurse found Mrs. Luna and her mother-in-law in the family compound. Mrs. Luna's systolic and diastolic pressures had risen from the previous day. Mrs. Luna's mother-in-law was not only the matriarch of the family, but also was recognized throughout the village as a knowledgeable practitioner of the native medicine. The mother-in-law informed the nurse that they understood that the doctors wanted to "cut-the-baby-out." She went on to explain that according to the "Indian way," once a woman demonstrated she was able to deliver "normally," as Mrs. Luna had done with her four previous pregnancies, any interference, such as that suggested by the doctors, would be considered "unnatural." Under no circumstances would a cesarean delivery be acceptable. Because Mrs. Luna and her mother-in-law had demonstrated receptiveness to diabetic therapy in the past, the nurse focused the discussion on Mrs. Luna's diabetes and its potential affect on the fetus. The mother-in-law agreed to allow Mrs. Luna's hospitalization for diabetic control.

The above case illustrates a potential source of misunderstanding between nurses and patients of other cultures—the locus of power or authority for making health-related decisions.

DECISION MAKING

It is generally accepted in the American culture that health-related decisions are the responsibility of the individuals involved, or in the case of minors, a mutually agreed-upon decision between parents, or one made by legal guardians. This is not always so within subcultures. Leininger notes, for instance, that the kinship system of Spanish-Americans is patriarchal with major decisions made by the father.[42] Under certain circumstances, the eldest son has authority over younger siblings. Aamodt reports that in matrilineal societies, such as that of the Hopi Indians, the mother's brother assumes disciplinary authority over nieces and nephews.[43] In matters concerning group behaviors, individual preferences may be considered secondary to those of the group as a whole. Since group affiliation and social interaction influence the individual's self-esteem, participation in activities not sanctioned by the group is unlikely. It is essential that community health nurses identify both formal and informal leaders of subcultural groups when planning programs directed toward group members, because they have the authority and power to influence the group's acceptance or rejection of the program. Immunizaion efforts, hypertension screening, and genetic screening programs for sickle cell disease or Tay-Sachs disease are examples of activities that require group acceptance and support. The latter two are of particular significance because they may be viewed as discriminatory. Native practitioners can also be included in the health care team as has been done with Native Americans. It must be accepted that patient responses and compliance may be optimized in the treatment of certain disorders if native practitioners are consulted in decisions of diagnosis and treatment.

FOOD AND CULTURE

The ingestion of food serves functions beyond those related to nutrition and physical survival. Specific foods may be perceived as having curative, causative, or preventive properties relating to health or illness. Hot chicken soup is the treatment of choice by millions of Americans for the common cold. Various subcultures within the American society similarly place therapeutic value on foods. For instance, Campbell and Chang report that the Chinese categorize diseases according to "hot" and "cold" classifications.[44] This also occurs among Native Americans and Mexican-Americans.[45] Illnesses falling into the "hot" category are treated with "cold" food, and vice versa. In other subcultures, pregnant women may be encouraged to eat specific foods to ensure a healthy child or a child of a particular sex. Still other foods may be consumed to restore or increase sexual potency.

Dietary practices are not infrequently related to the spiritual or religious doctrines of the subcultures. The dietary laws developed by the ancient Hebrews prohibiting pork and certain seafoods were essentially public health measures to prevent disease. Members of The Church of Jesus Christ of Latter-Day Saints (Mormons) abstain from all drinks containing caffeine, such as tea, coffee, and soft drinks, and also alcohol and tobacco. While other aspects of the social and psychological components of the Mormon life-style must be considered as contributing factors, it is significant to note that mortality rates from cancer and cardiovascular diseases in Mormons is considerably lower than the national average.[46]

Not all cultural food patterns are symbolic of health or spiritual practices, but a matter of preference based on exposure. We tend to prefer to eat those foods we are familiar with, enjoy, and can afford. However, community health nurses must be cognizant of food patterns and the beliefs and values associated with food preferences. If scientifically defined therapeutic diets are to be complied with, they must be compatible with cultural canons and patient potential. Campbell and Chang present an excellent example of poor patient potential: Instructing a hypertensive patient of Oriental heritage to eliminate soy sauce from the diet completely represents a change in life-style so drastic that compliance would probably be minimal.[47] A diabetic can use a substitute for sugar, but there is no substitute for soy sauce. Counseling directed at reducing the amount of soy sauce used and focusing on sodium restriction in other, less-valued components of the diet, increases the potential for compliance without negatively affecting the therapeutic goal.

COMMUNICATIONS

Caregivers and patients who do not speak the same formal language obviously present problems in communicating. Therefore, if services are offered to non-English speaking patients, these services should include translators. Using friends, family members, or other patients in interpreter-roles is not advisable (unless specifically requested by the patient) for two reasons: (1) it represents a breach of patient confidentiality, and (2) there is no assurance that the message is being translated accurately, regardless of the well-meaning intentions of the interpreter. Physicians, nurses, or paraprofessionals fluent in the language of the client group and possessing some medical knowledge and insight into the cultural tenets of the client group are preferable. Pharmacy labels, health education pamphlets, and clinic signs or posters should also be in language that is familiar to the clients.

Effective communication implies more than exchanging messages in the same tongue. The manner in which the message is delivered and the choice of words must also be considered. Health professionals tend to speak in the vocabulary of their profession when describing body functioning or anatomic parts. Terms such as void, buttocks, vagina, immunization, or carbohydrates may not be understood. The patient might not ask for clarification feeling that this might be rude. Nurses are instructed in the value of eye-to-eye contact and touching in developing a trusting rapport with patients; however, direct eye contact to members of some subcultures, such as certain Native American tribes, might be viewed as dominant behavior and in conflict with their cultural standard of interpersonal relationships, which are based on humility and respect. In her discussion of Mexican-American folk beliefs, Abril states that children are believed to be at particular risk for illnesses caused by the "Evil Eye" or "Mal Ojo." It is believed that if someone, especially a woman, admires someone else's child (looking at the child without actually touching him) the child may fall ill from "Ojo."[48]

Long waiting-periods in clinics, home visits that have not been pre-arranged, speaking in harsh or rapid fashion, insensitivity to a patient's sense of modesty are all factors that communicate to persons of all cultures, a lack of respect by the caregivers for the client system.

The cultural canons of a people influence their perceptions of illness and health and define behaviors appropriate to resolving the former and maintaining the latter. Community health nurses must be cognizant of these differences when nursing interventions are planned. Interventions that are imposed or are perceived to threaten strongly held beliefs will be rejected by the client. However, as noted by Dougherty, ". . . behavior changes can be made if they are consistent with established patterns, beliefs, and values."[49] Leininger adds that ". . . nursing care practices should become more tailor-made to fit the needs of different cultures or subcultures, rather than the past trend of having nursing and medical care fit with the dominant Anglo-American values and practices."[50] This philosophy seems more relevant than ever today in light of increased interest in tracing one's "roots" and re-establishing bonds with one's ethnic heritage. The risk is not in the "belonging" to a particular cultural group but in the failure of health care providers to develop health-care delivery programs, which attract rather than repel potential users.

There are a few words of caution, however. Banks writes that "We should not exaggerate the extent of cultural pluralism in the United States, and should realize that widespread cultural assimilation has taken place in America. To try to perceive cultural differences where none exist may be as detrimental as ignoring those which are real."[51] Mechanic adds that "it is imperative to differentiate between behaviors which are the result of cultural conditioning as opposed to those which are the result of innate inability, physiological defect, or inconsistent or haphazard childrearing."[52] We might add lack of knowledge or education to Mechanic's list. Both writers suggest "starting where the learner is." Do not stereotype. Through observation, interviewing, research and listening, the nurse must gain an accurate perception of the client's posture as it relates to cultural values and health behaviors.

Many years ago, as a young student nurse at a large metropolitan medical center, I was exposed to a patient care situation, which at the time, unfortunately, held little more than a curious interest for me. An elderly man in the terminal stages of a malignant disease was admitted to the medical unit where I was assigned. He was a patriarch to the gypsy community in the city. Much to the chagrin of the nursing staff, the hospital administration permitted his followers, a few at a time, to remain with him around the clock and to bring in specially prepared foods and "medicinals." Several times a day, the curtains would be drawn around his bed and the sounds of chanting would drift throughout the ward. The granting of such privileges 20 years ago, particularly to a ward patient, was indeed unique. The patient expired 3 or 4 days later. Today, I am acutely aware of the cultural significance of the episode and appreciate the insight demonstrated by that particular hospital administration.

COMMUNITY RISK FACTORS

Since communities are composed of people living or interacting within the same environmental boundaries it is tempting to limit this discussion to the simple statement that "communities at risk equal all of the above." However, the point must be stressed that identification and assessment of community risk factors relating to health status are multidimensional and complex. Morbidity and mortality data in and of themselves are insufficient in determining real or potential risk. Characteristics of the physical environment, the availability and accessibility of health-related services, the age, sex, and racial composition of the population, the predominant cultural influences, and the social and economic conditions all have an impact on the overall health status of a given community, whether or not the community is being defined in a narrow context, such as a school, neighborhood, or census tract, or in the broader context of a city, county, state, or nation. The community health nurse must focus on the boundary of orientation; that is, data regarding health status and resources in an affluent, predominantly White suburb are of little productive value to the community health nurse in planning for the health needs of an urban, predominantly Black neighborhood. The following information then is presented as a guide to community health nurses in assessing degrees of risk in order to develop nursing priorities and participate in program planning and goal development at agency, community, and governmental levels.

PHYSICAL ENVIRONMENT

Communities may be at risk by the mere fact that they exist in a certain geographic area and are susceptible to earthquakes, floods, tornadoes, hurricanes, volcanoes, extremes of temperature, or flow of air currents that influence retention of air pollutants.[53]

Man-made variables influencing the physical environment include types of industry, quality and density of housing volume and patterns of traffic, crime rates, and food and water sources.

Obviously it is not within the realm of community health nursing to control acts of nature, however, it is essential that community plans exist that address the physical and emotional needs of populations threatened by such calamities, whether natural or man-made. Questions the community health nurse may ask in relation to disaster risks include the following:

1. Is there a disaster plan developed for the community? Does the plan identify areas of responsibility by specific agency, either governmental, voluntary, or volunteer. Which agency, for instance, is responsible for food and water supplies to shelters; who is accountable for staffing first-aid stations or shelters; who coordinates communication and evacuation or transportation needs? Are there, in fact, designated shelter areas that are known to the public at large?
2. Is the nurse's agency of employment involved in the disaster plan? If so, are the agency's responsibilities clearly defined to staff? Is there an effective "alert" or "on-call" system developed to ensure prompt agency response? Are periodic in-service programs developed to update personnel skills in meeting the physical and emotional needs of communities traumatized by disaster?
3. Do all of the agencies and governmental bodies involved meet periodically to review, update, or revise disaster plans and areas of responsibility? Are there arrangements made for community-based "mock disaster" drills at regular intervals to identify and correct any program deficiencies?
4. Do mechanisms exist for the identification of persons more susceptible to adverse weather conditions and are resources available to meet their needs? Because elderly persons (especially those with pulmonary and circulatory disorders) have increased intolerance to cold and heat, prolonged periods of cold weather combined with limited or costly fuel supplies might necessitate the establishment of communal living arrangements ("cold" shelters) or low-cost provisions of heat. Air pollution persisting over days or weeks can further debilitate or prove fatal to persons with chronic pulmonary disorders. These persons are generally advised to stay indoors and limit activity; therefore, assistance in shopping or obtaining medications may be required. Resources to provide additional oxygen equipment or temporary air conditioning might be developed.

Again it is stressed that answers to these questions will not control the weather or prevent the occurrence of a natural or man-made disaster. However, absence of a disaster-preparedness program increases the risk of death and of physical and emotional disabilities, which remain after the disaster is over.

POPULATION CHARACTERISTICS

The process of identifying populations at risk to focus limited resources on those in greatest need involves the knowledge and ability to relate the demographic variables of the population to a variety of data, such as birth rates, morbidity and mortality data, communicable disease reports, and community economic profiles. The nurse must keep up with current research findings regarding the health-risk probabilities for different races, cultural or ethnic groups, economic levels and both sexes. Continuous observation and a familiarity with other allied-health and social-service agencies is also needed. Participation on community task forces, councils, committees and advisory boards is an excellent means of contributing to the identification and resolution of population health problems.

The process of planning for populations at risk is a team responsibility. The following sources might be useful in gathering assessment data.

1. City or county planning offices generate statistics on income levels by census tracts or planning districts.
2. Hospital emergency rooms gather data on accidents and other causes of trauma, including poisoning.
3. School records can provide information on immunization levels, absenteeism, and known adolescent pregnancies.
4. Vital statistic's offices at local or state levels maintain data on infant mortality, births, and therapeutic abortions. Abortion and birth data by age can prove extremely useful in identifying adolescents at risk.
5. Local and state health departments are sources of information on reportable communicable diseases and various environmental hazards.
6. Regional health systems agencies gather a variety of data, including information on the availability and types of resources in the area.
7. Research reports in various journals.
8. Area offices on aging, Meals-on-Wheels, or other agencies dealing with the aged and handicapped.
9. Community mental-health centers and local mental-health and mental-retardation service boards.
10. Social service agencies, both public and voluntary.

This list is by no means all-inclusive but is provided as a guide to community resources. The nurse should be aware that state and federal legislation may limit the type of information that can be shared. Information on specific patients is generally not released without the patient's written consent.

The following case study illustrates the type of programs that can be developed for clients as a result of nursing assessments:

> Several of the community health nurses working in an urban health department were meeting for a case conference. The family under discussion consisted of a 20-year-old mother, two children, aged 2 and 8 months, and a father, aged 21. The family had lived in the area for less than a year. The husband was in the military and assigned to a nearby naval base, however, during the past year his ship had only been in port for 4 months. The case conference was being held to discuss the many problems this mother was having with her role as a parent. The children were receiving pediatric care at the health department clinic and were both healthy and developing normally. The mother, however, was often concerned with toilet training, discipline, sleep and eating habits, and was obviously frustrated by her own perceived inability to deal with these situations. As the conference progressed, the nurses began to notice similarities between this family's problems and other families living in the area near the clinic. Many of the parents, particularly the mothers, had little factual knowledge about growth and development of children, their personal self-esteem was low, and they had few support systems, with husbands being away for long periods of time, if present at all. The mobility in the neighborhood was high, therefore, friendships were difficult to establish. Relatives were either nonexistent or too geographically distant to be of assistance. The nurses felt more information was needed about the neighborhood in general and contacted a social service agency to determine problems that they might have identified with the same population. The social service report revealed that the five census tracts surrounding the clinic had the highest incidence of child abuse in the city and that their social workers would be most interested in collaborating with the nurses in the development and implementation of a program to address the problem.

The nurses and social workers felt a preventive approach to child abuse should be considered, but decided their first step should be to determine what assistance, if any, parents would be interested in receiving. Questionnaires were developed to conduct an informal survey of parents obtaining services at the clinic and the social service agency. Responses revealed needs for information related to childhood growth and development, nutrition, and discipline, in addition to parental needs of sharing parental experiences and feelings about childrearing. Objectives and a course outline were prepared for a "Parenting Program" to be conducted by nurses and social workers, and to include opportunities for parents to meet together to discuss mutual concerns. The children, all preschoolers, would attend and receive a developmental assessment and appropriate stimulating activities according to their stage of development. Time was also allowed for parents and children to "get together" at the end of the 2-hour session for socializing and a review of the child's activities. A local church donated space, and other community organizations contributed play equipment. The initial parenting class was scheduled for once a week, however, parental reactions were so positive that applications for attendance increased to the point where within 6 months, three sessions per week were being held.

COMMUNICABLE DISEASES

Little has been mentioned thus far regarding the impact of communicable diseases, especially those that are preventable. With the exception of sexually transmitted diseases, these diseases have shown a dramatic decline in incidence and their overall impact on the health of the nation as a whole is minimal. This is not to imply that communicable disease control is no longer a community health concern. On the contrary, recent statistics show that despite the availability of vaccines to prevent polio, rubella, mumps, rubeola, diphtheria, tetanus, and pertussis, these conditions still exist and overall immunization levels, particularly in children, are less than optimal. In 1975, an estimated 32% of the children between the ages of 1 and 4 were not adequately protected against measles, 25% were at risk for DPT (diphtheria, pertussis, and tetanus), 38% were not protected against rubella, and 35% had not been fully immunized against polio.

More recent data indicate that there is a significant shift in the age of risk for susceptibility to rubella and rubeola.

The majority of rubella and rubeola cases are no longer occurring in the preschool and early elementary school populations. In 1977, more than 60% of reported measles cases occurred in children 10 years of age or older with 20% of these in the 15 to 19-year-old age group. In the same year, 70% of reported cases of rubella occurred in adolescents and young adults 15 years of age or older. The susceptibility of a community to outbreaks of communicable diseases such as rubella, rubeola, and others must be considered a community-risk factor because the overall health and economic impact of these diseases is not limited to the striken individual. The effects of a rubella infection in a woman in her first trimester of pregnancy are well-documented.

Most states have legislation requiring minimal levels of immunizations for children entering school. Many of these laws, particularly those specifically addressing rubella and rubeola, were enacted after the present adolescent population entered school, therefore, they were exempted from providing proof of immunization status. Many of these children may have been immunized prior to 12 months of age. It is now recognized that persisting maternal antibodies present in infants interfere with seroconversion, therefore, older children and young adolescents immunized prior to 1 year of age may be susceptible to infection. Both factors probably contribute to the rubella and rubeola patterns now being encountered.

Guidelines for community health nurses and preventable communicable disease include the following:

1. Identification of underimmunized and nonimmunized infants, children, and adolescents through monitoring of clinic and school health records.
2. Development and implementation of community-based educational programs that focus on recommended ages for immunizing, sources of care, state legislation requiring specific immunizations

at certain times such as school entrance and health risks from delay or omission of vaccine administration. Educational efforts should be directed toward completing the basic series of DPT, polio vaccine, and receiving MMR by 15 months of age.

3. Reporting immediately to the local health department cases of actual or suspected communicable diseases. This is particularly relevant to nurses functioning in school health, occupational, or military settings where rubella or rubeola is suspected.
4. Counseling of adolescents, particularly females who are sexually active, about the effects of rubella or rubeola infections during the first trimester of pregnancy. If their immunization status is unknown, or appropriate vaccines were not received at the appropriate age, information about resources for blood titer determinations, immunizations, or reimmunizations should be made available to them. Family planning clinics, sexually transmitted diseases clinics, secondary schools, colleges and universities, military bases and occupational sites provide unique settings for reaching the adolescent-aged population.
5. Identifying persons at risk for pulmonary disorders. This includes persons over 65 years of age and persons over age 2 with chronic illnesses such as emphysema, diabetes, cystic fibrosis, cardiovascular disorders, and so forth. Vaccines are now available to prevent pneumococcal pneumonia and various strains of viral influenza.

Gonorrhea ranks first among reportable communicable diseases in the United States, followed by chickenpox and syphilis. While incidence rates for syphilis appear to be leveling, rates for gonorrhea continue to climb, especially among teenagers. The lack of a serologic test for gonorrhea as is available for syphilis often makes diagnosis difficult, because approximately 80% of females and 12% of males are asymptomatic. There also remains the social stigma attached to venereal diseases, which undoubtedly leads to underreporting and treatment.

The key factors involved in the control of sexually transmitted diseases include prevention, early detection, prompt treatment, and follow-up of contacts. One form of prevention is the prophylactic use of ophthalmic ointment or drops with newborns. This is required by law in some states. Other methods include careful selection of sexual partners (whether heterosexual or homosexual), the use of condoms, and of course, abstinence.

The community health nurse can prove most valuable in the educational processes by addressing disease transmission problems, prevention, and treatment. Intensified public education, particularly for teenagers and young adults, is in order. Frank discussions of the consequences of sexual activity during adolescence should be included in the curriculums of schools no later than the junior high-school level. This would require the support and approval of parent groups who are also in need of accurate information. School nurses are again in unique positions to initiate or politick for these kinds of programs.

Many states have passed legislation allowing persons under 18 years of age to consent to their own treatment for venereal diseases. Teenagers should be made aware of this, because fear of parental reaction can interfere with teenagers seeking assistance if they suspect that they are infected. Contact investigations must be conducted discreetly, especially if involving adolescents or homosexuals for the same reasons. Educational and screening programs in family planning, adolescent, maternity, or other type clinics, where sexually active teenagers are under care, need to be developed if they are not available in the community. It should be noted that the term "sexually transmitted diseases" is not limited to syphilis and gonorrhea. The following diseases are also included in this classification: nongonococcal urethritis, trichomoniasis, genital herpes, vulvovaginal candidiasis, *Hemophilus vaginalis* vaginitis, pediculosis pubis, scabies, genital warts, chancroid, lymphogranuloma venereum, granuloma inguinale, and hepatitis B.

Tuberculosis while not as prevalent, as in the past remains a community health concern especially with the poor, those with alcohol debilitation, and the elderly. Many cases in the elderly are the result of infections acquired when they were young and often undiagnosed at the time. Chronic diseases and a generalized lowered resistance reactivates the bacilli. The nurse's role in the management of tuberculosis includes the following:

1. Referral for early diagnosis and treatment. Close

monitoring may be required to ensure the patient is faithful to the medication regimen.
2. Identification of the source and evaluation of close contacts through skin testing and x-rays.
3. Providing the patient, family, and contacts with information on the etiology of the disease, modes of transmission, and possible side effects of medication.
4. Surveillance to encourage continued medical supervision.
5. Instruction of the patient and family in methods of preventing the spread of the disease.

AVAILABILITY OF HEALTH SERVICES

Of particular importance when determining risk factors of a community is the availability and accessibility of health care and related services. What kinds of health-and-illness services exist in the community and what barriers are evident to deter use? Physicians, hospitals, clinics, dental services, pharmacies, home-care services, school and occupational health programs, emergency medical services, mental health programs, and social services must be considered in light of population needs. If services exist, are they provided in a manner that is culturally acceptable to the client system? Is transportation provided or obtainable? Are services provided at hours consistent with the life-style of consumers? Is babysitting or child care available? And are the services affordable?

The economic factors have long been the greatest barrier to obtaining health care particularly for the poor population. Recent studies, however, indicate that the health care utilization rate for the poor is increasing and average numbers of physician contacts per year are as high or higher than those of the more affluent population.[54,55] Medicaid and Medicare have to a great extent made health care more accessible to the poor, however, this is not to imply that the health status of the economically disadvantaged is equal to that of the non-poor population. The poor suffer in greater proportions from both acute and chronic illnesses, therefore, their need for health care is greater. Removing the financial barriers to care increases their perceptions of need for medical attention. However, even with Medicaid and Medicare, not all poor or indigent persons are eligible for coverage. Overall, 77% of the population is covered by some form of public or private health insurance.[56] It is estimated that in 1978, 18 million persons in this country will have no protection against health care expenses.[57] The uninsured tend to be relatively young with 44% being 17 years of age or younger, poorly educated, with low incomes, and dwell in urban areas.[58]

Eighty percent of the population report a regular source of medical care, especially children under 15 years of age and persons 65 years of age or older.[59] Young adults, especially males, are least likely to have a regular source of care. The most common source of care is a physician's office or group practice particularly for higher income groups and children. Blacks and other minorities, and families with incomes below $5000 per year rely on hospital outpatient clinics and emergency rooms in proportionately greater numbers than the White and higher income populations. Residents of rural areas tend to have fewer encounters with a health source than urban dwellers. This suggests continued inequities in the quality of care received and reflects the unequal distribution of private health-care resources. Urban ghettos and rural areas do not attract the private medical-entrepreneur primarily because of economic conditions although the need in these areas is obviously tremendous in scope.

Women of childbearing age and low-income families most often report difficulties in obtaining care.[60] In addition to financial barriers—inconvenient office hours, trouble getting an appointment, and transportation are cited as frequent problems. Transportation also appears to be a significant barrier to the elderly.

SUMMARY

With the exception of those risk factors controlled by nature, virtually all individual and community risks discussed can be modified by individual and social actions. Noise, water, and air pollution can be reduced; exposure to teratogenetic, mutagenic, and other disease-producing chemicals can be managed; seat belts for adults and safety seats for children can be used during automobile rides; smoking can be stopped; alcohol and other substance abuse can be eliminated. Equities in education, employment opportunities, housing and access to quality medical care can be achieved if society is willing to shoulder the financial responsibility. Yeracaris and Kim warn, ". . . socieconomic inequities in our society continue to contribute wasted lives—a social by-product a democratic and human society can no longer afford."[61]

Technology exists for the elimination of death and disability from childhood communicable diseases. Unwanted children need never be conceived if appropriate family planning methods are used by both sexes; the list is endless. Control of even a few of these factors would undobutedly contribute toward the reduction of disease-producing stressful stimuli, which influence the number and quality of our years on this planet.

Implications for community health nursing are complex. In addition to those already identified, nursing actions should include the following:

1. Promotion of a nutritionally sound diet and exercise program thoughout the life cycle.
2. Thorough assessment of all patients' employment histories to identify real or potential health hazards.
3. Thorough assessment of patient and family coping mechanisms used to deal with stressful situations in their social and physical environment.
4. Early detection of handicapping conditions in children, which have the potential for interfering with achievement of their full physical, emotional, and social potential. This includes detection and treatment of the wide range of learning disabilities, in addition to physical and emotional disorders.
5. Research directed toward the identification of nursing strategies that will prove effective in modifying patient and family behavior in positive directions.

Nurses as individuals and as the single largest subsystem in the health-care delivery system must assert their political power in supporting public health issues such as,

1. Control of chemical and nuclear waste disposal.
2. Establishment and strict enforcement of air, water, food, and noise control standards.
3. Support of a more equitable system of financing health care.
4. Alternatives to institutional care for the disabled elderly.
5. Introduction of Family Life Education programs during the elementary school years that go beyond the teaching of anatomy and physiology and venereal disease control. Content should include the pnysical, emotional, and financial preparation for parenthood, growth and development of children, and the art and skills of parenting.

How many, if any, of the previous issues will be acceptable to any given community is open to speculation. People resent it if they feel they are being told what to do. As noted by the National Science Foundation, ". . . the public seems clearly willing to suffer a much larger risk (or higher probability of hazard) if that choice is in the individual's hands than if a surrogate decision-maker arrives at the decision for him."[62] Hence, the failure of prohibition and the resistance now to the 55 mile per hour speed limit. The greater the perceived benefit to the group at large, the greater the acceptable risk society is willing to assume. Therefore, the economic benefits brought to a community by a chemical-producing industry may overshadow the probability of health hazards, which might not become evident for 20 to 30 years.

HEALTH HAZARD APPRAISALS

Traditional health education efforts directed toward changing life-style behaviors have had limited success. A notable exception appears to be the reduction in mortality rates from cardiovascular disorders because of increased public awareness of the effects of diet, exercise, and smoking on the cardiovascular system. People are perceiving themselves to be at risk and in control of those factors that reduce or increase the probability of illness.

A relatively new approach in persuading persons to change their life-styles is called risk-analysis or health hazard appraisal. The **health hazard appraisal (HHA)** usually consists of a series of questions about an individual's personal and family health history, physical measurements, blood pressure and behaviors related to smoking, exercise, and drug and alcohol abuse. Based on probability tables developed from U.S. mortality rates, a risk assessment is then calculated from the personal profile along with a goal that would result in risk reduction. For instance, a 35-year-old male who drinks heavily, smokes, and leads a sedentary life might have a "risk age" of 40 years (*i.e.*, within the next 10 years he has the same chance of dying as a person 5 years older). By altering his behavior he might be able to reach an "achievable age" of 33. It has been found, though, that this information alone is insufficient to produce change. Counseling and follow-up are also needed to reinforce the data. Several studies have demonstrated substantial changes in participants' life-styles and related drops in risk age.[63] Should further studies confirm the usefulness of this type of risk assessment, community health nurses might play a pivotal role in the counseling and educational phases of the program.

REFERENCES

1. Sakalep J: The meaning of health and illness. In Mitchell P (ed): Concepts Basic to Nursing Practice. New York, McGraw-Hill, 1973
2. Suchman E: Sociology and the Field of Public Health, New York, Russell Sage, 1963
3. Carter C O: An ABC of Medical Genetics, p 1. Boston, Little Brown, 1969
4. Ibid
5. Center for Disease Control: Ten Leading Causes of Death in the United States. Atlanta, 1975
6. Eckholm E P: The Picture of Health, p 19. New York, W W Morton, 1977
7. National Foundation, March of Dimes: Genetic Counseling. New York, 1972
8. National Research Council: Genetic Screening Programs, Principles and Research, p 11. Washington, D C, National Academy of Sciences, 1975
9. National Foundation, March of Dimes, op cit
10. Hendin D, Marks J: The Genetic Connection. New York, William Morrow, 1978
11. Ibid
12. Carter C O, op cit
13. Holtzman N A: Newborn Screening for Genetic-Metabolic Diseases, p 7. DHEW Publication No. 77-5207, 1977
14. Riccardi V M: Health care and disease prevention through genetic counseling: a regional approach. Am J Public Health Vol. 68, No. 3:268–272, 1976
15. The National Foundation, March of Dimes, op cit
16. Riccardi V M, op cit
17. The National Research Council, op cit, p 3
18. Auger J R: Behavioral Systems and Nursing, p 118. Englewood Cliffs, Prentice-Hall, 1976
19. Ibid
20. Tyroler H A, James S A: Blood pressure and skin color. Am J Public Health Vol. 68, No. 11:1170–1172
21. Health Resources Administration: Health United States—1976–77. DHEW Publication No. (HRA) 77-1232, 1977
22. Harburg E, Gleiberman L, Roeper P, Ozgoren F, Schork MA: Skin color, ethnicity, and blood pressure I: Detroit Blacks. Am J Public Health Vol. 68, No. 11:1177–1188, 1978
23. National Institute of Enivronmental Health: Basic Concepts of Environmental Health. DHEW Publication No. 77-1254, 1977
24. Health Resources Administration, op cit
25. National Institute of Environmental Health, op cit
26. Burton L E, Smith H H: Public Health and Community Medicine, 2nd ed. Baltimore, Williams & Wilkins, 1975
27. Ibid, p 440
28. Ibid
29. Health Resources Administration: Health United States, 1975, DHEW Publication No. (HRA) 76-1232, 1976
30. Metropolitan Life Insurance Company: Mortality from Leading Types of Accidents. Statistical Bulletin, pp 9–12. (59) 1978
31. Environmental Protection Agency. Noise: A Health Problem. Washington, D C, 1978
32. Krech D, Crutchfield R S, Ballachey E L: Individuals and Society, p 346. New York, McGraw-Hill, 1962
33. Ibid, p 380
34. Aamodt A: Culture. In Clark A (ed): Culture, Childbearing, Health Professionals. Philadelphia, F A Davis, 1977
35. Leininger M: The Cultural Context of Behavior: Spanish Americans and Nursing Care. In Spradley BW (ed): Contemporary Community Nursing, pp 159–174. Boston, Little Brown, 1975
36. Mechanic D: Medical Sociology, p 52. New York, Free Press, 1968
37. Parsons T: Social Structure and Personality, p 274. London, Free Press, 1970
38. Ibid, p 274
39. Ibid
40. Blaine M, Willis T, Chanety M: Social factors in the diagnosis of alcoholism: Part I. Quarterly Journal on Alcohol, 24:640–664, 1963
41. Leininger M: Transcultural nursing: A promising subfield of study for nurses. In Reinhardt, A Quinn M (eds): Current Practice in Family-Centered Nursing, pp 36–50. St. Louis, C V Mosby, 1977
42. Leininger M, op cit
43. Aamodt A, op cit
44. Campbell T, Chang B: Health care of the Chinese in

America. In Spradley BW (ed): Contemporary Community Nursing, pp 189–197. Boston, Little Brown, 1975
45. Abrit I F: Mexican-American folk beliefs: How they affect health care. In O'Connor AB (ed): Nursing in Community Health Settings, pp 72–81. New York, American Journal of Nursing, 1978
46. Henry J P, Stephens P M: Stress, Health and the Social Environment. New York, Springer-Verlog, 1977
47. Campbell T, Chang B, op cit, p 194
48. Abril I F, op cit, 74
49. Dougherty M C: A cultural approach to the nurse's role in health care planning. In Spradley BW (ed): Contemporary Community Nursing, pp 439–445. Boston, Little Brown, 1975
50. Leininger M, op cit, p 39
51. Banks J: Pluralism and the schools. In Weiser M (ed): Ethnic America, pp 163–166. New York, H W Wilson, 1978
52. Mechanic D: op cit, p 32
53. Freedman B: Sanitarian's Handbook, 4th ed. New Orleans, Peerless, 1977
54. Andersen R: Health status indices and access to medical care. Am J Public Health 68:458–463, 1978
55. Skinner E A, German P S, Shapero S, Chase G A, Zauber A G: Use of ambulatory health services by the near poor. Am J Public Health Vol. 68, No. 12:1195–1201, 1978
56. Health Resources Administration, op cit, 1976
57. Health Resources Administration, op cit, 1977
58. Ibid
59. Ibid
60. Ibid
61. Yeracaris C A, Kim J H: Socioeconomic differentials in selected causes of death. Am J Public Health Vol. 68, No. 4:342–351, 1978
62. National Science Foundation: Chemicals and Health: Report of the Panel on Chemicals and Health of the President's Science Advisory Committee, p 184. Washington D C, 1977
63. Milsum J H: Health, risk factor reduction and lifestyle change. In Faber M (ed): Family and Community Health 3:1–13, 1980.

PART V

STRENGTHENING AND EXTENDING COMMUNITY HEALTH NURSING IN VIEW OF CHANGING HEALTH NEEDS

12

Strengthening and Extending Community-Health Nursing Services

Sheila Spelman

CURRENT AND FUTURE TRENDS

Nursing, society, and the health-care system are all in the midst of an evolutionary period that promises to alter the values and focus of professional practice in significant ways.

NURSING

Despite generations of debate, the question of the exact nature of nursing and the minimal educational requirements necessary for entry into the profession remain unanswered and even more confusing than ever. Nurses are prepared in 2- and 3-year diploma programs, 2-year associate-degree programs, and 4-year baccalaureate programs. Recently, yet another type of program has been initiated in which graduates receive an ND, or doctorate in nursing, degree as their basic educational preparation.

In 1960, the American Nurses' Association's (ANA) House of Delegates adopted a resolution designating baccalaureate programs as the basic educational foundation for professional nursing. The ANA expanded this concept in 1965 by advocating two levels of nursing preparation and practice: the baccalaureate education for "professional" nurses and the associate degree education for "technical" nursing practice. In 1978, the ANA's House of Delegates established goals for the implementation of their proposals: the two levels of practice were to be clearly defined and competencies for each level identified by 1980, and by 1985, baccalaureate preparation for "professional" nurses would become a reality. They also called for greater flexibility in designing educational programs to permit the majority of practicing registered nurses, who do not have baccalaureate degrees, to advance their careers. The ANA's proposals have not been universally embraced by the nursing profession.

Community health nursing has a tradition of recognizing baccalaureate preparation as the desirable level of entry into practice. The required skills of a community health nurse go beyond the technical, curative procedures that are essential to the care of the acutely ill. The community health nurse is a teacher, coordinator, planner, counselor, facilitator, and evaluator, as well as caregiver and consumer advocate. The focus of service is to individuals, families, and groups through independent and multidisciplinary approaches. The essence of community health practice revolves around human systems, in illness and in health, within a physical, social, and emotional environment. Knowledge of the concepts derived from social, behavioral, organizational, educational, as well as the biologic sciences is a necessity in developing competency in community-health nursing practice. Competence, as defined by the Association of State and Territorial Directors of Nursing is ". . . the quality of being functionally adequate in performing activities and assuming the role of a specified position with the requisite knowledge, ability, capability, skill, judgement, attitudes and values."[1] The Public Health Nursing section of the American Public Health Association recommends the title Public Health Nursing ". . . as descriptive of this special area of practice because the essential knowledge needed for practice is the synthesis of public health science and professional nursing theories."[2]

Nurse Practitioners. The federal government defines a nurse practitioner as ". . . a registered nurse who has successfully completed a formal program of study designed to prepare registered nurses to perform in an expanded role in the delivery of primary health care. . . ."[3] The components of this expanded role include physical assessment, medical history taking, instruction and counseling services and coordination of care to individuals and families. Nurse practitioners are generally required to function under the medical direction of a physician with clearly defined protocols defining the scope and limitations of their activities. As with the rest of the nursing profession, there is little uniformity in the basic educational preparation of nurse practitioners, therefore, practitioners may have baccalaureate or master's degrees, or be graduates of diploma programs. Specialized fields for nurse practitioners include anesthesiology, family practice, family planning, obstetrics and gynecology, pediatrics, school health and geriatrics.

The emergence of the role of the nurse practitioner as a member of the public health team has unlimited potential especially in areas where access to physicians is limited, as in rural, school, and occupational settings.

QUALITY ASSURANCE

The escalating costs of health care combined with increased public concern for quality service and cost containment have not gone unnoticed by governmental bodies controlling fiscal resources. The Social Security Amendments of 1972 (P.L. 92-603), and the Health Maintenance Organization Act of 1973 (P.L. 93-222), both contain mandates for the implementation of quality control mechanisms. The theme is repeated in SECTION 1502 of the National Health Planning and Resources Development Act of 1974 (P.L. 93-641), in which, "The promotion of activities to achieve needed improvements in the quality of health services . . ." is listed as a national health priority.[3]

Appproaches to the assessment of quality in health care frequently focus on one or more of the following criteria: structure, process, or outcomes.[4,5]

Structure criteria address organizational characteristics such as funding sources, licensure, accreditation, philosophy, policies, type of personnel, equipment and other elements commonly referred to as resources.[6]

Process criteria deal with the actual delivery of patient care and encompass all four phases of the nursing process: (1) assessment of the client's status of well-being and identification of problem areas, (2) goal planning for the resolution of the problems identified, (3) implementation of the care plan, and (4) evaluation of the progress toward problem resolution with revisions in the plan as needed and determined by the patient's progress.[7] Process criteria are oriented toward the activities of the care provider.

Outcome criteria deal with the results of the care provided and are oriented toward the actual changes or alterations in the client's health status or behavior. Ideally, outcome criteria should also reflect client satisfaction with the services received.[8]

The distinction between these three measures may be clarified by the following example:

1. Childhood immunizations (DPT, polio, MMR) will be provided at no cost to persons 18 years of age or under at all health department clinics. (Structure)
2. The nurse will discuss possible reactions to MMR vaccine with parent/guardian prior to administration (Process)
3. By age 15 months, the children will have been immunized against measles, mumps, and rubella. (Outcome)

Structure criteria are assessed when agencies are evaluated for licensure, accreditation, or certification. For instance, the accreditation of home health agencies and community nursing services, a service cosponsored by the National League for Nursing and the American Public Health Association, is based on four sets of structure criteria: organization and administration, program, staff, and future plans. "The criteria . . . test administrative practices and conditions, the underlying belief being that there is a relationship between quality of administration and quality of services delivered to the people."[9]

It is generally accepted that determination of quality of care can no longer be judged exclusively on the basis of structure alone. Appropriate resources are of course essential in defining the scope and boundaries of the organizations service potential, but sound fiscal management, adequate policies, and a clearly defined philosophy do not reflect actual nurse performance based on professional knowledge and skills.

In developing a quality assurance program, whether based on process criteria, outcome criteria, or both, several steps (Fig. 12–1) are suggested as follows:

1. Criteria should be written for specific patient populations that are representative of the agency's client system. Patient populations may be classified according to nursing diagnosis (inadequate mother–infant bonding); medical diagnosis (diabetes mellitus); developmental stage (infancy); symptom or syndrome (urinary incontinence); or concepts (family planning).[10,11] Further breakdown of the patient population may be necessary in order to focus on variations in need. For instance, the category of diabetes mellitus might be subdivided to establish criteria for adolescent diabetics and adult diabetics. Categories of criteria may therefore be combined (*e.g.*, medical diagnosis and developmental stage).
2. It is useful to organize criteria around a conceptual framework, such as, nursing theories, functional states or problems, or nursing diagnoses to assure that the client's physical or biologic, emotional, and social needs are addressed.[12] An example of this kind of criteria is presented by Taylor in relation to neurologic patient evaluations.[13] Based on Levine's four conservation principles of nursing intervention, which are the conservation of patient energy, and structural, personal and social integrity, common nursing problems were identified and specific outcome criteria developed.[14,15] Criteria should also be realistic, achievable, time-related and behaviorally oriented.[16,17] Nurse behaviors are addressed in process criteria, patient behaviors in outcome criteria. The time element is usually selected as the point where services are terminated; however, other time limits may be established. For instance, critical times for maternity clients may be identified according to trimesters.

   An example of criteria developed for diabetic patients might resemble the following:

NEED	PROBLEM	PROCESS CRITERIA	OUTCOME CRITERIA
Biologic	Inability to self-administer insulin	Nurse will instruct pt. in self-administration of correct dose of insulin using sterile technique	Pt. administers correct dose of insulin using sterile technique after 5 nursing visits

3. Standards of acceptable levels of nurse performance and patient outcomes must be established; the phamplet *Standards of Practice for Community Health Nursing* has been issued by the American Nurses' Association. Standards for patient outcomes may start with an anticipated 100% achievement. As data is gathered about actual achievement, the standard may be reduced if legitimate reasons for the reduction can be identified. For example, school nurses may establish a standard of 100% correction of visual defects by the end of the school year. The availability and accessibility of ophthalmology or optometric services in the community may make this standard unrealistic. Therefore, a revised standard of 80% might well be more realistic.
4. Standards and criteria should be developed and approved by those persons whose behavior and efforts are being evaluated. Representation from staff and supervisory nursing personnel play a central role in identifying and sanctioning criteria

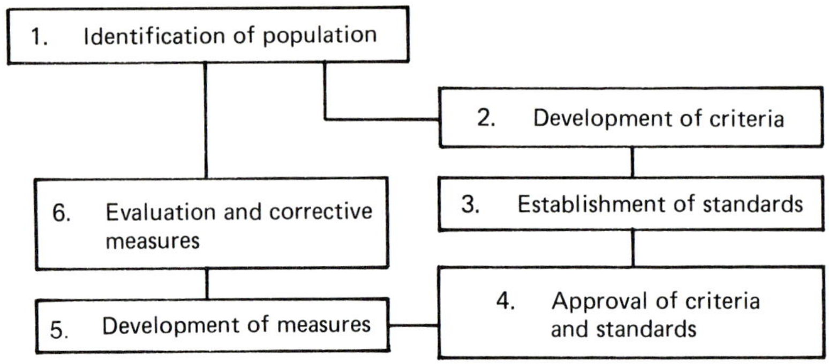

Figure 12–1
Quality assurance framework.

and standards, whether process or outcomes.[18] Input and approval from clients should also be sought through consumer advisory boards to the agency, or other feasible mechanisms.

5. Measures of attainment of the established standards and criteria are mandatory. This is usually accomplished through an audit or review of the patient/family record, concurrently or retrospectively. Concurrent audits are performed while the client system is still receiving care. Retrospective audits are conducted following discharge. An example of a process audit form for maternity patients is shown in Appendix E. This audit is performed retrospectively and the established standard for compliance is 100%. The actual auditing process is carried out monthly by a committee of staff and supervisory personnel. Deficiencies and discrepancies are reported to the Director of Nursing with recommendations for corrective actions. This type of audit is not designed to improve recording or to evaluate individual nurse performance, but its purpose is to identify strengths and weaknesses in the health-care delivery system and increase staff perceptions of acceptable levels of nursing practice.
6. As deficiencies or discrepancies are identified (differences between what is expected and what actually occurred), reasons for their occurrence must be analyzed. If unrealistic or unachievable criteria contribute to the problem, then revisions must be undertaken. Once established, criteria must not remain static, but must change as technology and knowledge improve. If appropriate, in-service programs, workshops, research, new equipment or policy changes may be initiated to decrease the gap between expectations and actual performance, or level of achievement. The implementation of solutions to correct inadequate patient care processes and improve health-status outcomes is the difference between quality assessment and quality assurance programs.

Process criteria, or those goal-directed activities performed by nursing in relation to identified patient needs, are thought by some to be the most valid measures of quality nursing care.[19,20] Others contend that outcome measures are more cogent.[21,22,23] Undoubtedly, the three sets of criteria are interrelated and each must be considered in the final analysis of cost-effective health-care delivery; however, action is currently being mandated on the development and refinement of outcome criteria. The underlying assumption is that the condition or behavior of patients themselves is the best indicator of efficient use of resources and effective application of nursing technologies. There are, however, several problems associated with the use of outcome criteria alone in quality assurance programs, especially in relation to community-health nursing practice. First, health status can improve despite inadequate process; therefore, deficiencies in nursing practice may go undetected and uncorrected. Diddie queries, "With clear conscience can it be said that that does not matter as long as the outcome is 'good'?''[24] Second, genetic predisposition and social and physical environmental influences beyond nursing's immediate control may negatively effect outcomes, even though excellent nursing care was provided. For instance, proper amounts of nutritional foods, accessibility and availability of medical care, and extremes of environmental temperature are controllable in institutional settings. This is not always the case in the community setting. Third, anticipatory guidance and counseling in preventive health measures are critical components of community-health nursing practice, yet there are no reliable methodologies existing today that provide measures of the long-term effects of these nursing activities. Outcomes may take years to become evident. Finally, the nature of "illness" today requires new and innovative strategies to address the restoration or maintenance of optimal levels of well-being. It also requires approaches to health care developed around multidisciplinary teams in which each discipline contributes to the outcome of care. Aside from "laying-on-of-hands" activities, such as, dressing changes, administering medications, and catheter insertions, the client's health status and alterations in behavior reflect the combined and mutually supportive efforts of the team, not just the nurse.

The previous discussion may be interpreted as an unjustifiable attack on the use of outcome criteria in favor of process criteria, but this is not intended. What is being proposed is the development of quality assurance criteria, combining both process and outcome criteria, which are adaptable to the concept of patient care and not just nursing care. Phaneuf also suggests the need for the "development of a holistic basis for quality auditing of process and outcomes that could be used without impairing or minimizing the accountability of each of the professions involved in patient care."[25]

NATIONAL HEALTH FOCUS

Between the years 1965 and 1979, national expenditures for health care rose from $39 billion to $212.2 billion, and the expenditures continue to rise. An estimated 40% of this increase is attributed to increased per capita use of services, and improved technologies. Barely 10% is the result of population growth, while the remaining 50% is attributed to increases in the cost of medical supplies, equipment, and personnel. During the 1979 fiscal year Medicare and Medicaid programs cost 29.3 billion and 21.7 billion respectively or 27% of all health care in the nation. Public expenditures account for more than 43% of all national health care spending.[26]

These data will undoubtedly be outdated by the time this book is in print, however, the intention of the message is still timely. Health, or actually sickness, since little of the previously noted expenditures was donated to preventive services, is an expensive business. Long-term chronic disorders can economically devastate families, and as has been said, lack of fiscal resources can influence one's perceptions of need for care. The old saying "the poor get sicker and the sick get poorer" continues to hold true.

The overwhelming economic aspects of health care, combined with the need to exert uniform controls over the environmental hazards of our industrialized society, have raised consumer interest in nationalized health-care programs and environmental control legislation.

For most of our national history, federal concern in health-related matters was devoted primarily to the provision of care to the military, coast guard, merchant marines, Native Americans, aliens, and Eskimos. The U.S. Department of Health and Human Services (formerly, The Department of Health, Education, and Welfare) was not created until 1953. However, since 1935 with the enactment of the Social Security Act, the federal government's role in financing health-care delivery systems, supporting research, funding medical and nursing education programs, and establishing standards for environmental control has been impressive. Following is a sampling of federal legislation in recent years that has influenced or will influence the scope and direction of community health nursing practice.

- *Social Security Act of 1935* (P.L. 74-241)—Provided assistance to states through grants-in-aid for program development and care to maternity patients, children, crippled children, the aged and the blind, and certain other disabled persons.
- *The National Cancer Institute Act of 1937* (P.L.

75-244)—Authorized the National Cancer Institute for research activities relating to cancer.

- *The LaFollette-Bulwinkle Act of 1938* (P.L. 75-540)—Provided grants-in-aid to states for venereal disease control activities.
- *The Nurse Training Act of 1941* (P.L. 77-146)—Authorized financial support to schools of nursing.
- *The National School Lunch Act of 1946* (P.L. 79-396)—Funding of a national school lunch program.
- *The National Dental Research Act of 1948* (P.L. 80-755)—Established the National Institute of Dental Research and funded dental research programs.
- *The Air Pollution Control Act of 1955* (P.L. 84-159)—Authorized assistance to states and localities in air quality control and research.
- *The National Health Survey Act of 1956* (P.L. 84-652)—Authorized the continuing study of illness and disability in this country.
- *Assistance to Migrating Workers Act of 1962* (P.L. 87-692)—Provided financial aid for clinical services to migrating farm workers and their families.
- *Civil Rights Act of 1964* (P.L. 88-352)—"No person in the United States shall, on the ground of race, color, or national origin, be excluded from participating in, be denied the benefits of, or be subjected to discrimination under any program or activity receiving Federal financial assistance."[27]
- *Food Stamp Act of 1964* (P.L. 88-525)—Established the Food Stamp Program.
- *Social Security Amendments of 1965* (P.L. 89-97)—Established hospital and medical insurance (Medicare) for aged social security beneficiaries and certain categories of disabled under Title XVIII. Medicare is managed directly by the federal government. Also established medical assistance programs to medically indigent families with dependent children, or who are aged, blind or disabled under Title XIX (Medicaid). Medicaid is managed by state governments within federal guidelines.
- *Aircraft Noise Abatement Act of 1968* (P.L. 90-411)—Amended Federal Aviation Act to deal with noise hazards.
- *Radiation Control for Health and Safety Act of 1968* (P.L. 90-602)—Provided for enforcement of safety standards for x-ray equipment, microwave ovens, television sets, and other electronic products.
- *Public Health Cigarette Smoking Act of 1970* (P.L. 91-222)—Prohibited cigarette advertising on television or radio.
- *Comprehensive Alcohol Abuse and Alcoholism Prevention, Treatment, and Rehabilitation Act of 1970* (P.L. 91-616)—Authorized assistance to states and localities and established the National Institute of Alcohol Abuse and Alcoholism.
- *Lead-Based Paint Poisoning Prevention Act* (P.L. 91-695)—Provided financial aide for communities for lead-based hazards.
- *Occupational Safety and Health Act of 1970* (P.L. 91-596)—Authorized the establishment of safety and health standards in working environments, and the enforcement of the standards.
- *National Sickle Cell Anemia Control Act of 1972* (P.L. 92-294)—Authorized funding for research and control programs.
- *Noise Control Act of 1972* (P.L. 92-574)—Established programs for noise research and control activities.
- *Federal Water Pollution Control Amendments of 1972* (P.L. 92-500)—Expanded program to ensure proper disposal of sewage and improve water quality in rivers, streams, and drinking water sources.
- *Social Security Amendments of 1972* (P.L. 92-603)—Established the Professional Standard Review Organization Program (PSRO) for the purpose of evaluating the quality of medical care and need for care of clients receiving services through Medicare, Medicaid, and Maternal-Child Health Programs.
- *Child Abuse Prevention and Treatment Act of 1974* (P.L. 93-247)—Established the National Center on Child Abuse and Neglect; provided demonstration grants for research and program development.
- *Social Security Amendments of 1974* (P.L. 93-647)—Title XX provides financial support to states for a variety of health and social programs including family planning services, family counseling, protective services for children and aged or disabled adults, home health care, homemaker services, day care for children and adults, and so forth.
- *National Health Planning and Resources Devel-*

opment Act of 1975 (P.L. 93-641)—Authorized major reorganizations of federal health-planning programs; authorized the establishment of local areawide Health Systems Agencies (HSA). HSAs are mandated to develop long-range regional Health Systems Plans and Annual Implementation Plans based on analyses of health care needs and resources. HSAs also review certain categories of proposed financial expenditures by hospitals and other health care facilities. SECTION 1502 identifies the National Health Priorities.
- *Developmentally Disabled Assistance and Bill of Rights Act of 1975* (P.L. 94-103)—Provides funding to states for developmentally disabled services such as day care, transportation, diagnosis, treatment, education, and so forth; also includes guidelines for protection and advocacy.
- *The National School Lunch Act and Child Nutrition Act Amendments of 1975* (P.L. 94-379)—Amended school lunch program and funded the supplemental food program for poor pregnant and lactating women, infants, and children to age 5 (W.I.C. program).
- *Education for All Handicapped Children Act of 1975* (P.L. 94-142)—Mandates a "free appropriate public education" to all handicapped children ages 3 to 18 years in the "least restrictive" environment, *i.e.*, as much as possible with non-handicapped children. Federal funding is contingent on compliance.[28]

The federal legislation listed represents a mere sampling of the government's areas of interest, which reflect consumer concerns. We are well into a system of national health insurance for specific categories of persons, primarily indigent pregnant women, infants, children, the aged, and the disabled. Regardless of income level, the public is now demanding equity in access to health care providers for all. The issue of whether health care is a "right" or a "privilege" is no longer debatable: Health care is a right. The unresolved problem is the agreement upon the extent or scope of care included in this right and the fiscal management of an equitable program.

NATIONAL HEALTH INSURANCE

There are several bills before Congress proposing a variety of national health insurance plans. Differences in the proposals are primarily in identifying the target population, scope of benefits, methods of financing, reimbursement to providers and administration of the programs.

Even though the concept of health care as a right is established, can we afford to provide equal access to health care for all during these inflationary times? The opposition's point of view is, of course, can we afford not to? Medicare and Medicaid do not cover all poor or nearly poor persons, or all indigent elderly or disabled persons. One approach to a national program, therefore, is to expand existing Medicare and Medicaid programs to include services now limited or not covered and to revise eligibility criteria in order to spend limited financial resources on the most needy.

Medicaid, Medicare, and even private health-insurance programs provide limited or no coverage for certain kinds of services. With the exceptions of the Early Periodic Screening, Diagnosis, and Treatment program under Medicaid, and Family Planning Services under Titles XIX and XX, preventive health-care services are not covered by either federally funded program. Dental care is not available under Medicare; neither are homemaker services or medications if the person is not hospitalized. Therefore, a major issue in defining the scope of services is whether to include coverage for "well-care" and "maintenance care," in addition to "sick care." It should be noted that Health Maintenance Organizations, (HMOs), which are a form of group medical practice providing comprehensive primary care to those enrolled, do provide preventive services. The federal government, through the provision of the Health Maintenance Organization Act of 1973, has already committed substantial sums toward the continued expansion and development of these prepaid group practices.

Should the entire population be guaranteed coverage for eyeglasses, mental health care, cosmetic surgery, or abortions? Should nurses be reimbursed for care provided that is *not* physician ordered? Are health education activities to be considered as an essential component of the scope of services and should they be reimbursable? Should assistance in the event of "catastrophic illnesses" be limited by family income?

The term "insurance" implies prepayment for all or substantial portions of services available.[29]

For example, many private health-insurance programs and Medicare require the individual to pay a certain amount of the cost of hospital care before the insurance program assumes responsibility (*i.e.*, you must meet the required "deductible" fixed-rate out of your own pocket). This type of co-payment arrangement is called cost sharing. Should a national health-insurance program incorporate cost-sharing features based on income levels? If so, what should be the limits of the eligibility criteria in order to assure equal access to services?

Who will finance a national health insurance program? Obviously the taxpayer, but by what means? If financing is established through employer–employee co-payment mechanisms, then how will coverage be available to the unemployed or self-employed? Or, is an indirect financing mechanism more conducive to equity of services? Indirect financing is a premium or tax based on risk factors or income level.[30] Should reimbursement to providers be handled directly by the government or contracted through a private health-insurance company or branch of state or local government?

There are no obvious answers to these questions. They are presented to increase community health nurses' perceptions of themselves individually and as a group, and also as consumers, providers, and consumer advocates. Nurses must remain cognizant of the political environment influencing health care and use this knowledge as a power base for the promotion of professional and consumer interests. The implementation of a national health-insurance program can be expected to increase the demand for covered services. Community health nurses must be prepared to meet the challenge, and more importantly, to participate in defining those services most beneficial to client well-being and the profession as a whole.

NATIONAL HEALTH PRIORITIES

The National Health Priorities, established under SECTION 1502 of Public Law 93-641, are as follows:

> SEC. 1502. The Congress finds that the following deserve priority consideration in the formulation of national health planning goals and in the development and operation of Federal, State, and area health planning and resources development programs:

1. The provision of primary care services for medically underserved populations, especially those which are located in rural or economically depressed areas.
2. The development of multi-institutional systems for coordination or consolidation of institutional health services (including obstetric, pediatric, emergency medical, intensive and coronary care, and radiation therapy services).
3. The development of medical group practices (especially those whose services are appropriately coordinated or integrated with institutional health services), health maintenance organizations, and other organized systems for the provision of health care.
4. The training and increased utilization of physician assistants, especially nurse clinicians.
5. The development of multi-institutional arrangements for the sharing of support services necessary to all health service institutions.
6. The promotion of activities to achieve needed improvements in the quality of health services, including needs identified by the review activities of Professional Standards Review Organizations under part B of Title XI of the Social Security Act.
7. The development by health service institutions of the capacity to provide various levels of care (including intensive care, acute general care, and extended care) on a geographically integrated basis.
8. The promotion of activities for the prevention of disease, including studies of nutritional and environmental factors affecting health and the provision of preventive health care services.
9. The adoption of uniform cost accounting, simplified reimbursement, and utilization reporting systems, and improved management procedures for health service institutions.
10. The development of effective methods of educating the general public concerning proper personal (including preventive)

health care and methods for effective use of available health services.[31]

REGIONALIZATION

Priorities number 5 and number 7 of the previous section introduce a concept that was briefly mentioned in the discussion of genetic influences, that of regionalization of health-care delivery systems.

Within any given geographic area, population needs vary according to the socioeconomic, age, sex, cultural, and educational variables of the population; availability and accessibility of health care services also may differ. In an effort to focus planning, financial allocations, and limited resources toward more specific and clearly defined problem areas, emphasis is being placed on decentralization of administrative controls and maximization of resources based on geographic boundaries. For instance, the Department of Health and Human Services has regional offices through the country, each responsible for a particular section of the country. Health systems agencies also focus on need assessment and planning for a limited geographic area where it is presumed that consumer needs would be similar. Direct patient care is also being organized along similar structural guidelines. For example, regionalized networks of perinatal care to high-risk mothers and infants are already established in many parts of the country. The system generally consists of four components. The first is the clinic or private provider of prenatal care of the client's choice in her immediate community. The second component is termed a Level I hospital, again usually in a small community facility near the patient's home. Level I hospitals are capable of meeting the needs of normal, uncomplicated deliveries and healthy newborns. Level II hospitals are generally larger, urban-based institutions better equipped to handle complications of the mother and noenate. Level III facilities are designated as the Regional Perinatal Centers and are responsible for the management of the most severe complications, such as, extreme low-birth-weight infants or certain congenital anomalies.[32] The Regional Center coordinates services with Level I and Level II facilities including consultative services, transportation of high-risk mothers and neonates, professional staff education and outreach and communications programs. The patient enters the system at the most convenient facility and as needs are identified can be transferred to the location where the services are most appropriate. The community health nurse plays a pivotal role in follow-up care, facilitating exchange of information between hospitals and providing guidance and support to families in the event of the birth of a defective child or an infant death. The entire approach to this system of care is based on multidisciplinary teamwork directed toward achieving positive patient outcomes. This is just one example of regionalized health care. Other kinds exist and are being developed. Depending upon the agency affiliation of the community health nurse and the assignment, the nurse's community boundaries may be expanding or contracting.

FUTURE DIRECTIONS

Community health nursing is confronting a future of challenge filled with opportunities for innovation. The population is changing with more persons living longer and birthrates declining slowly, thereby increasing the percentage of older Americans. Because women outlive men, an increase in the number of widowed elderly can be expected. The rising cost of fuel and limited supplies of other energy sources may precipitate a population influx back to the cities, further aggravating already overcrowded living conditions. Inflation in general may dictate revisions in life-styles. More women will return to the work force out of financial necessity, dietary habits may be altered in light of meat prices, and consumer demands for quality of all services, including health care, will increase. Unless an equitable national health-insurance program is adopted, people may not use their limited incomes for health care, unless an acute episode or crisis occurs. Environmental stresses, both physical and social, may accelerate with resulting increases in mental disorders and self-destructive behavior.

As the population ages, there will be an increase in chronic diseases and more emphasis on care of the terminally and chronically ill, both having implications for home-based nursing care and support services needed to maintain the elderly at home.

The national health priorities suggest restructuring of the health-care delivery system itself.

Emphasis on primary sources of health, especially in medically underserved areas may effect use of and reimbursement of nurse practitioner skills. Group practices, such as Health Maintenance Organizations, are being encouraged to reduce fragmentation of care and foster a primary care system of health-care delivery, which focuses more on preventive services. Coordination of services among institutions may tend to decrease the differences in services between voluntary and nonvoluntary agencies, proprietary and nonproprietary agencies. Public health as a distinct entity directed toward prevention may become less clearly defined as sharing of services develops.

What are the implications for nursing? Counseling in preventive health behavior and the promotion of preventive health services have already been identified as national health priorities. Much research is needed in perfecting teaching strategies and measuring outcomes, particularly in young populations.

One unique approach to preventive health behaviors and health maintenance is the "activated" or motivated teaching model.[33] The "activated patient" is "one whose clinical skills and understanding of his health are such that he becomes an active participant in his own health care in contrast to the passive role traditionally assigned him."[34] Through the sharing of medically relevant knowledge, the consumer develops a sense of power or control over his or her own health status and changes behaviors accordingly. The educational program consists of a series of workshops designed at teaching patients basic self-help measures, such as, taking vital signs, including blood pressure; simple first aid; the Heimlech maneuver; use of health resources more efficiently and effectively; medical terminology; medication purchasing, storage, administration and possible side effects; interpretation of clinical symptoms such as a sore throat or chest pain; nutrition, exercise, and substance-abuse facts; and may include a Health Hazard Appraisal. Specific content can be altered to meet client needs. Suggested content is detailed in Schnert's book *How to Be Your Own Doctor (Sometimes)*.[35]

Nursing should also address itself toward the identification and development of services needed to support persons, especially the handicapped young and elderly populations, in their homes.

With a larger number of elderly, chronically ill clients, the demand for home health services will accelerate. These services go beyond needs for skilled nursing, physical or occupational therapy, and medical social work. Homemaker services to aid in housekeeping, shopping and food preparation at a reasonable cost cannot be overlooked as a basic component to home health care. Public funding for such programs is limited at present. Day-care centers for adults is also a viable alternative to institutionalization, yet again the availability of such services is not widespread.

A new dimension to home health, which combines professional care with consumer self-care, is the Hospice concept. The word "hospice" can be traced back to medieval days in Europe and meant a way station for travelers. The medieval hospices evolved into hospitals where care was administered by members of religious orders. Modern use of the term developed in 1967, in England, when Dr. Cicely Saunders founded St. Christopher's Hospice for the care of the terminally ill and their families.

Hospice is a program of coordinated home-based and institutional care for the terminally ill and their families emphasizing a multidisciplinary approach in the delivery of medical, spiritual, psychological, and social services. A key concept to the Hospice philosophy is the control of pain, both preventively and through the use of drugs. Emphasis is placed on the home care component of the program and, if appropriate, and desired, the patient is allowed to die at home in the company of family and friends. Hospitalization is used primarily when the patient has no family, symptoms must be closely monitored, or the family requires respite from the stresses associated with patient care. Services, home-based and institutional, are available daily, around the clock. Hospice care should be ordered by the physician. Coordination of the care is the responsibility of the community health nurse. In addition to providing physical care to the patient, the nurse instructs the family in basic nursing skills to the degree that they are comfortable with it. Participation in the care of the loved one reduces feelings of guilt, following the patient's demise. The nurse participates by assisting the patient with pain prevention and in alleviating other discomforts through fear-reduction, relaxation techniques, and the use of pain-relieving medications. The patient's and family's spiritual leader is an integral part of the team and can be supportive of both the client and the nurse in dealing with dying, through all its stages.

Volunteers are also an integral part of the Hospice program. Carefully selected, trained volunteers assist families with shopping chores, provide family members with a rest period, assist in planning funeral arrangements, babysit or listen attentively to patient or family members needing the opportunity to ventilate their problems.

The nurse must deal with her own attitudes toward dying to assume a supportive role for the patient and his or her family. Assessment of emotional states and the need to discuss feelings openly must be handled as skillfully as the performance of physically related tasks. Continued support for the family is provided after the patient's death, throughout the bereavement period. This represents family-centered community nursing in its purest sense.[36]

REFERENCES

1. Association of State and Territorial Directors of Nursing: Position Paper. May, 1980
2. American Public Health Association. The definition and role of public health nursing in the delivery of health care. APHA Newsletter June, 1980
3. Federal Register, 42-229, p 60886. Nov 29, 1977
4. Donabedian A: The quality of medical care. Science Vol. 200, No. 26: 856–864, 1978
5. American Nurses' Association. Quality Assurance Workbook. Kansas City, American Nurses Association, 1976
6. Ibid.
7. Hegyvary S T, Haussmann R K D. Monitoring nursing care quality. J Nurs Admin Vol. 5, No. 5: 17–26, 1975
8. Donabedian A, op cit
9. Council of Home Health, Agencies and Community Health Services: Accreditation of Home Health Agencies and Community Nursing Services, pp 1–2. New York, National League for Nursing, Publication No. 21-1306, 1976
10. American Nurses' Association, op cit, p 14
11. Zimmer M J: Guidelines for the development of outcome criteria. Nurs Clin North America Vol. 9, No. 2: 317–321, 1974
12. Ibid
13. Taylor J W: Measuring the outcomes of nursing care. Nurs Clin North America Vol. 9, No. 2: 337–348, 1974
14. Ibid, p 341
15. Levine M E: Introduction to Clinical Nursing. Philadelphia, F A Davis, 1969
16. American Nurses' Association, op cit. p 16
17. Taylor J W, op cit, p 340
18. Zimmer M J: Quality assurance for outcomes of patient care. Nurs Clin North America 9(2), Vol. 9, No. 2: 305–315, 1974
19. Hegyvary S T, Haussmann R K D, op cit
20. Phaneuf M C, Wandelt M A: Quality assurance in nursing. Nurs Forum, Vol. 13, No. 4: 328–344, 1974
21. Zimmer M J, op cit
22. Taylor J W, op cit
23. Donabedian A, op cit
24. Diddie P J: Quality assurance—A general hospital meets the challenge. J Nurs Admin Vol. 6, No. 6: 6–16, 1976
25. Phaneuf M: The Nursing Audit—Profile for Excellence, p 113. New York, Appleton-Century-Crofts, 1972
26. Health Care Financing Administration: Health Care Financing Review, p 1. Summer 1980
27. Civil Rights Act of 1964. Public Law 88-352, 88th Congress, 1964
28. The Children's Defense Fund. Your Rights Under the Education for All Handicapped Children Act—P.L. 94-142, p 5. Washington, DC, 1975
29. Boaz R F: Equity in paying for health care services under a national insurance system. Milbank Memorial Quarterly Vol. 53, No. 3: 337–350, 1975
30. Ibid
31. National Health Planning and Resources Development Act of 1975, op cit
32. Graner S N: Perinatal health promotion: An overview. Family and Community Health Vol. 1, No. 3: 1–11, 1978
33. Wang V L, Recter H, Lentz G, Whaples G C: An approach to consumer patient activation in health maintenance. Public Health Reports Vol. 90, No. 5: 449–454, 1975
34. Sehnert K W: How to be Your Own Doctor (Sometimes), p 326. New York, Grosset & Dunlop, 1975
35. Ibid
36. Department of Health, Education, and Welfare: Medicare and medicaid hospice projects. Federal Register, pp 50376–50378. Friday, Oct 27, 1978

APPENDICES

Appendix A

FAMILY ASSESSMENT GUIDE

INTERNAL CHARACTERISTICS

- Members of the Household

Name	Birthdate	Sex	Relationship to Head	Occupation

- Ethnic Background
  ______ Caucasian ______ Black ______ Oriental
  ______ Mexican ______ Other
- Religious Background
  ______ Protestant ______ Catholic ______ Jewish ______ Other
- Health Status
  What is the current health status of each member? Are they within appropriate ranges of growth and development—physically, mentally, psychologically? Is illness present in any member? What are the past significant illnesses and accidents of members? Are any members taking medications? What is the immunization and dental status of members? Do members use alcohol, tobacco, or other drugs? Are there allergies? Do members use prostheses or other appliances such as glasses? Describe the health of each member using the above and any other appropriate data.

INTERNAL DYNAMICS

- Patterned Role Behaviors
  Who is assigned to what tasks?
  Adults
  Children
- Patterned Relationships
  How do members get along together?
  Adult–Adult (Husband–wife, unmarried couple of opposite or same sex)
  Adult–Children (Father–child, Mother–child, or parent substitute–child).
  Children–Children (Siblings or unrelated)
- Patterned Decision-Making Behavior
  Who makes decisions? How are decisions made?
  Decisions affecting adults.
  Decisions affecting children.
  Decisions affecting whole group.
- Sleeping Patterns
  Which members sleep together? Alone?
  What sleeping facilities are available for the above (bed, couch, adequate covers, pillows)?
  Where do they sleep (bedroom, living room)?
  What are the usual hours of sleep?
  - Adults
  - Children
- Eating Patterns
  Which meals are eaten at home?

Breakfast	Adults
	Children
Lunch	Adults
	Children
Dinner	Adults
	Children

  Are members adequately nourished based on assessment?
  - Adults
  - Children

  Are meals nutritionally balanced and consisting of required vitamins, minerals, protein, carbohydrates, and fat?
  Yes _____ No _____
  Basis of decision: _____ 24-hour food intake list _____ history _____ observations.
  Is food bought in quantity?
  Is there adequate storage space for foods?
  What is the weekly amount of money spent on food?
- Activity Patterns
  What are the usual activities of members?
  - Adults
  - Children

  How much time is devoted daily to leisure activities?
  Are these group or individual activities?
- Family Planning Patterns
  Do members use family planning methods?
  Are they interested? What are the implications for health?

- Patterned Values
  What are the values and goals of the group?
  - Adults
  - Children
  - Total group

  How are these values reflected in:
  - Type of home
  - Type of furniture
  - Reading material present
  - Neighborhood
  - Health patterns and behavior
  - Other
- Family Developmental Patterns
  At what stage of family development is this group?
  Are they meeting the tasks and patterns successfully?
  If not, what are the blocks?
- Human Needs Patterns.
  Where is the group in relation to Maslow's Hierarchy of Needs?
  Physiological ______
  Safety ______
  Love ______
  Esteem ______
  Self-actualization ______
  Can nursing help them move to a higher level of need fulfillment?
  Identify ways.
- Internal Patterns and Negentropy
  Are family members flexible and able to change role behaviors and relationships to facilitate growth of members or the family as a group? Describe.
  What techniques (feedback) are used by members to facilitate change?
  Do these techniques indicate maturity on the part of family members? Which members?
- Internal Patterned Behaviors and Health
  Are any of the internal dynamic patterns of behavior detrimental to the health of individual members or the group as a system? Describe and identify patterns.

GROUP EXCHANGE WITH NON-HUMAN ENVIRONMENT

- Housing
  Type of housing: ______ Apartment ______ Single family house
  ______ Duplex
  Rent ______ Own ______
  Number of rooms ______ Describe ______________________________
  ____
  Furnishings adequate ______ inadequate ______
  Toilet facilities: adequate ______ inadequate ______
  Heating: adequate ______ inadequate ______
  Ventilation: adequate ______ inadequate ______
  Lighting: adequate ______ inadequate ______
  Water supply: city ______ well ______ other ______
  Sewage: city ______ septic tank ______

Garbage collection: adequate _____ inadequate _____
Flies: present _____ absent _____
Rodents: present _____ absent _____
Accident hazards present: unlighted halls _____ open fireplaces _____
unprotected stoves _____ medications and cleaning supplies left out _____
stairs in poor repair _____ loose carpets _____ slippery bath tub _____
other _____
Describe other, if checked ______________________________
______________________________.

- Housing and Health
  Are any of the exchanges with the non-human environment of the home potential health hazards. Describe.
  ____

EXCHANGES WITH THE COMMUNITY

- Economic Subsystem
  Describe the current and past occupational history of each working member.
  Do these occupations present potential threats to the health of members such as chemical exposure, extremes of temperature, and so forth?
  What is the total family income $_____ per week/month/year?
  What is the source of income?
  Does the income adequately meet the needs of members? Yes _____ No _____
  If no, is the deficit due to inadequate income _____ or improper budgeting _____?
  Does the group have a savings account?
- Educational Subsystem of Community
  Describe the educational level of each member.
  What are the implications of educational levels for health patterns and health teaching?
  Do members want further education?
  If so, what plans have been made?
  Is the educational level of members adequate to meet their economic goals?
- Religious Subsystem of Community
  What is the religious affiliation of the family?
  Attendance: weekly _____ monthly _____ yearly _____
  less frequent _____
  Are the places of worship accessible?
  Yes _____ No _____
- Social Subsystem of the Community
  Who do the family members interact with on a social basis in the community?
  Describe.
  Friends ______________________________
  Neighbors ______________________________
  Church ______________________________
  Extended Family ______________________________
  Occupational Cohorts ______________________________
  Clubs ______________________________
  Other ______________________________
  Are family members active in civic and professional groups in the community?
  Describe.
  ____
  ____

- Transportation Subsystem of Community
  What is the means of transportation for the group?
  own car _____ buses _____ street cars _____
  If members must use public transportation, is it accessible for:
  Work: Yes _____ No _____
  Health care: Yes _____ No _____
  Social activities: Yes _____ No _____
  Professional obligations: Yes _____ No _____
  Religious activities: Yes _____ No _____
- Health Subsystem of Community
  What is the usual source of family health care?
  Describe.
  How is this care financed?
  Do members receive immunizations as recommended?
  Do members receive periodic dental care?
  What is the families knowledge and attitudes regarding health and health care?
  What do they see as their health problems?
  What does the family expect from the community health nurse?
  Are these expectations realistic?
  What resources have families used in the past to cope with crises or illness?

SUMMARY OF FAMILY HEALTH

- Identify unmet health needs resulting from internal characteristics.
- Identify unmet health needs resulting from internal dynamics.
- Identify unmet health needs resulting from exchanges with the non-human environment.
- Identify unmet health needs resulting from exchanges with the community.
- Set priorities for the family health problems based upon the family and nurse's assessment.
- Which of these problems can be resolved using nursing knowledge and skill?
- Which of these problems should be referred to other community resources because they fall outside the nurse's scope of competence?
- Set priorities for the nursing needs identified.

Appendix B

COMMUNITY NURSING ASSESSMENT GUIDE

Community ______________________ Date ____________________

INTERNAL CHARACTERISTICS

- Typography and Climate
  - Describe:
    - terrain
    - climate including seasonal variations in temperature, humidity, and rainfall
    - unusual typographical features
- History of Study Area
  Write a brief historical account of the settlement date, developmental events, and the key people involved.
  Write a brief historical account of health related activities in the study area. Include dates of establishing major hospitals, institutions, health departments, non-governmental health agencies and nursing organizations. Also include dates of epidemics, disasters and important court decisions and laws affecting health.
- Boundaries
  Specify the study area boundaries (school, industry, census tract, community)
  Area in square miles __________

- Economic Subsystem
  Employment distribution

	NO. IN COMMUNITY	% OF TOTAL POPULATION
Employed persons		
Manufacturing		
White collar		
Wholesale & retail		
Local government		
Federal government		
Unemployed persons		

Leading industries

Name Address No. employees Mgt

Family income

		COMMUNITY	STATE	NATION
	Median income			
Percent of population	Under $3000			
	3001–5999			
	6000–9999			
	10,000 & over			

Governmental Budget

	COMMUNITY TOTAL IN DOLLARS	% OF TOTAL
Education		
Transportation		
Welfare		
Health		
Police		
Fire		

- Education Subsystem
  Number of educational facilities

	COMMUNITY	
	PUBLIC	PRIVATE
Total		
Elementary		
Junior high		
Senior high		
Jr. Colleges		
Colleges		
Special schools		

Educational level of population

	COMMUNITY	STATE	NATION
Less than 5 years			
H.S. graduate			
Some college			
College graduate			
Median school completed			
Currently			

Health manpower facilities

	NUMBER	# GRADUATED YEARLY
Total		
Medical schools		
Nursing schools		
Dental schools		
Physical therapy		
Social workers		

- Communications Subsystem
  Newspapers

Name	Frequency	Circulation
______	______	______
______	______	______
______	______	______

Radio stations

Name	Address	Audience (No. & kind, *i.e.*, young–old, black–white—social class group
______	______	______
______	______	______
______	______	______

Television

Name	Address	Audience
______	______	______
______	______	______
______	______	______

Key community leaders/decision makers influencing subsystem

Name	Affiliation
______	______
______	______
______	______

Health coverage
Adequate ____ Inadequate ____
If inadequate: List media as follows with deficits

Name	Deficits
______________________	______________________
______________________	______________________
______________________	______________________

Quality
Good _____ Poor _____
If poor: List media below with deficits

Name	Deficits
______________________	______________________
______________________	______________________
______________________	______________________

Is there a speakers' bureau for health subjects?
Yes _____ No _____
List community organizations which have active health programs for the public.

Agency	Type of program	Qualified personnel Yes	Qualified personnel No
__________	______________	_____	_____
__________	______________	_____	_____
__________	______________	_____	_____

Health materials in schools
Is health integrated into the school curriculum at all grades?
Yes _____ No _____
If no, discuss deficits.
____

Discuss areas of health covered by grade levels
____
____
____

Is the information adequately covered?
Yes _____ No _____

- Political Subsystem

Political parties and leadership
Major party ______________________________
Key leaders ______________________________
Minor party ______________________________
Key leaders ______________________________
Major Issues over last five years which influence health

	YES	NO	PARTY FAVORING	IMPLEMENTED ACTIONS
Housing				
Transportation				
Health facilities				
Water & sewage				
Immunizations				
Fluoridation				
Communications				

- Recreation Subsystem
  Number and location

	TOTAL NO.	PUBLIC	PRIVATE
Central community			
North			
East			
South			
West			

Recreation type, age group, and frequency of use

	TYPES	AGE GROUPS	NO. USING DAILY
Central			
North			
East			
South			
West			

Leadership available during recreation

AREA	TYPE LEADERSHIP
1. ______	______
2. ______	______
3. ______	______
4. ______	______

- Religion Subsystem
  Religious distribution

	COMMUNITY TOTAL NO.	% OF TOTAL
Protestant		
Catholic		
Jewish		
Other		

Key leaders in religion (List)

Leaders	Phone no. or address
______	______
______	______
______	______

- Transportation Subsystem
  Routes and services
    Describe major transportation routes
    Services available on these routes (buses, trains)
  Future plans
  Transportation and health services
    Are transportation routes adequate for population getting to health facilities?
      Yes ______ No ______
    If no, discuss specific deficits

- Welfare Subsystem
  Agencies
  List agencies, location, area served, and service
  ____
  ____
  ____
  ____

  Are these services adequate to meet population needs?
  Adequate _____ Inadequate _____
  If inadequate, discuss agency and inadequacies
  ____
  ____
  ____

- Families Subsystem
  Population characteristics
  Population at last census _______________
  Population density _______________
  Population changes over 10 year period _______________
  Age distribution _______________

	COMMUNITY			STATE		
Age Group	*% of Total*	*Population 10 yrs ago*	*% of Total*	*Population*	*Percent*	*National Population %*
0–5 5–14 15–24 24–34 35–44 45–54 55–64 65 +						

Sex and race distribution

CATEGORY		COMMUNITY		STATE	NATION
Race	*Sex*	*Current No./%*	*10 yrs. ago No./%*	*No./%*	*No./%*
White	Male				
	Female				
Non-White	Male				
	Female				

Vital statistics

CATEGORY	COMMUNITY		STATE	NATION
	Current No./%	*10 yrs. ago No./%*	*No./Rate*	*No./Rate*
Live births				
Neonatal deaths				
Infant deaths				
Maternal deaths				
General deaths				

Social problems

PROBLEM	COMMUNITY	
	Number	*% of Total*
Illegitimate births		
Venereal diseases		
Syphilis		
Gonorrhea		
Narcotic users		
Suicide		
Alcoholism		

Health Problems
Communicable Disease Incidence

DISEASE	NO. OF CASES	
	Current year	*5 years ago*
Diphtheria		
Encephalitis		
Infectious hepatitis		
Influenza		
Measles		
Tetanus		
Tuberculosis		
Typhoid		
Other		

Immunization Level for Acute Communicable Diseases

DISEASE	PERCENT IMMUNIZED BY AGE			
	Under 1	*1–5*	*6–15*	*Over 15*
Diphtheria				
Poliomyelitis				
Smallpox				
Tetanus				
Measles				
Whooping cough				

Leading causes of death

CAUSE OF DEATH	COMMUNITY		STATE		NATION	
	No.	*Rate*	*No.*	*Rate*	*No.*	*Rate*
1.						
2.						
3.						
4.						
5.						
6.						
7.						
8.						
9.						
10.						

Chronic diseases

DISEASE	COMMUNITY		STATE		NATION	
	No.	*Rate*	*No.*	*Rate*	*No.*	*Rate*
Cardiovascular						
Cancer						
Diabetes						
Other						

- Health Subsystem
  Hospital Services

HOSPITAL SERVICES	BED CAPACITY	ADEQUATE	INADEQUATE
Medical			
Surgical			
Maternity			
Psychiatric			
Communicable disease			
Pediatric			
Rehabilitation			
Chronic disease			

Nursing home services
  Adequate _____ Inadequate _____
Ambulatory services
  Adequate _____ Inadequate _____
Occupational health services
  Adequate _____ Inadequate _____
School health services
  Adequate _____ Inadequate _____
Health department services
  Adequate _____ Inadequate _____
Discuss any inadequacies ____
____
____

Health manpower

CATEGORY	BUDGETED POSITIONS	% UNFILLED
Physicians		
Nurses		
Social workers		
Psychologists		
Aides		
Sanitarians		
Physical therapists		
Other		

- Community Health Nursing Services
  Community health nursing agencies
  Name ____
  Address ____
  Purpose ____
  Accredited Yes _____ No _____

Services provided
Total # clients seen in home ______
% of these for home care ______

Types of services in home

CATEGORY	# CASES	# VISITS	% OF TOTAL
Cancer			
Heart disease			
Diabetes			
Tuberculosis			
Venereal disease			
Other diseases			
Maternity			
Infant			
Preschool			
School			
Adult			

Clinic services

TYPE	MONTHLY ATTENDANCE	PURPOSE

School services

TYPE	MONTHLY VISITS TO NURSE	PURPOSE

COMMUNITY DYNAMICS AS THEY AFFECT FAMILIES

- Protection

Fire protection: Adequate ______ Inadequate ______
If inadequate—describe ______
Police protection: Adequate ______ Inadequate ______
If inadequate—describe ______
Health services: Adequate ______ Inadequate ______
If inadequate—describe ______
Environmental services: Adequate ______ Inadequate ______
If inadequate—describe ______

Transportation services: Adequate ______ Inadequate ______
If inadequate—describe ________________________________
Social services: Adequate ______ Inadequate ______
If inadequate—describe ________________________________
Community nursing services: Adequate ______ Inadequate ______
If inadequate—describe ________________________________
Ambulance services: Adequate ______ Inadequate ______
If inadequate—describe ________________________________
Hospital services: Adequate ______ Inadequate ______
If inadequate—describe ________________________________
Educational services: Adequate ______ Inadequate ______
If inadequate—describe ________________________________

EXCHANGES WITH NON-HUMAN ENVIRONMENT

- Housing Condition

TYPE OF DWELLING	GOOD		FAIR		POOR*	
	No.	%	*No.*	%	*No.*	%
*Substandard housing						

Housing complaints—Numbers

PROBLEM	CURRENT YEAR	5 YEARS AGO
Heating		
Lighting		
Ventilation		
Nuisances		
Other		

Sanitation

AIR CONTAMINANTS THAT ARE SOURCE OF PROBLEM COMPLAINTS			
Smoke	Yes ______	No ______	
Gases	Yes ______	No ______	
Odors	Yes ______	No ______	
Vapors	Yes ______	No ______	
Pollens	Yes ______	No ______	
Others	Yes ______	No ______	Specify:

SOURCES OF AIR CONTAMINANTS		
Industry	Yes ______	No ______
Vehicles	Yes ______	No ______
Homes	Yes ______	No ______
Incinerators	Yes ______	No ______
Other—Specify	Yes ______	No ______

Water supply

SOURCE	NO.	%	ADEQUATELY TREATED—%
Public Private			

Sewage disposal

SOURCE	NO.	%	% WITH ADEQUATE RX
Public Private			

Solid waste disposal

Adequate ______ Inadequate ______

Vector control program

PROGRAM	ADEQUATE	INADEQUATE
Mosquitoes Insects Rodents Other (Specify)		

Food and milk

FOOD SOURCE	NUMBER	% SALE	% USAGE
Restaurants Stores			

EXCHANGES BEYOND THE COMMUNITY

- Health threats

  Present ______ Absent ______

  If present, describe ____

  ____

  Programs to reduce threat ____
- Health resources

  List available sources

  Manpower ____

  ____

  Money ____

  ____

  Equipment ____

  ____

SUMMARY OF COMMUNITY HEALTH

- Identify unmet health needs resulting from the internal characteristics.
- Identify unmet needs resulting from the internal dynamics.
- Identify the unmet health needs resulting from exchange with the non-human environment.
- Identify the unmet needs resulting from exchanges beyond the community.
- Set priorities for the community health problems.
- Which of these problems can be resolved using nursing knowledge and skill?
- Which of these problems should be referred to other community resources because they fall outside the nurse's scope of competence?
- Set priorities for the nursing needs identified.

Appendix C

SELF-EVALUATION GUIDE FOR COMMUNITY HEALTH NURSES

- Preparation for visit (home, school, industry, clinic, or office).
  - How well do I plan before visits in relation to:
    - reviewing data and planning visit?
    - obtaining orders if indicated?
    - agency policies regarding the particular problems?
    - reviewing necessary scientific knowledge?
    - obtaining necessary literature and equipment?
- The Visit
  - How well do I carry out nursing procedures in relation to:
    - scientific principles and effectiveness?
    - anticipation of system's needs and wishes?
    - physical and mental comfort of the system?
    - organization of the procedure?
    - prevention at all levels of intervention?
    - improvising as necessary in the setting?
    - planning for care between visits?
  - How well do I relate to patients and families in relation to:
    - putting them at ease?
    - being friendly and courteous?
    - liking them as people?
    - adjusting to the situation?
    - understanding them?
    - being sincere and honest?
    - gaining and holding their confidence and respect?
  - How well do I promote learning in relation to:
    - recognizing teaching opportunities?

being an active listener and directing conversation into productive channels?
using teaching materials constructively?
teaching by example and demonstration?
using good judgment in giving and withholding suggestions?
being aware of emotional factors as they influence learning?
applying general principals of learning?
encouraging self-directed activity?
evaluation of learning that has taken place?

How well do I apply systems concepts to the family in relation to:
recognizing the family as a unit?
recognizing the relationship of the patient's health to the family and community?
recognizing environmental and psychological factors that influence or are influenced by illness?
using community resources with the family?
the economic implications of health and illness?
considering the influence of religious, racial, social, political, and other forces acting on the system?
considering myself as a member of the community subsystem of health and interpret its policies and programs?

- After the Visit

How well do I record the visit in relation to:
constructive use of the records?
including significant data?
clear, concise, and well-organized sentences?
completeness, accuracy, legibility, and promptness of recording?
using the problem-oriented format?
my awareness of the value of records and reports to the organization?

What are my relationships within the organization in relation to:
interest and friendliness with others?
respecting the viewpoint of others?
working cooperatively with others?
initiating and participating in group discussions?
taking initiative in contacting community resources?
keeping others informed when appropriate?
being overly dependent on or overly protective of others?
encouraging and supporting others?

(Modified from A Guide for the Public Health Nurse in evaluating her growth and progress from Public Health Nursing Supervisors' Manual, Virginia State Health Department, Richmond, Virginia)

Appendix D

CRITERIA FOR THE ASSESSMENT OF CARE FOR THE MATERNITY PATIENT

	YES	NO
• Assessment Criteria		
In addition to identifying data is the following included in the right upper hand corner: The source and reliability of history.		
Chief Complaint:		
Length of gestation		
Expected date of confinement		
History of Present Illness:		
Date of last menstrual period		
Where and when pregnancy was diagnosed		
Where patient is receiving pre-natal care, and frequency of visits		
When pre-natal care was begun		
Satisfaction with pre-natal care		
Any medications or vitamins the patient is taking and if they were prescribed by a doctor		
Pre-pregnancy weight and present weight		
Have high-risk factors that *relate to this pregnancy* been identified. These should be discussed in greater detail under past personal history.		
The patient's feelings about her pregnancy		
The father's feelings toward the pregnancy		
Discomforts of pregnancy that patient is presently experiencing		
Attitudes and expectations of labor and delivery		

YES | NO

Patient Profile:
- Date and place of birth
- Sex and race
- Marital status and relationship
- Family composition
- Education and achievement
- Occupation and employment history
- Patient's life patterns—examples
  - Sleeping habits
  - Diet
  - Hobbies
  - Exercise
  - Alcohol
  - Caffeine
  - Tobacco
  - Drug use
  - Home environment
  - Adequacy & source of income
- Some of the previous items may have been included in the family history sheet—if so, is this clearly stated?

Past Personal History:
- Have *relevant* factors about the patient's childhood been included?
- Examples:
  - growth and development
  - past diseases
  - allergies
  - injuries
  - hospitalizations
  - immunizations, esp. rubella
- Is there a thorough history of past pregnancies included? Does it contain all medical and social factors that may influence the outcome of this pregnancy?
- Have high risk factors been identified?
- Examples:
  - under 15
  - over 35
  - single
  - over para 5
  - 2 or more induced or spontaneous abortions
  - previous abnormal labor
  - previous ABO or RH sensitized fetus
  - positive serology
  - hypertension
  - abnormal pelvic measurement
  - malnourished, obese
  - emotional problem
  - infection with Herpes Zoster, Type II
  - previous stillborn
  - previous premature
  - anomaly
  - diabetes
  - pre-eclampsia
  - anemia
  - poverty
  - child abuse
  - any others

Family History

Has information about congenital or genetic disease and health status for all close relatives (including maternal and paternal) been included?

Has a *complete* Review of Systems been included?

Has a physical screening been included which contains nursing observations such as:
- general appearance
- skin color
- blood pressure
- TPR
- presence of edema
- varicosities
- condition of breasts
- fetal heart tones

Are these noted on subsequent encounters?

	YES	NO
Has the patient's specific problem been identified, prioritized and recorded on problem list?		
• Planning Criteria		
Are goals mutually set with patient and family? Are they time related, realistic and measurable? Are they stated in behavioral terms which are patient oriented?		
• Implementation Criteria		
In following through on identified problems, have the following educational and counseling areas been discussed, *as relevant to this patient?*		
The physiological changes of pregnancy as related to conception, pregnancy, labor and delivery and postpartum period		
The importance of good nutrition		
Explanation of clinic procedure		
Community resources, if applicable:		
financial — Red Cross classes		
mental health — Lamaze		
day care — W.I.C.		
The importance of regular medical care		
The development of the fetus		
The importance of rest and exercise		
Proper clothing		
Danger signals and instructions on what to do if they occur		
Signs of labor		
Hospital procedures during labor, delivery and postpartum period		
Instructions on what to pack for hospital for mother and baby		
Instructions on personal hygiene, including the use of douching, feminine sprays, vaginal suppositories, etc.		
Importance of not taking any "over-the-counter" drugs		
Discussion of sexual intercourse during pregnancy		
Instruction on breast care whether breast feeding or not		
A description of the appearance of a normal newborn with some emphasis given to the possibility of physiological jaundice and the need for a PKU test		
Discussion of infant feeding methods—if breast feeding was preferred, was mother advised to inform hospital personnel of her decision?		
Instruction on care of the newborn, for example: Feeding, cord, and circumcision care, bathing, normal habits of sneezing, etc., that are common in infants		
Discussion of planning for help with care of the infant during the first few days home		
Instruction on family planning—including an explanation of the process of conception, methods of birth control, and location of family planning clinics		
Inclusion of the father of the child in discussion and instructions, if possible		
Methods of preparing family members for the arrival of a new baby		

	YES	NO
• Evaluation Criteria		
Is progress or lack of progress toward goal attainment evaluated? Are new priorities and goals developed as needed? Are alternative actions identified and mutually agreed upon?		
Is termination of service based on reassessment of patient/family needs and mutually agreed upon?		
(Adapted from Norfolk Health Department, Division of Nursing)		

Appendix E

THE CODE FOR NURSES

1. The nurse provides services with respect for human dignity and the uniqueness of the client unrestricted by considerations of social or economic status, personal attributes or the nature of health problems.
2. The nurse safeguards the client's rights to privacy by judiciously protecting information of a confidential nature.
3. The nurse acts to safeguard the client and the public when health care and safety are affected by the incompetent, unethical, or illegal practice of any person.
4. The nurse assumes responsibility and accountability for individual nursing judgements and actions.
5. The nurse maintains competence in nursing.
6. The nurse exercises informed judgement and uses individual competence and qualifications as criteria in seeking consultation, accepting responsibilities, and delegating nursing activities to others.
7. The nurse participates in activities that contribute to the ongoing development of the profession's body of knowledge.
8. The nurse participates in the profession's efforts to implement and improve standards of nursing.
9. The nurse participates in the profession's efforts to establish and maintain conditions of employment conducive to high quality nursing care.
10. The nurse participates in the profession's effort to protect the public from misinformation and misrepresentation and to maintain the integrity of nursing.
11. The nurse collaborates with members of the health professions and other citizens in promoting community and national efforts to meet the health needs of the public.

(Published by The American Nurses' Association, Kansas City, and reprinted with permission)

Appendix F

THE PATIENT'S BILL OF RIGHTS

It says that the patient has the right:

1. To considerate and respectful care.
2. To obtain from the physician information regarding his diagnosis, treatment and prognosis in terms that are understandable to him.
3. To give informed consent before any procedure or treatment is started.
4. To refuse treatment to the extent permitted by law based upon a knowledge of the medical consequences of this action.
5. To privacy concerning his medical care program.
6. To expect confidentiality regarding all records and communications of his treatment.
7. To expect reasonable compliance to a patient's request for service.
8. To information about the relationships of the hospital with other health and educational institutions regarding his care.
9. To refuse to participate in research.
10. To expect continuity of care.
11. To examine and question the hospital and medical bill.
12. To know the hospital rules and regulations pertaining to patient's conduct.

(The American Hospital Association, Chicago, 1975)

Index

Numerals in *italics* indicate a figure; "t" following a page number indicates a table.